EAT BETTER LIVE LONGER

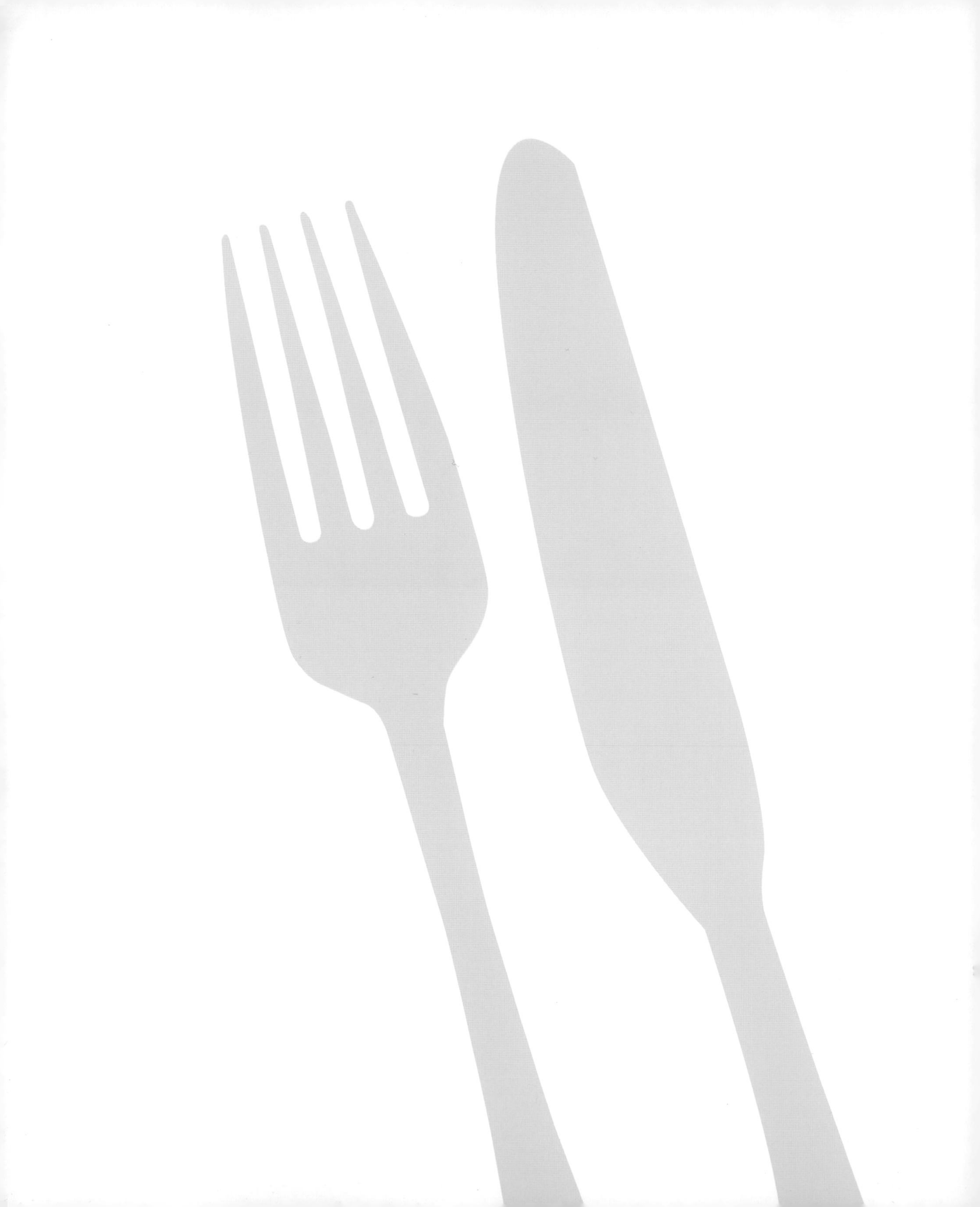

EAT BETTER LIVE LONGER

UNDERSTAND WHAT YOUR BODY NEEDS TO STAY HEALTHY

DR. SARAH BREWER
JULIETTE KELLOW RD

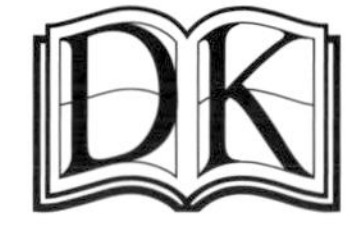

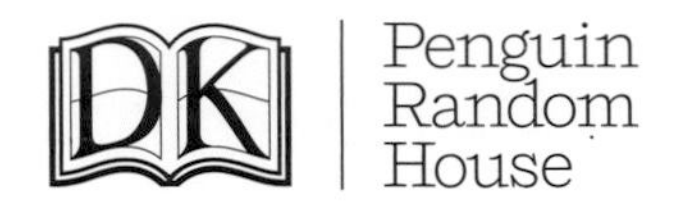

Senior Editor Nikki Sims
Senior Designer Saffron Stocker
Editor Claire Wedderburn-Maxwell
Designer Jade Wheaton
Illustrator Keith Hagan
Recipe Photographer Tara Fisher
Prop Stylist Robert Merrett
Food Stylist Maud Eden
DTP Designers Satish Gaur, Rajdeep Singh
Pre-production Producer Robert Dunn
Producer Luca Bazzoli
Jacket Designer Saffron Stocker
Jacket Co-ordinator Laura Bithell
Creative Technical Support Tom Morse
Managing Editor Dawn Henderson
Managing Art Editor Marianne Markham
Art Director Maxine Pedliham
Publishing Director Mary-Clare Jerram

US Editor Kayla Dugger
US Executive Editor Lori Hand

Recipes with photographs developed and written by Anne Harnan. All other recipes by Juliette Kellow.

First American Edition, 2018
Published in the United States by DK Publishing
345 Hudson Street, New York, New York 10014
Copyright © 2018 Dorling Kindersley Limited
DK, a Division of Penguin Random House LLC
18 19 20 21 22 10 9 8 7 6 5 4 3 2 1
001–307517–May/2018
All rights reserved.
Without limiting the rights under the copyright reserved above, no part of this publication may be reproduced, stored in or introduced into a retrieval system, or transmitted, in any form, or by any means (electronic, mechanical, photocopying, recording, or otherwise), without the prior written permission of the copyright owner.Published in Great Britain by Dorling Kindersley Limited

Disclaimer, see page 224.

A catalog record for this book is available from the Library of Congress.
ISBN 978-1-4654-6852-9

DK books are available at special discounts when purchased in bulk for sales promotions, premiums, fund-raising, or educational use. For details, contact: DK Publishing Special Markets, 345 Hudson Street, New York, New York 10014
SpecialSales@dk.com

Printed and bound in China
All images © Dorling Kindersley Limited
For further information see: www.dkimages.com

A WORLD OF IDEAS:
SEE ALL THERE IS TO KNOW
www.dk.com

Contents

-PART-

{3} THE LONGEVITY EATING PLAN

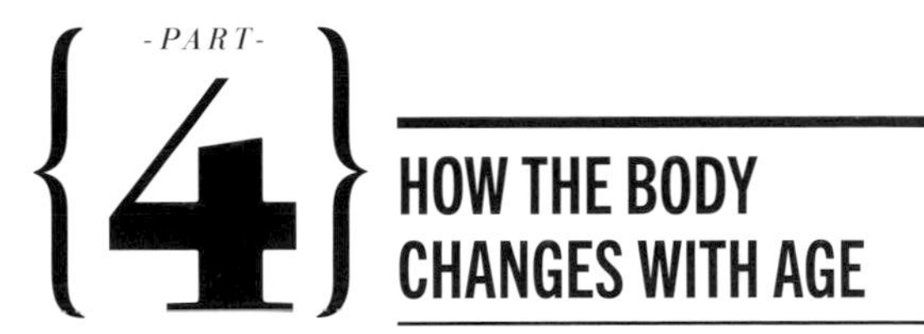

Foreword

Eat Better, Live Longer is your fad-free food guide for adding extra years to your life. It confirms what medics and nutritionists have known for many years: that the secret elixir to aging well doesn't come in a pill, potion, or lotion; instead, it can be found in your very own kitchen! Together with not smoking and exercising regularly, eating a healthy, well-balanced diet is one of the most important things you can do to extend the number of healthy years you live.

But just what should an age-defying diet consist of? This book starts by identifying 10 common eating habits or principles that are seen among the longest-lived communities around the world. These principles are the foundation for protecting against many diseases common in the Western world, including obesity, heart disease, cancer, type 2 diabetes, dementia, and arthritis—all conditions that hinder quality of life and often cut lives short.

The 28-day longevity plan moves you closer toward achieving these principles on a week-by-week basis. Interspersed throughout the plan, you'll find delicious, nutrient-packed recipes, together with in-depth information on the anti-aging benefits of 20 longevity "wonderfoods" or "supergroups" of foods. These confirm it's not weird and wonderful ingredients you need to support a longer and healthier life, but normal everyday foods you can buy at your local supermarket. You'll also find detailed information on how the body ages, along with advice on specific foods to help address the aging process.

The advice in this book is designed to reinforce what you may already know, and to build on this knowledge with the most up-to-date research based on science fact rather than science fiction. With new ideas and practical information, it couldn't be tastier or simpler to eat your way to a happier, healthier, and longer life.

Juliette Kellow

Juliette Kellow, author and registered dietitian

Sarah B.

Dr Sarah Brewer, consultant

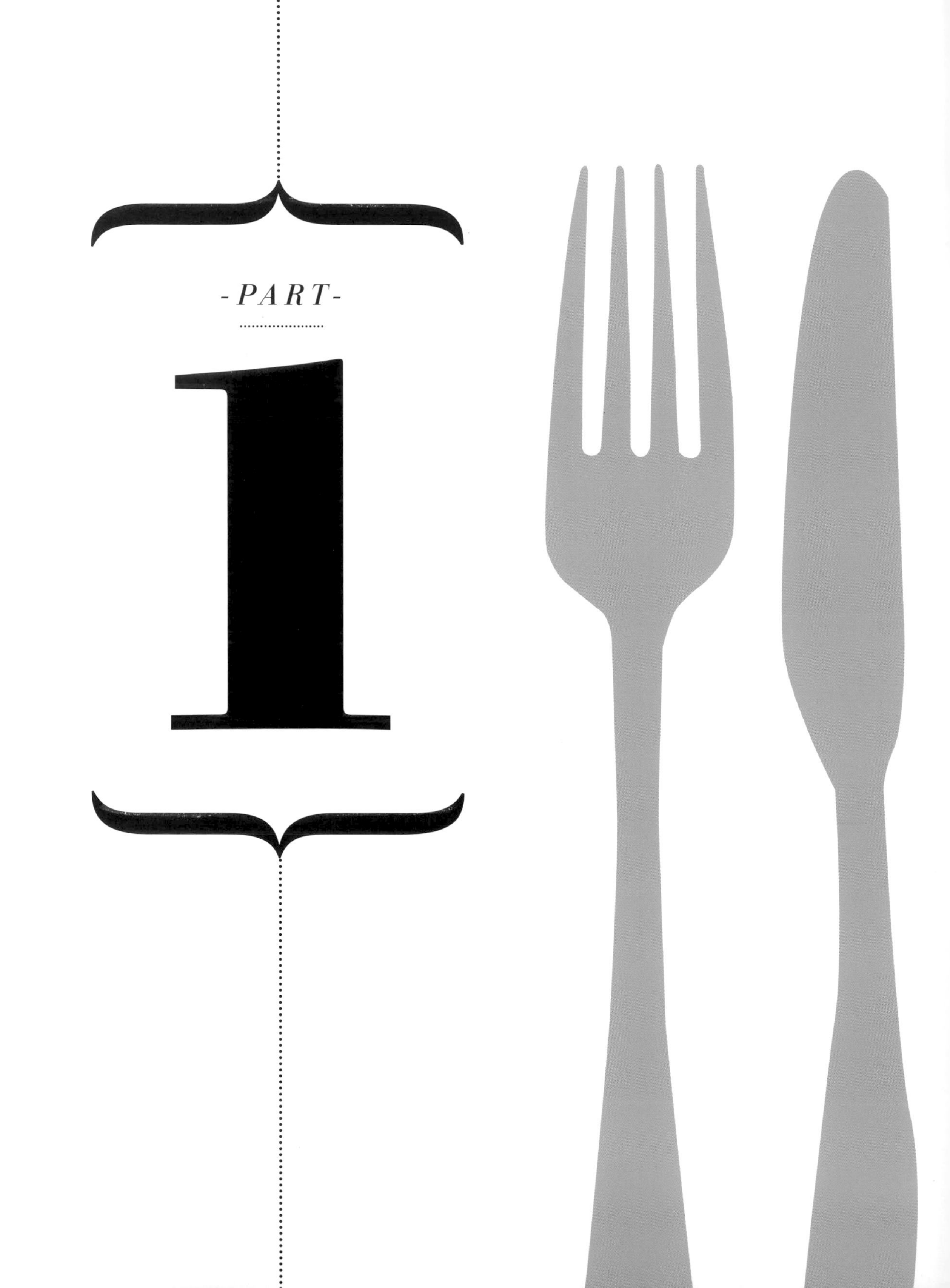
-PART-
1

What is aging?

Explore aging and the aspects of life that can influence how fast you age. Plus, see what lessons you can learn from the world's longest-lived communities.

Theories of aging

Experts are beginning to reach a consensus on why we age, and we're closer than ever to understanding the mechanisms involved. This knowledge is crucial for understanding what causes many of the health problems commonly seen in later life.

Fortunately, the idea that aging is programmed into us at a genetic level—such that we can't do anything about it—is outdated. Instead, many theories seem to support the idea that cell damage is central to the aging process.

> **Experts agree that lifestyle plays a significant part in how quickly—or how slowly—we age.**

Cellular wear and tear

The longer we live, the more damage our cells suffer simply because they have been working for a longer time. As a result of this damage, our organs and tissues begin to function less effectively, until eventually they stop working. Cell damage, loss, or change seems to be an inevitable part of aging, but our lifestyle probably has a role to play in both the process and the speed at which it occurs.

By leading a healthy lifestyle, our cells should only need to perform their normal functions and not go beyond the call of duty, thereby wearing themselves out. If you constantly race and neglect a car, it will deteriorate far quicker than if you drive sensibly and maintain it; the body is the same.

A growing consensus

Scientists have reduced hundreds of theories of aging to just a few significant ones that all support each other. We don't yet know definitively what causes cell damage, but we are closer to understanding the underlying mechanisms. There are now four dominant theories aiming to explain age-related damage to cells and to DNA.

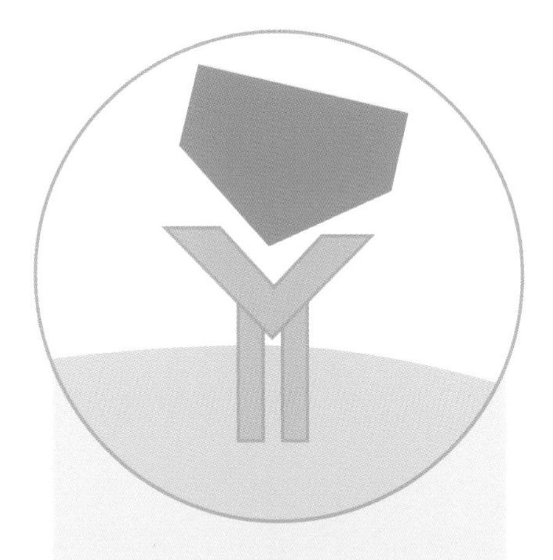

1

AGEs FORMATION

AGEs (advanced glycation end-products) form in the body when sugars combine with proteins. AGEs stick to other proteins, forming cross-links that stiffen the proteins so they no longer function normally and damage surrounding cells. Studies show this process may be responsible for everything from wrinkles to Alzheimer's. AGEs are also found in sugary foods, red and processed meat, and grilled foods.

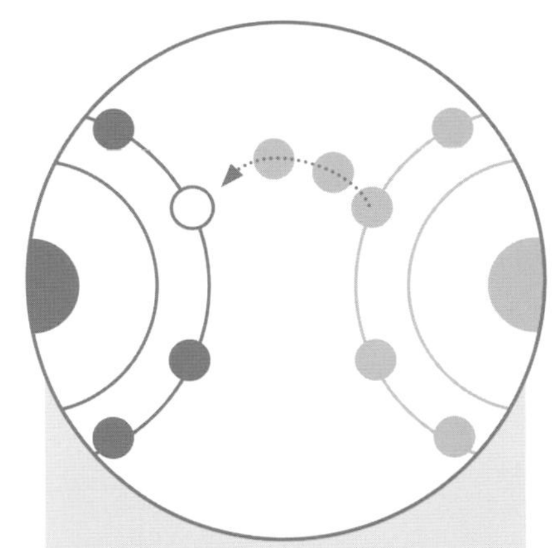

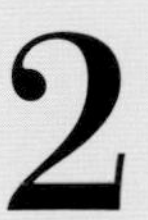

FREE RADICALS

Free radicals are unstable atoms produced naturally from body functions, such as breathing and digestion. Most are neutralized by antioxidants, but any that escape can cause oxidative damage to DNA, proteins, and mitochondria (the "batteries" of our cells). Free radicals also come from external factors, such as pollution, tobacco, drugs, alcohol, stress, and a poor diet that's high in unhealthy fats and sugars.

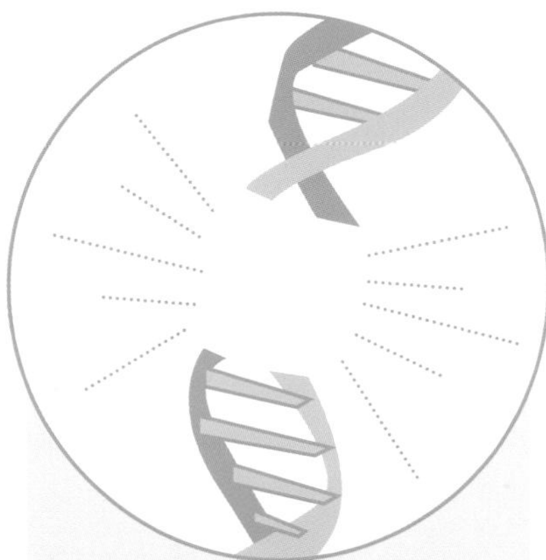

3

DNA DAMAGE

Mistakes in replication and external factors, such as toxins and free radicals, cause damage to DNA, and this may also contribute to the aging process. DNA damage happens in every cell of our body thousands of times a day, and we have evolved an armory of repair mechanisms to cope. Not all damage is corrected, however, and this results in mutations that amass with age, until cells malfunction and die.

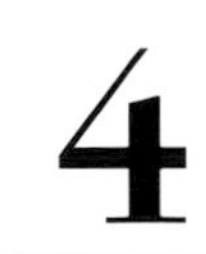

TELOMERE SHORTENING

Telomeres are caps on the ends of chromosomes (coiled molecules of DNA), which stop DNA unraveling. Telomeres shorten each time a cell divides, until they get so short the cells can't replicate and may die off or no longer be capable of repair—factors that contribute to aging. More research is needed, but it's becoming clear that bad habits, such as poor diet, seem to speed up this telomere shortening.

What affects how we age?

Physical aging is inevitable, but how we live our lives has a big impact on just how quickly—or slowly—this happens. Making a few simple lifestyle changes could be all it takes to keep your body and brain younger.

While we are not programmed to live a certain number of years or age in a specific way, genes do still play a role in the aging process, albeit a fairly small one. Studies of families, and especially twins, suggest genetic make-up accounts for only around 25 percent of lifespan. Our genes give an indication of how long we could live, but how we fare in the aging game is largely determined by the way we lead our lives. Here are the top 10 lifestyle changes to help you stay healthy and slow down the aging process, potentially adding years of life.

75%
of human lifespan is attributable to lifestyle and environment.

Changing habits, changing outcomes

The importance of lifestyle over genetics is clear when you look at residents of Okinawa in Japan, an island famous for its high number of centenarians. Recent generations who've swapped traditional habits for a more Western way of life are not living as long as previously. Studies also show when Okinawans leave the island and adopt the eating habits of their host countries, they succumb to the same health problems as their adopted nation.

ADOPT A HEALTHY DIET

What we eat can have a major impact on our health. Poor diets are a risk factor for many chronic diseases, including cancer, obesity, cardiovascular disease, type 2 diabetes, osteoporosis, and dementia. While all these conditions become more likely as we get older due to the natural aging process, unhealthy eating habits can accelerate their progression. According to one large global study, a poor diet was found to be the highest risk factor for premature death. Fortunately, making some simple dietary changes can dramatically increase your life expectancy.

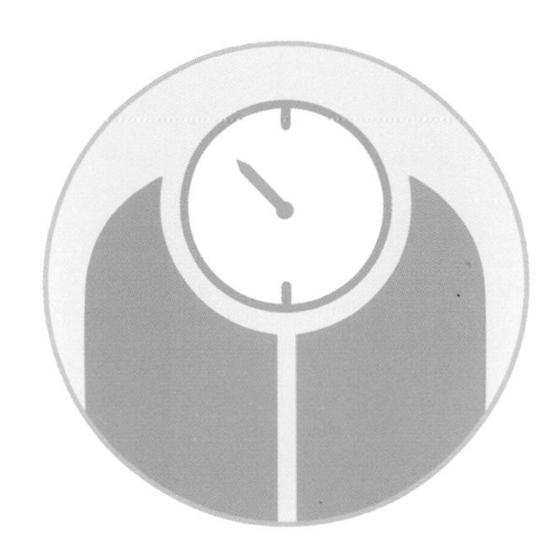

STAY A HEALTHY WEIGHT

Weighing too much kills an estimated 3.4 million adults worldwide. In one study, people who were obese at the age of 40 shortened their lives by 6.5 years. Excess weight raises blood pressure and cholesterol, which increases risk of heart disease and stroke. It also leaves us more prone to developing type 2 diabetes, metabolic syndrome, asthma, osteoarthritis, liver and kidney disease, sleep apnea, and depression. Obesity is the second biggest preventable cause of cancer, according to the World Health Organization.

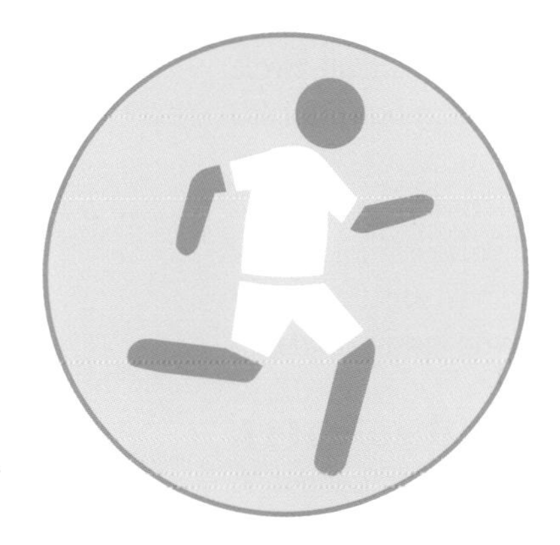

GET ACTIVE

According to a major study, inactivity is responsible for almost 1 in 10 early deaths. Exercise benefits every part of the body: it strengthens the heart, lungs, bones, joints, muscles, and immune system; it lowers the risk of diseases such as type 2 diabetes, high blood pressure, stroke, and colon cancer; it releases mood-boosting endorphins, helping to ease or prevent stress and depression; it helps keep our weight steady; it improves sleep; and it helps us stay flexible and maintain good posture and balance, so that we can continue with everyday activities as we age and reduce the risk of falls.

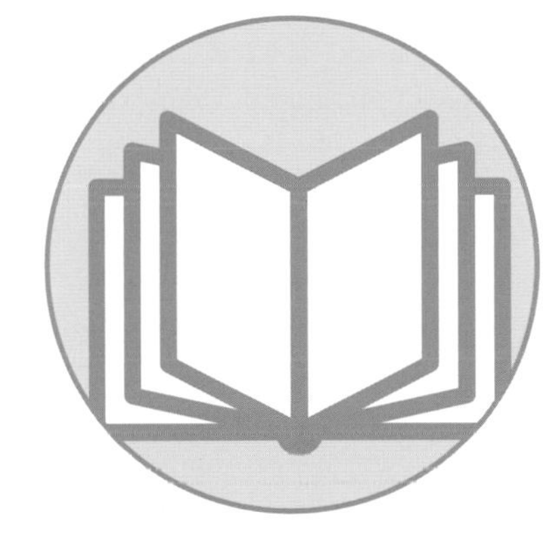

KEEP SHARP

In the same way that the body loses strength and vitality if we don't exercise it, so, too, does the brain. Encouraging an active mind is shown to slow the decline in mental ability as the years advance. One study found 70- and 80-year-olds who stayed mentally active by reading, playing games, and doing crafts were up to half as likely to suffer with memory loss as those who didn't do such activities. The benefits don't just start in later life, either. The same study found people who in midlife enjoyed reading and had active social lives had a 40 percent reduced risk of memory loss when they were older.

CONTINUED

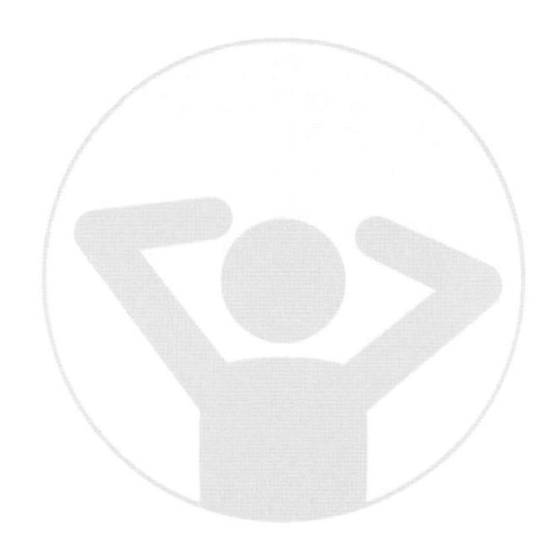

DEAL WITH STRESS

Chronic stress is a cause of wrinkles and can lead to unhealthy habits, such as poor diet, drinking too much alcohol, and smoking. Stress can upset the digestive system and affects how well we sleep. It lowers immunity, making us more prone to infections. It increases blood pressure and the risk of heart disease and stroke. It destroys cells in an area of the brain responsible for memory—indeed, studies show a link between stress and Alzheimer's. Recent studies suggest stress even shortens the length of our telomeres (see page 11), potentially speeding up the aging process.

BE HAPPY

According to a 5-year study of adults aged 52 to 79 years, those who reported feeling happy on a typical day were 35 percent less likely to die during this time. Other studies show happier people suffer with fewer wrinkles, aches, pains, and health problems, and have lower heart rates and blood pressure, less heart disease, and stronger immune systems. Making positive connections with other people is a great way to stay happy. One review found people with good social relationships had a 50 percent lower risk of dying than those who were more isolated.

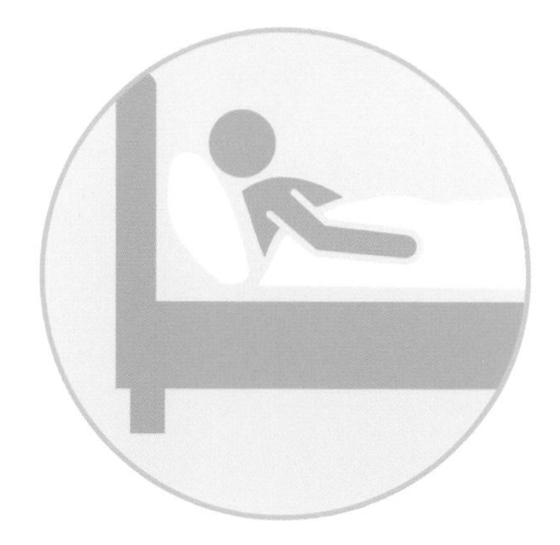

GET ENOUGH SLEEP

Lack of sleep—or poor-quality sleep—has been linked to many diseases, including heart disease, stroke, type 2 diabetes, and Alzheimer's. It may reduce the body's immunity—one study found people who had less than 7 hours sleep a night were three times more likely to develop a cold than those who had more than 8 hours. Sleep deprivation can also wreak havoc with mood, concentration, mental ability, and memory, and it may be a factor in depression. It can lead to poor eating habits and weight gain, and leave a person too tired to exercise.

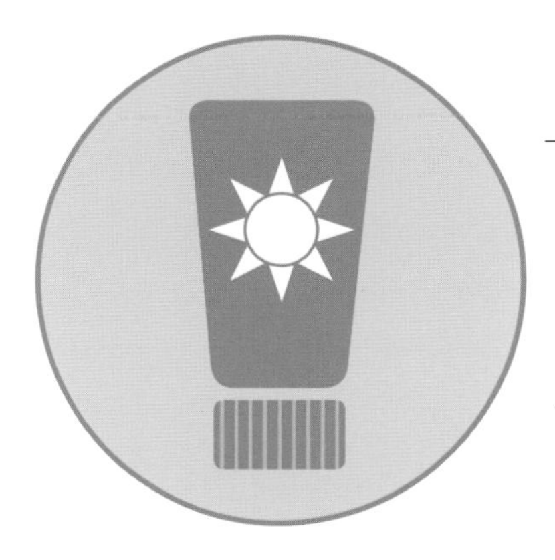

STAY SAFE IN THE SUN

A little sunlight is good for us—it creates vitamin D in our body, vital for muscle function, bone health, and immunity (see pages 36–37). But too much sun can age us fast. One study found the sun's UV rays caused 80 percent of wrinkles, skin pigmentation, and discoloration, with the effects more apparent as we age. The sun's UV rays are also linked to all forms of skin cancer—a study found 86 percent of malignant melanomas in the UK were caused by sunlight. To stay safe, avoid getting burned, use sunscreen, and keep out of the sun during the hottest part of the day.

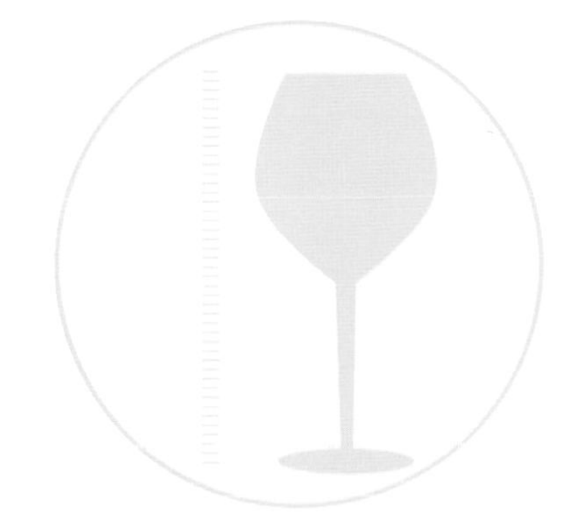

REDUCE ALCOHOL

Regularly drinking too much alcohol hastens the aging process. Externally, the skin suffers with redness, puffiness, and premature wrinkles. Internally, excessive alcohol increases the risk of liver disease, cirrhosis, pancreatitis, type 2 diabetes, high blood pressure, heart disease, stroke, seven types of cancer, osteoporosis, dementia, and depression. Alcoholic drinks are high in calories, and excessive drinking can cause unwanted weight gain while draining the body of nutrients. Alcohol can also have a detrimental effect on the quality of sleep.

AVOID SMOKING

Smoking is one of the biggest causes of visible aging, estimated to age skin prematurely by up to 20 years. And it's not just looks that suffer. Smoking kills around 7 million people every year and is the single most preventable cause of death worldwide. Smokers are more likely to have health problems that shorten life, including asthma, emphysema, chronic obstructive pulmonary disease, heart disease, high blood pressure, stroke, osteoporosis, dementia, and cancer. And it's not just lung cancer—smoking increases the risk of leukemia and many other cancers.

Diet lessons from around the world

Look at the countries with the longest life expectancies and you'll find a diverse range. It's a similar story when you compare those with the greatest proportions of centenarians. The reasons are many and varied, but research shows that diet and eating habits play a key role, and some communities and areas of the world are particularly significant.

Rank—Country	Years
1st—Japan	**83.7**
2nd—Switzerland	**83.4**
3rd—Singapore	**83.1**
4th—Australia and Spain	**82.8**
5th—Iceland and Italy	**82.7**
6th—Israel	**82.5**
7th—Sweden and France	**82.4**
8th—Republic of Korea	**82.3**
9th—Canada	**82.2**
10th—Luxembourg	**82**

YEARS

Who lives the longest in the world?
This chart shows the countries with the top 10 highest life expectancies, according to the WHO. Diet and eating habits can play a significant role in longevity, as well as environment, healthcare, and lifestyle.

SEVENTH-DAY ADVENTISTS

Studies have shown members of this Christian denomination from California have better health and higher life expectancy than the average American (which ranks 31st). Much of the advantage in this self-contained group can be attributed to their mainly plant-based eating.

What they eat
- At least nine servings of fruits and vegetables per day
- Lots of legumes, nuts, and seeds
- Whole grains
- Plant-based milks, e.g. soy
- Small amounts of eggs and low-fat dairy
- Some fish

What they limit
- Red meat and poultry
- Fatty, sugary, and processed foods, and those with a lot of additives
- Alcohol (93 percent reported as abstinent)
- Drinks containing caffeine

Eating habits
- A mainly vegetarian diet is promoted for bodily health
- Gluttony and excess, even of good things, are discouraged
- Meals are appreciated and food is respected

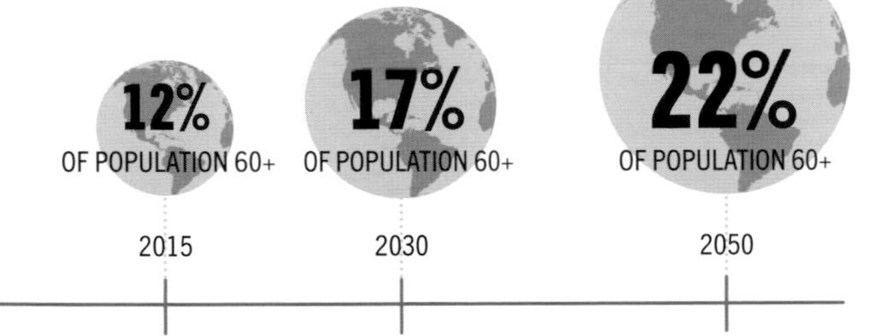

The world's aging population
The United Nations has projected that the percentage of those aged 60 and over will almost double by 2050. It's never been more important to eat for a healthier long life.

NORDIC NATIONS

Scandinavian countries rank highly in the life expectancy stakes—Sweden, Norway, Denmark, Finland, and Iceland sit in the top 30. While healthcare is key, diet also has a part to play. Long-term studies have linked traditional Nordic diets (whole-grain bread, fish, cabbage, oats, root vegetables, and fruits) to healthier and longer lives.

What they eat

- Whole grains (rye, oats, and barley)
- Leafy greens, root veggies, peas, beans, seaweed, and mushrooms
- Fruits, especially berries
- Nuts
- Oily fish
- Canola oil

What they limit

- Red meat, except for small amounts of game meat
- Processed foods (although fish products are often dried, smoked, salted, or pickled)

Eating habits

- Breakfast tends to be a good-sized meal with some protein
- Families eat together at the table
- On-the-go snacking is rare, as food is expensive, discouraging impulse buys

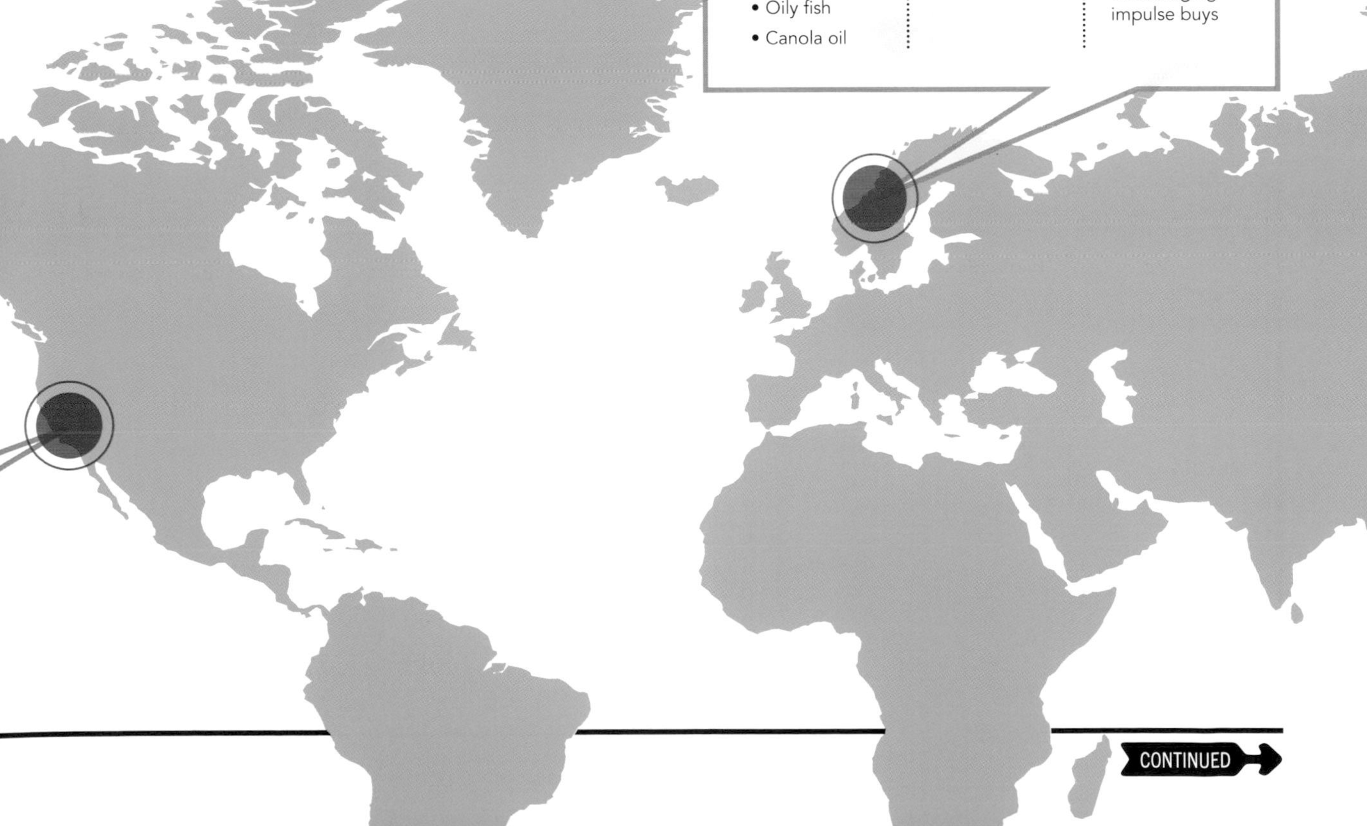

CONTINUED

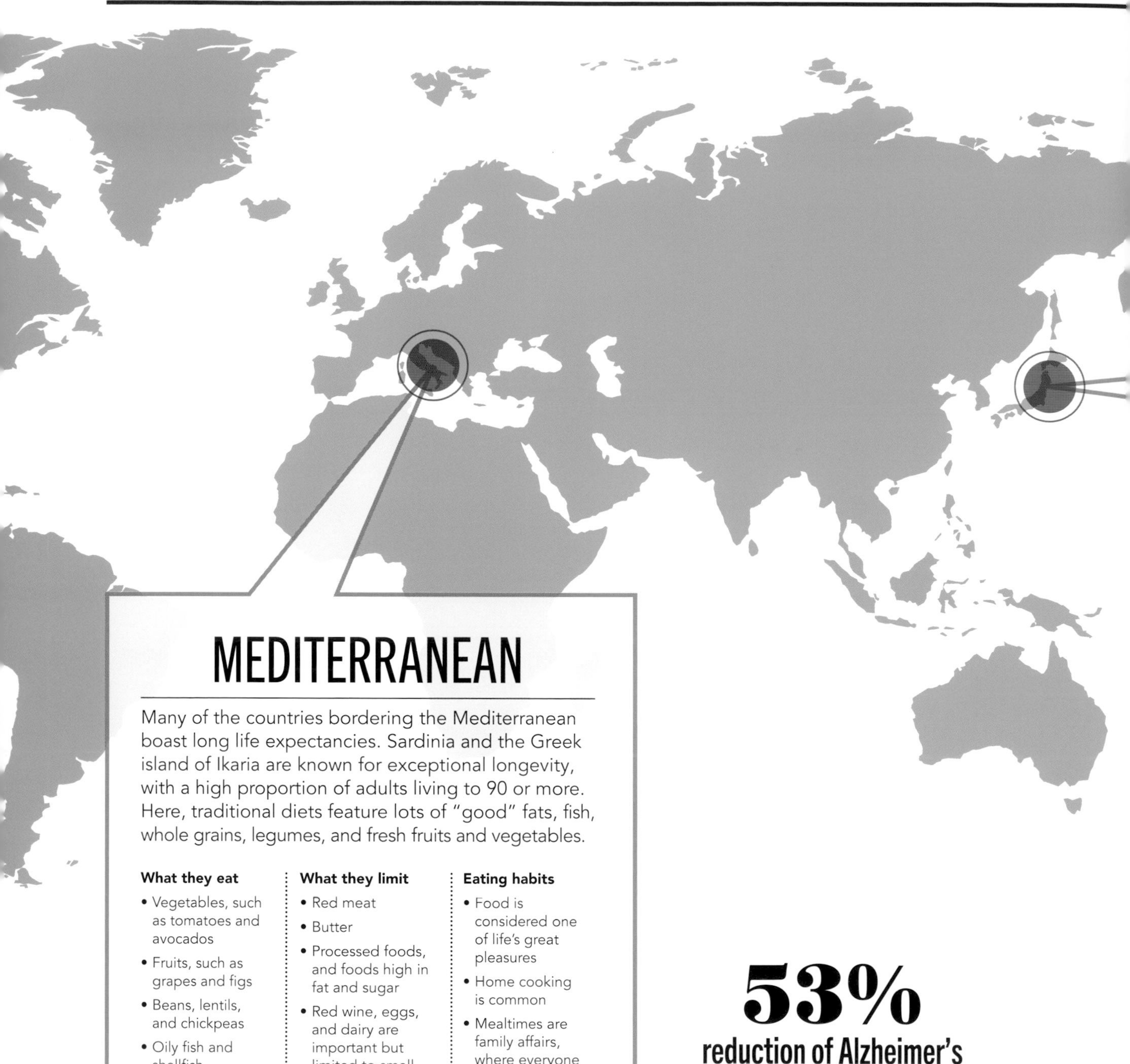

MEDITERRANEAN

Many of the countries bordering the Mediterranean boast long life expectancies. Sardinia and the Greek island of Ikaria are known for exceptional longevity, with a high proportion of adults living to 90 or more. Here, traditional diets feature lots of "good" fats, fish, whole grains, legumes, and fresh fruits and vegetables.

What they eat

- Vegetables, such as tomatoes and avocados
- Fruits, such as grapes and figs
- Beans, lentils, and chickpeas
- Oily fish and shellfish
- Nuts
- Olive oil
- Herbs and garlic

What they limit

- Red meat
- Butter
- Processed foods, and foods high in fat and sugar
- Red wine, eggs, and dairy are important but limited to small amounts

Eating habits

- Food is considered one of life's great pleasures
- Home cooking is common
- Mealtimes are family affairs, where everyone eats together at the table

53%

reduction of Alzheimer's risk in people who follow a combined Mediterranean and blood pressure diet.

JAPAN

Japanese people are the longest-living in the world, and the island of Okinawa especially is famous for its large number of centenarians. Eating habits across Japan remain unique when compared with many other parts of the world and are thought to make a major contribution to the nation's longevity.

What they eat

- Rice and noodles
- Leafy greens, root veggies, mushrooms, and bean sprouts
- Seaweed
- Soy products
- Plenty of fish, including oily fish
- Fermented foods
- Green tea

What they limit

- Meat—small amounts of pork and poultry are eaten occasionally
- Butter
- Dairy products
- Processed foods that are high in fat and sugar

Eating habits

- Okinawans follow a mantra of "hara hachi bu": eating until 80 percent full
- Breakfast is often the largest meal, involving hot food with protein and vegetables

JAPANESE WOMEN LIVE 6.3 YEARS LONGER THAN MEN

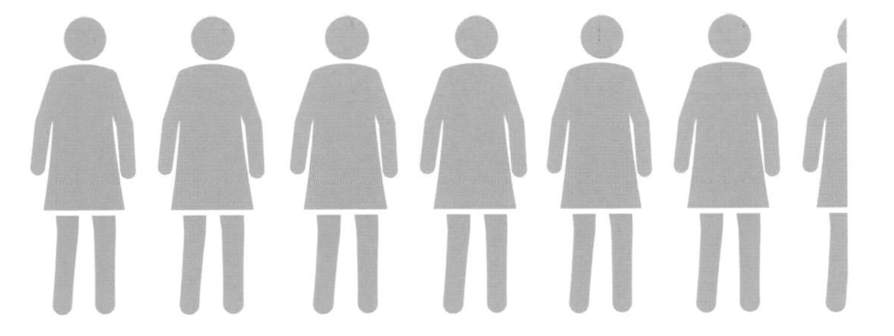

Life expectancy—the gender divide
In every country, women live longer than men; women are more health conscious and biology helps, too. And in Japan, for instance, a diet rich in soy, fish, and green tea provides a powerful combination of nutrients for longevity.

NUMBER OF CENTENARIANS PER 100,000 PEOPLE

Country	Centenarians per 100,000
Japan	45.3
France	31
Italy	28.6
Switzerland	24
UK	22.9
New Zealand	21.7
Spain	21.6
Sweden	20.4
Canada	19.5
USA	19.4
Norway	19.2
Portugal	19.2
Germany	18.4
Greece	17.8
Australia	16.8
Argentina	13.8
Israel	12.4
Netherlands	11.8
Mexico	8.7
Thailand	7.3

Top 20 nations for centenarians
Diet has a part to play in reaching old age, as Japan's, Mediterranean, and Nordic countries' rankings show in estimates compiled by the UN.

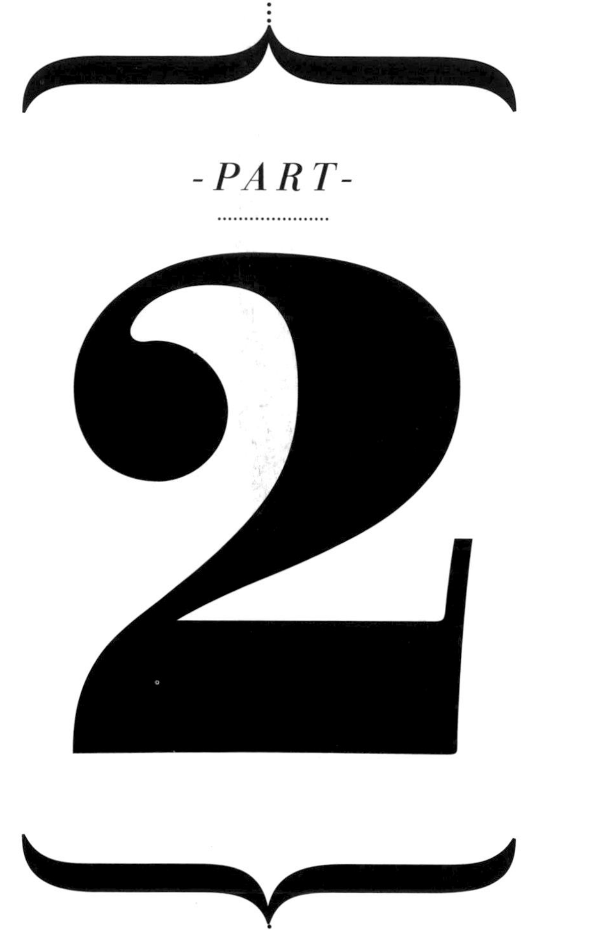
-PART-
2

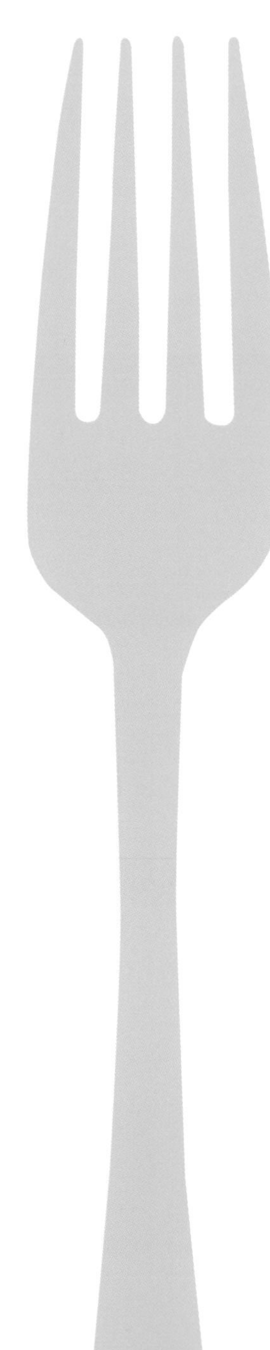

Principles of a long and healthy life

Transform your life for longevity with these 10 simple but meaningful adaptations to what you eat and how you eat.

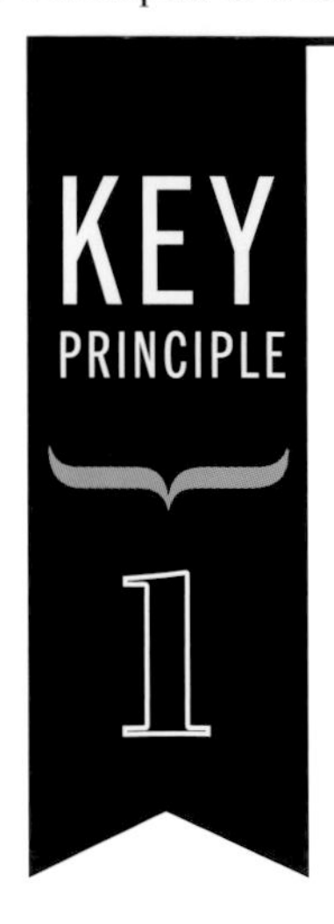

Downsize your meals as the day goes on

Skipping breakfast, nibbling at lunch, and gorging in the evening is rare in long-lived communities. Follow their lead of starting the day with food aplenty to lower the risk of obesity, heart disease, and type 2 diabetes.

"Breakfast like a king, lunch like a prince, and dine like a pauper"—scientists believe that such eating can confer major health benefits.

Insulin body clock

Scientists are looking at how the circadian rhythm—or our internal body clock—affects metabolism, nutritional intake, and the way the body responds to food. Studies certainly show we have an increased risk of metabolic syndrome, obesity, and type 2 diabetes when the circadian rhythm is disrupted. Other research provides evidence to suggest that we're more sensitive to the effects of insulin in the morning and so need less of it to control blood sugar levels. At night, this sensitivity is reduced, so more insulin is needed after eating to lower blood sugar. Over time, this eating pattern can lead to insulin resistance, a precursor for type 2 diabetes. The bottom line is: our bodies cope better when we eat more at the start of the day and less as the day wears on.

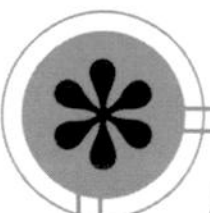

Skip breakfast at your peril

Not only does eating breakfast mirror what many centenarians do, but research also shows that skipping breakfast can spell disaster for your health. Many studies show that people who skip this meal are more likely to be overweight or obese and also have an increased risk of heart disease, stroke, high blood pressure, and type 2 diabetes.

Our bodies cope better, in terms of insulin sensitivity, when we eat more at the start of the day.

A vicious cycle

In Western societies, many of us miss breakfast, grab a small lunch, have a huge dinner, and snack during the evening. Studies confirm that such eating patterns are linked to obesity. Eating lots of food in the evening also means we're less likely to feel hungry the next morning, so we skip breakfast—and the cycle repeats.

Better eating habits

To ensure that you can make the switch to healthier eating for the long term, the longevity eating plan (see page 44) offers a transition toward "breakfasting like a king." The month-long plan is a nutritionally designed menu that leads you to downsize calories through the day without noticing.

THE BIG BREAKFAST BOOST

A study exploring the idea of how 1,400 calories were consumed across the day looked at overweight women with metabolic syndrome. After 12 weeks, group B (those eating half their calories at breakfast) had results that were significantly better than group A's in every respect.

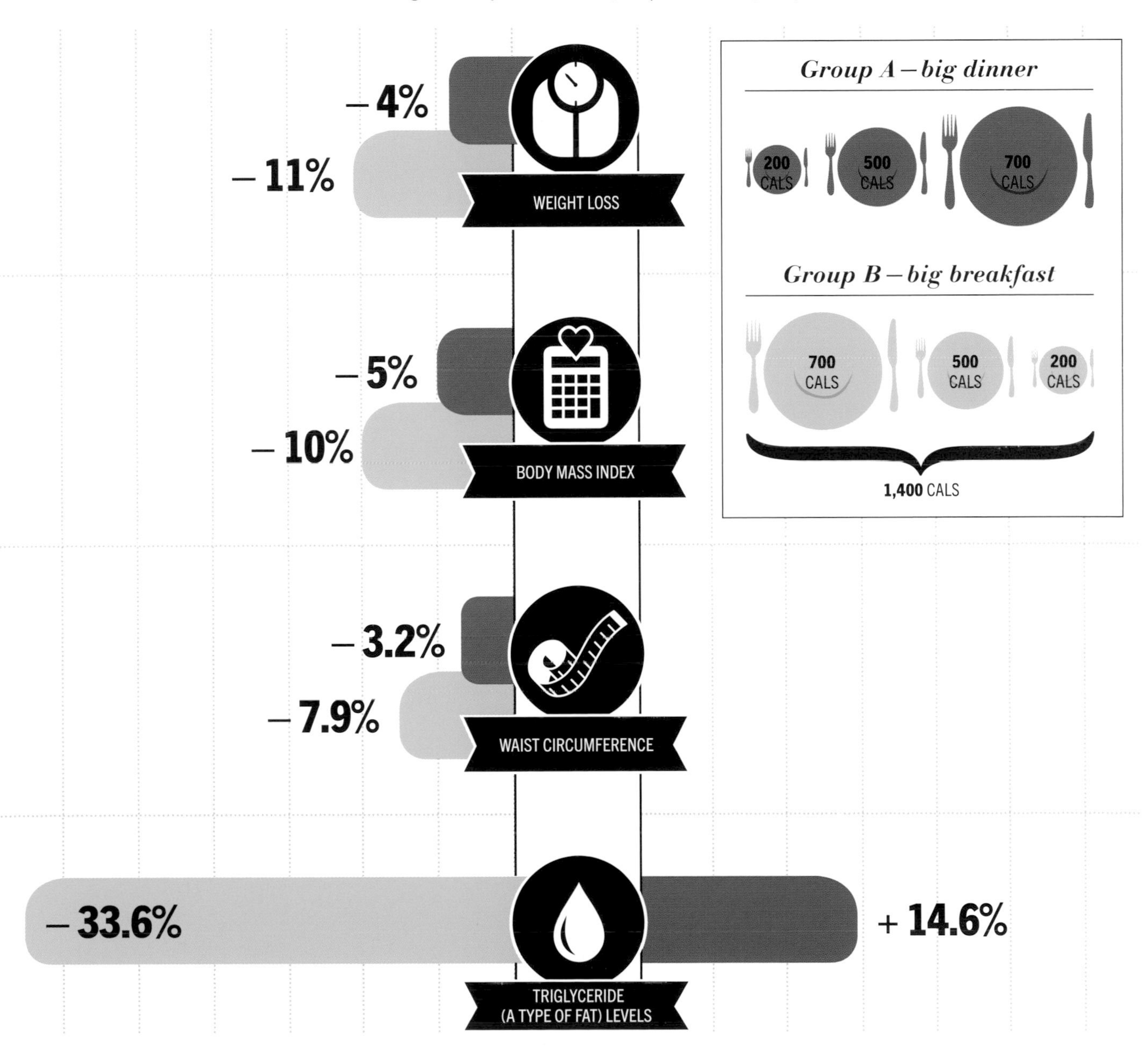

Know how much is enough

The more overweight we are, the shorter our lives: fact! Experts agree one of the best things we can do to live longer is to stay a healthy weight. And for many people, that means breaking a lifelong habit of overeating.

In 2016, a study confirmed that weighing too much shortens lives. Looking at 3.9 million adults worldwide, the study found that being overweight or obese is directly linked to a higher risk of dying early from conditions such as respiratory disease, heart disease, stroke, and cancer. And it was found the risk increases the heavier we get: being overweight reduces life expectancy by 1 year, while obese people lose 3 years of life.

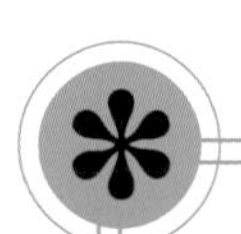

Calculate your BMI

Body mass index (BMI) can identify if you are a healthy weight. To calculate, use this formula: weight in pounds ÷ height in inches^2 x 703. For example: 154lb ÷ 70^2 x 703 = 22.1. A BMI of 18.5 to 24.9 indicates a healthy weight; 25 to 29.9 means you are overweight; and over 30 is a measure of obesity.

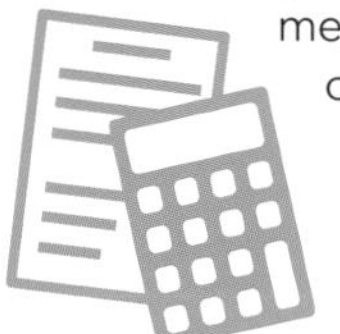

Studies show that severely obese people can expect to live 10 years less than people of a healthy weight.

Inevitably heavier?

Statistics reveal that weight gain becomes more common with age. In the UK, for example, 39 percent of 16–24-year-olds are overweight or obese, but this increases to 71 percent of 45–54-year-olds. Yet middle-aged spread doesn't have to be a fact of life. Yes, our metabolism slows down a little with age and we lose muscle mass, but it is changes (or lack of) in our lifestyle that are mainly responsible for an increase in our waistline as we age.

Learning from Japan

Only 4 percent of adults are obese in Japan, and the life expectancy is the highest in the world—almost 84 years (see also page 16). In contrast, 38 percent of Americans and 27 percent of Brits are obese, with an average life expectancy of 80 years.

80 percent full

The elders of Okinawa, who are renowned for their long and healthy lives, practice something called "hara hachi bu," which translates as eating until they are 80 percent full. It's impossible to know when we've reached 80 percent fullness, but the important message is to stop eating at the point when we could still eat a little more—and well before we are "stuffed"!

STRATEGIES TO PREVENT OVEREATING

The science behind becoming overweight is simple: if we take in more calories from food and drink than we use up, they're stored as fat, and we put on weight. While increasing exercise levels has a role to play in burning more calories, the key factor in reducing weight is to avoid overeating.

Choose smaller plates

Average plate size has risen over 20 percent since the 1960s, with a similar increase in meal size. With a visual trick, we perceive identical portions of food as reduced in size on a large plate compared with a small plate.

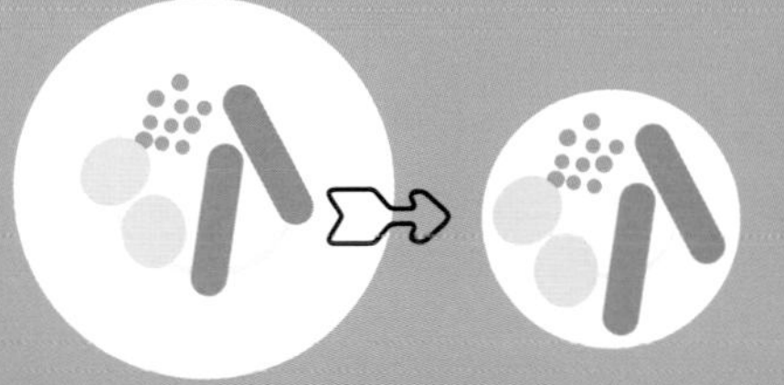

Eat more slowly

It takes 15 to 20 minutes after food is first eaten for our brain to get all the signals it needs to register a full stomach. Reducing the speed at which we eat therefore gives us a truer sense of when we've had enough.

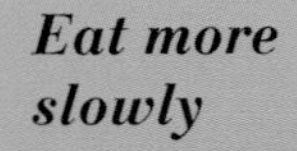

Scale down portions

A fifth less food on your plate should leave you feeling 20 percent less full than normal. Serious overeaters may need to drop down by another fifth. Your aim is to finish meals feeling satisfied but not stuffed.

Focus on the food

Pay attention to every mouthful and avoid distractions: no TV, no computer, no smartphone, and no magazines when you're eating. Concentrating on a meal will help you better identify when you're starting to feel full.

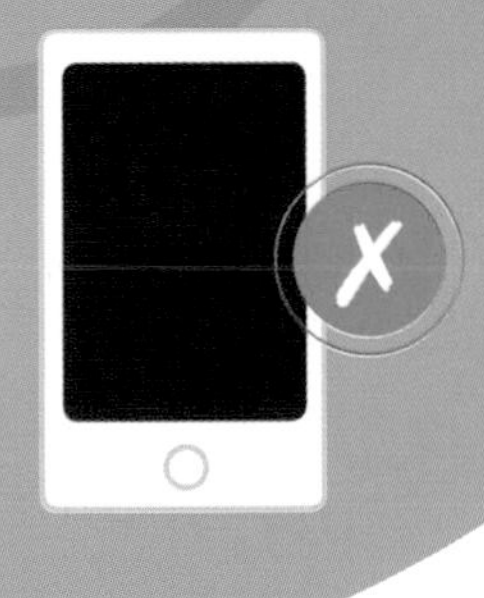

Eat more plants

Look at the communities in the world with the longest life expectancies and one of the key things they share is a mainly plant-based diet with plenty of fruits and vegetables. Skewing your diet toward plants seems to protect against many age-related conditions, including heart disease, cancer, obesity, and type 2 diabetes.

Studies show that diets based mainly on plants are linked to a reduction in mortality, and from cardiovascular disease especially. And you don't need to be 100 percent vegetarian to benefit: a 2015 study found that diets comprising 70 percent plant-based foods cut the risk of cardiovascular disease by 20 percent, so the priority is to obtain most nutrients from plants.

Health promotion

Good intakes of fruits and vegetables seem to help lower the risk of many other conditions, too, such as respiratory problems, dementia, arthritis, and age-related macular degeneration. Such emphasis is core to the longevity eating plan (see page 44).

Double the benefits

Experts agree the health benefits of plant-based diets are twofold. First, by eating more plant foods, we "crowd out" animal foods and reduce our intake of the nutrients they contain that are linked to poorer health. Second, most plant-based foods come with built-in beneficial nutrients, many of which are unique to plants.

Fiber provider

Only plants contain fiber, which plays an important role in keeping us full and regular. When we eat fiber-rich foods, we are less likely to overeat, making it easier to stay a healthy weight. And fiber also has body-wide benefits relating to heart disease, colon complaints, and certain cancers (see opposite).

↓24%

reduced risk of heart disease from eating 1¾lb (800g) of fruits and veggies a day.

Phytochemical magic

Fiber isn't the only nutrient unique to plants; they're also rich in naturally occurring chemicals known as phytochemicals, many of which act as antioxidants and help prevent inflammation. In lab

Is five-a-day enough?

The World Health Organization recommends eating 14oz (400g) of fruits and vegetables a day, or roughly five portions. A 2017 study found that every 7oz (200g) increase in fruits and vegetables offered health benefits, and 1¾lb (800g) a day—about 10 portions—was optimal. That said, 10 portions has been criticised as unrealistic, so aim for five but more is better.

FIBER-BASED BENEFITS

Fiber can only be obtained from plants, so a plant-based diet will naturally be high in fiber. Fiber cannot be digested by the body; it comes as two main types: soluble and insoluble. Soluble fiber forms a gel in the intestine and helps control blood sugar, while insoluble fiber increases the bulkiness and softness of stools. Find out how fiber benefits health and longevity below.

Heart disease

Whole grains—a good source of fiber—are linked to better heart health. Soluble fiber helps lower cholesterol, too.

Stroke

A study in 2013 showed that increasing fiber intake by 7g a day may be associated with a 7 percent fall in the risk of stroke.

Diabetes

Soluble fiber slows sugar absorption into the blood. Better blood sugar control helps to protect against insulin resistance and type 2 diabetes.

Cancer

According to the World Cancer Research Fund, a high-fiber diet may help to reduce the risk of colon cancer.

Colon complaints

Fiber protects against diverticular disease and constipation by helping stools pass quickly. It also feeds gut bacteria.

studies, phytochemicals have been linked to everything from boosting immunity and slowing down or stopping the growth of cancer cells, to delaying cognitive decline and helping to lower cholesterol. For a detailed look at phytochemicals, see pages 38–39.

Holistic nutrition

Studies suggest it's the unique overall package of nutrients in plant foods that protects health. When vitamins or antioxidant compounds are consumed in isolation, they often don't offer the same benefits and may even be harmful in some cases: vitamin E and beta-carotene supplements, for example, may have been found to increase the risk of certain cancers. Ultimately, most experts agree it is better to gain plant-derived nutrients from plants themselves.

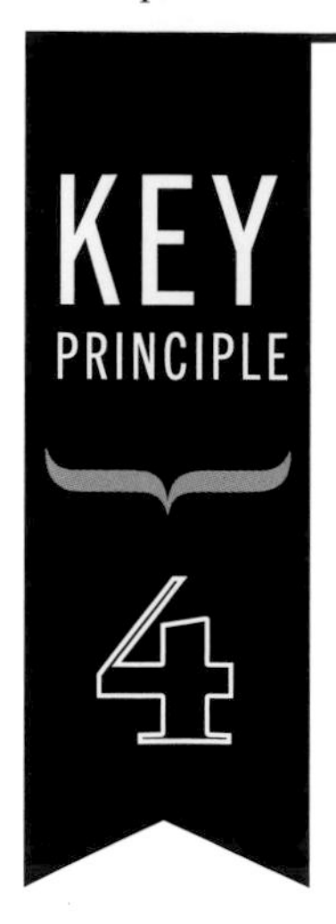

Eat the right carbs

Carbohydrates get a lot of bad press, and many people have jumped on the low-carb, high-protein bandwagon in search of magical weight loss and health gains. But, in longevity terms, carbs continue to be the main event in long-lived communities, while protein-rich foods play more of a supporting role.

Carbohydrates are the main raw material needed to power our bodies. Yet high carb intakes have been blamed for the rising incidence of numerous health problems, including obesity, heart disease, type 2 diabetes, and even dementia. So the idea of putting carbs firmly on the menu may seem controversial. Interestingly, however, a carb-based diet is far more aligned to the traditional eating habits of people from long-lived communities, such as the Seventh-Day Adventists and on the Greek island of Ikaria (see pages 16 and 19). In these areas, it's legumes, potatoes, sweet potatoes, fruits, and vegetables, along with mainly nonwheat whole grains, such as oats, rice, barley, and quinoa, that are the carb "stars."

Long-lived peoples around the world still eat plenty of carbs, but in smaller portions and mainly as whole grains.

Ditch the sugar

High intakes of sugar (a simple carbohydrate) are linked to weight gain and associated health issues.

- **Avoid fakes**—Calorie-free sweeteners won't get rid of a sweet tooth, so gradually cut down on sugar.
- **Check the label**—Sugar hides under names such as corn syrup, hydrolyzed starch, sucrose, glucose, fructose, and maltose.
- **Find alternatives**—Top yogurt and oatmeal with fresh fruit instead of honey, for instance.

Age-friendly carbs

Such star carbohydrates are naturally low in fat and packaged with other beneficial nutrients (such as vitamins and minerals).

Whole grains are a supergroup of wonderfoods that aid well-being and reduce the risk of age-limiting disease, and you'll see there are plenty to discover, from oats to wild rice (see page 74).

Quality, not quantity

People in traditionally long-lived communities tend to eat less food overall. Even though carbs form the bulk of what they eat, compared with Western diets the total carbs consumed is smaller—a serving of rice in a small bowl, for example, not most of a dinner plate! And the carbs tend to be served with other nutrient-rich ingredients, such as vegetables, beans, fish, and nuts, rather than lots of fat, meat, cheese, or processed foods. So for longevity, choose whole carbs, serve sensible portions, and partner with healthy ingredients.

PICK THE WINNING CARBS

All carbohydrates are energy-rich, but not all carbs offer the same benefits. Simple carbs tend to be refined sugars that burn fast, whereas complex carbs (refined or not) are starchy foods that break down more slowly. As you'll see, unrefined complex carbs top the list for optimum health.

5%

is the maximum percentage of daily calories that should come from added sugar, according to the WHO.

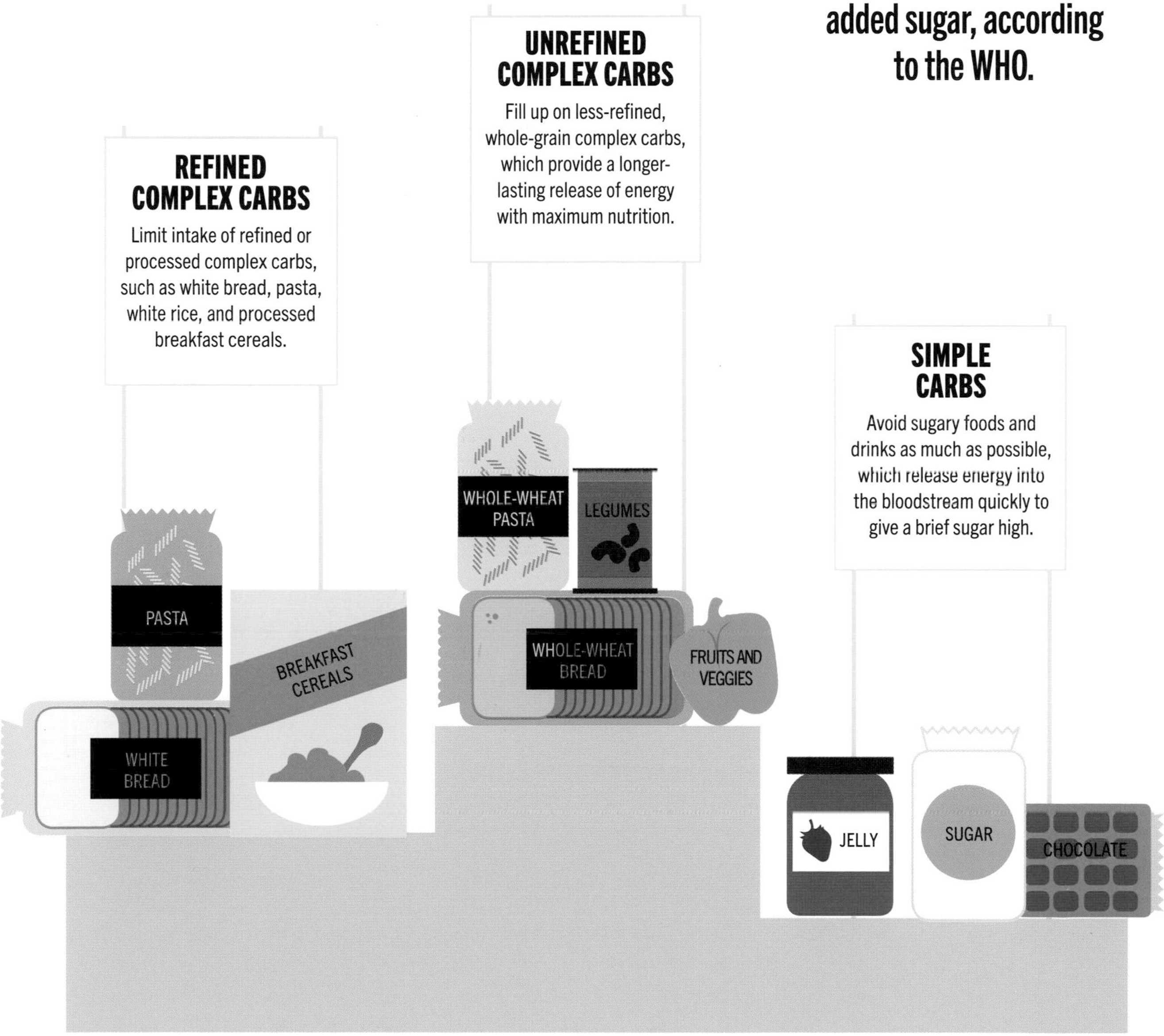

REFINED COMPLEX CARBS

Limit intake of refined or processed complex carbs, such as white bread, pasta, white rice, and processed breakfast cereals.

PASTA
BREAKFAST CEREALS
WHITE BREAD

UNREFINED COMPLEX CARBS

Fill up on less-refined, whole-grain complex carbs, which provide a longer-lasting release of energy with maximum nutrition.

WHOLE-WHEAT PASTA
LEGUMES
WHOLE-WHEAT BREAD
FRUITS AND VEGGIES

SIMPLE CARBS

Avoid sugary foods and drinks as much as possible, which release energy into the bloodstream quickly to give a brief sugar high.

JELLY
SUGAR
CHOCOLATE

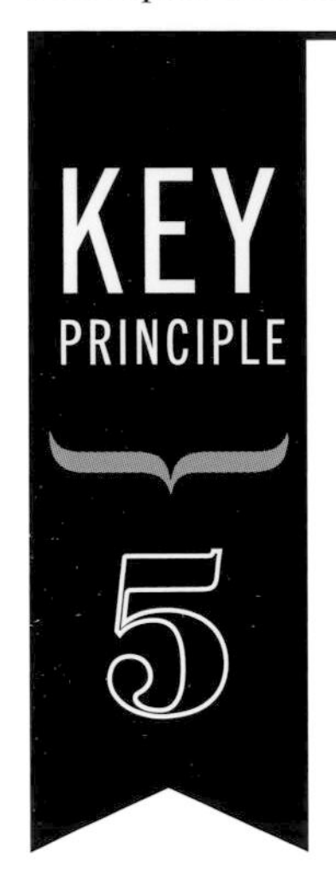

Swap red meat for fish

It's official: red meat should be off the regular menu if you want to live a long and healthy life. High intakes of red meat are unheard of in countries with the greatest number of centenarians. People aren't necessarily vegetarian, but fish takes pride of place at the dinner table, with meat featuring only now and then.

After a study by the International Agency for Research on Cancer concluded that every 3½oz (100g) of red meat eaten daily could increase the risk of colon cancer by 17 percent, the World Health Organization has now classified red meat as being "probably carcinogenic." Processed meat (any meat that's cured, salted, smoked, or preserved) fared worse as "definitely carcinogenic," alongside smoking and alcohol. Studies have also shown a link between higher intakes of red meat and a higher risk of heart disease.

But what if I'm vegan or vegetarian?

Even if you don't eat eggs and dairy, all the protein you need can come from a balance of legumes, nuts, and grains. Some plant-based foods offer short- chain omega-3 fats, which can be converted into the long-chain versions seen in oily fish, although the process is inefficient. Vitamin B12 is only found in animal foods, however, so a supplement may be wise.

The omega-3 factor

In contrast, good intakes of fish have been linked with a lower risk of overall death. It's unsurprising really, since fish is high in protein, low in saturated fat, and packed with a wide range of nutrients.

Many of fish's health benefits are attributed to its omega-3 fats. In a 2013 study of elderly people, those who had the highest levels of omega-3 fats in their blood lowered their risk of dying from all causes by 27 percent. And a 2016 review of studies found that eating the equivalent of three full portions a week was linked to a 12 percent reduction in dying compared with a fish-free diet. It's no surprise that many of the world's longest-lived communities, such as Okinawa in Japan and Ikaria in Greece, are located on islands or by the coast.

35%

lower risk of dying from heart disease for older adults with the highest levels of omega-3 fats.

Is all meat bad?

While white meat, such as poultry, is packed with nutrients, is lower in fat and saturates than red and processed meat, and doesn't seem to be linked to heart disease and bowel cancer, it does lack the omega-3 fats you get from fish.

What all these facts show is that eating lots of red meat is detrimental to longevity, and one good alternative to red meat is fish.

MAKE SMART SWAPS FOR LONGEVITY

A 2017 review of studies found that people who ate the most fish every day reduced their risk of death from all causes by 7 percent. In stark contrast, the highest intakes of red meat and processed meat actually made death more likely; see below. It's easy for meat to be the default option, but it's easy to make everyday switches from meat options to fish or seafood choices that will boost health and reduce your risk of dying.

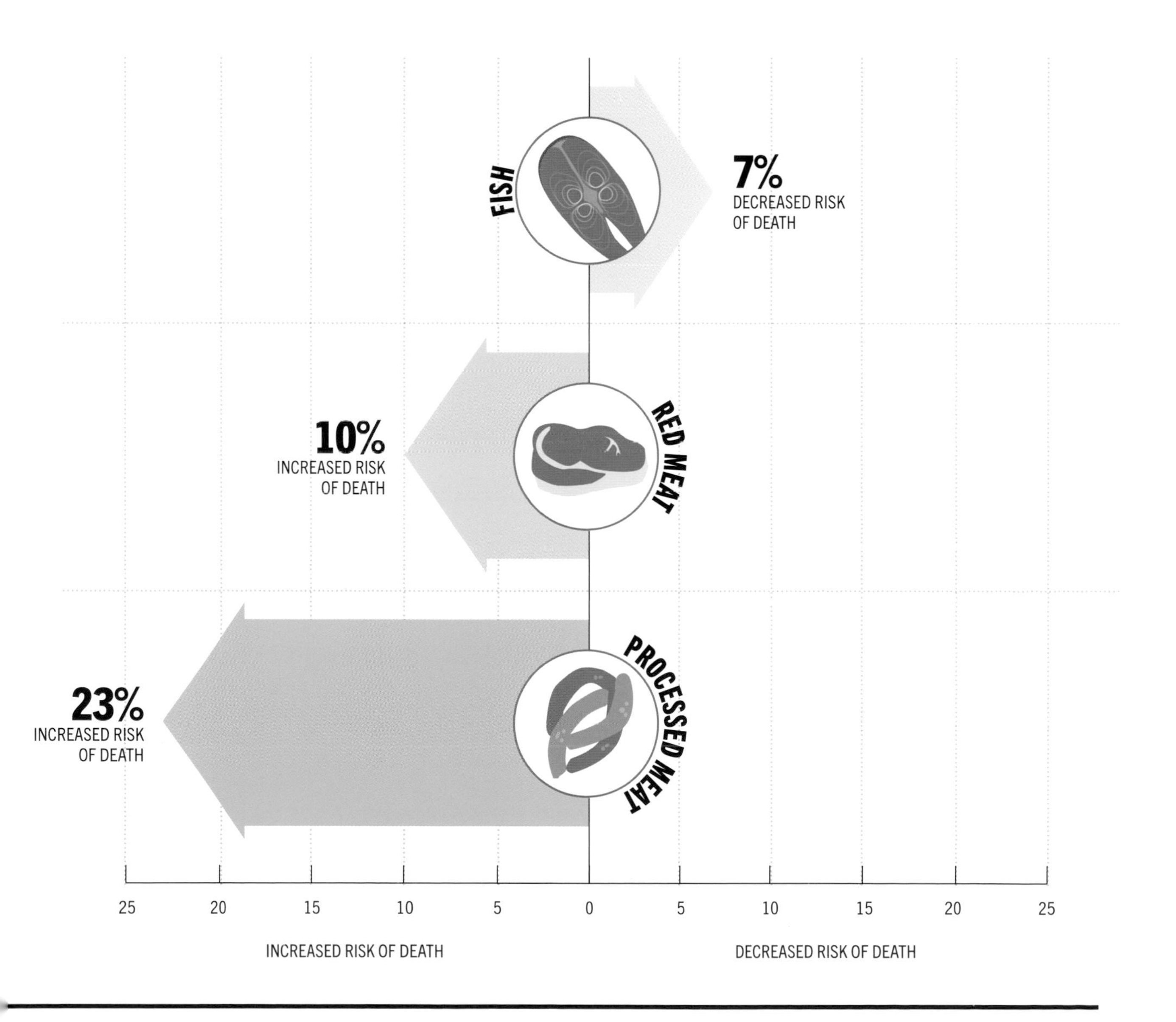

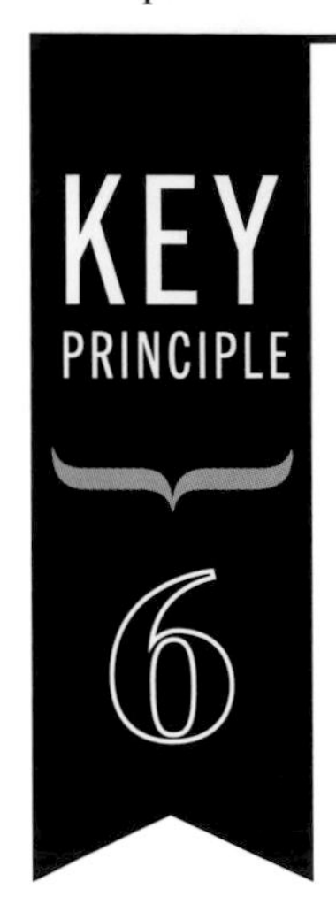

Eat as nature intended

Which kind of eating do you think will help you live a longer and healthier life: a diet of fresh food in its natural form or one based on artificial, processed, and refined ingredients? Yes, you've guessed right—eating as nature intended scores best in terms of health and longevity.

Take a look around a supermarket in the Western world and it's easy to find thousands of products that are completely unrecognizable from their natural state—from chicken nuggets and frosted cereal to instant mashed potatoes and spaghetti rings. But these types of foods don't feature in the traditional diets of those people living long and healthy lives, such as those in Japan or the Mediterranean. There, people are far more likely to "eat naturally" as a matter of course by choosing ingredients that are fresh; unprocessed; and have little, if anything, added to them. Put simply, it means they eat fresh fish rather than fish sticks, brown rice rather than white rice, and homemade curry rather than processed meals.

Boost nutrition

Most foods eaten in their natural form tend to be packed with health-giving fiber, vitamins, minerals, and antioxidants but low in health-sapping saturated fats, sugar, and sodium—all nutritional qualities that are linked to longevity. These stand in direct contrast to many processed or refined foods, which are low in nutrients but loaded with trans fats, saturated fats, sugars, and sodium.

58%

rise in fruit and vegetable consumption when people learn to cook meals from scratch.

Added extras

Many ready-made foods also include additives (flavors, colors, and preservatives). A good rule of thumb is: the more additives a product has, the more hidden fat, sugar, and sodium it also contains. So steer clear of the processed food aisles and embrace shopping for, and cooking with, natural ingredients.

Long-lived communities farm organically

Most experts generally agree the priority for health is to eat a mainly plant-based diet that contains plenty of whole grains, fruits, and vegetables—regardless of whether these are produced organically or not. But most of the food eaten by people in long-lived communities is produced organically, avoiding artificial pesticides, chemical fertilizers, and antibiotics.

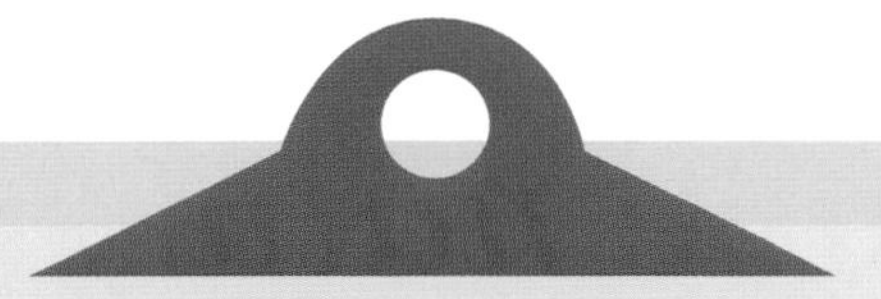

SMART CHOICES FOR FOOD SHOPPING

As well as cooking from the recipes in the longevity eating plan (see page 44), a few thoughtful choices on ingredient buying will help shift the balance from refined to fresh foods. Follow the advice below and you'll find that food shopping maximizes health and minimizes the "baddies."

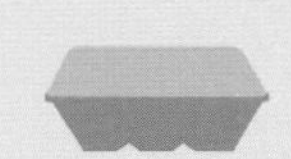

Choose sustainable

Buy meat, fish, eggs, and milk that are sustainably sourced and produced at high animal welfare standards.

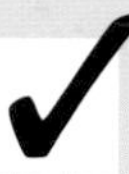

Source food locally

When shopping locally, you're more likely to find produce that tastes better and has been handled less.

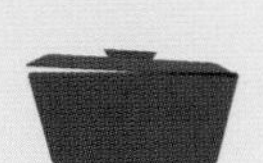
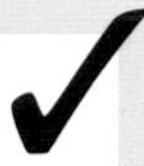

Cook from scratch

Making dishes yourself means you know exactly what goes into them. You can also boost vegetables and whole grains.

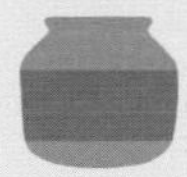
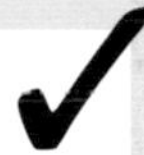

Get label savvy

Check ingredient lists. Don't buy a product if it has anything you don't recognize or wouldn't have in your own kitchen.

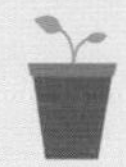

Grow your own food

Long-lived communities tend to grow most of the food they eat. Growing herbs is a good start and encourages cooking.

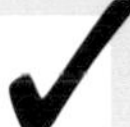

Drink tap water

Water is the best drink for health (see page 40). Tap water is free and plentiful, plus there's no packaging. It's win/win.

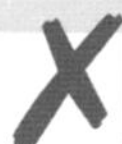

Limit all salt

Rock salt, sea salt, and Himalayan pink salt are all salt and bad for health. All forms of salt are high in sodium, which increases blood pressure.

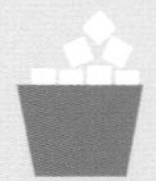
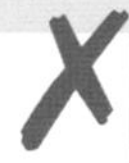

Cut down on sugars

Agave syrup, rice syrup, honey, and pomegranate molasses might sound healthy, but they offer few nutritional benefits and are as calorific as sugar.

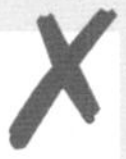

Skip "healthy" items

Foods labeled as "low fat," "low sugar," or "low sodium" are usually not very filling, contain few nutrients, and can be crammed with additives.

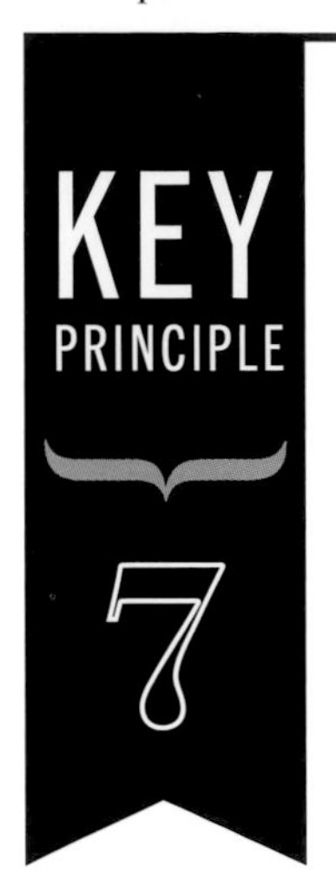

Choose naturally packaged fats

Whether it's following the low-fat diet of Okinawa, Japan, or the higher-fat diet of the Mediterranean, people who live longest get their fats from natural foods alongside a host of other wholesome nutrients.

Look at the traditional diets of people in long-lived communities and intakes of fat are well below international recommendations. The World Health Organization recommends that for health, total fat shouldn't exceed 30 percent of calories. But in terms of longevity, we should look to the traditional diets of the Mediterranean and Okinawa (see pages 16–19).

Figures certainly seem to support a low-fat diet for longevity. But if this is the case, then why do people from countries in the

THE SMART FAT STRATEGY

Being smart about including fat in your diet is as simple as 1, 2, 3. First, avoid trans fats in high-fat, processed foods. Second, limit your intake of saturated fats by cutting back on animal-based foods; research is ongoing to clarify saturated fat's role in heart disease, but health organizations advise cutting saturated fat intake. Third, choose more ingredients that naturally contain unsaturated fats, both monounsaturated fat and polyunsaturated fat.

LOSE

Trans fats

Artificial trans fats raise "bad" cholesterol and lower "good" cholesterol levels. Avoid such fats, mostly hidden in processed foods.

COOKIES AND CAKES

PASTRIES AND PIES

TAKEOUT FOODS

FRIED FOODS

LIMIT

Saturated fats

Saturated fats tend to be solid at room temperature and increase levels of cholesterol in the blood. Limit your intake of these foods.

RED MEAT

CHEESE

BUTTER

COCONUT OIL

31%

of all deaths worldwide were due to cardiovascular disease in 2015—equal to 17.7 million people.

Mediterranean—where fat intakes are much higher—live longer, too? Researchers believe the answer is down to the types of fat those people are eating and what other nutrients that fat comes with.

Traditional Mediterranean diets are high in fat, but they're reasonably low in saturated fats and trans fats (see below). Italy, for example, has one of the lowest intakes of trans fats in the Western world. Much of the fat Italians eat is unsaturated, coming from olive oil, nuts, seeds, and oily fish.

Get fat savvy

It's a similar picture in Japan. Yes, fat intakes are much lower to start with, but so are saturated fats. Just 15g of the daily fat in Japanese diets is saturated fat (compared with 26g in America; a healthy limit is no more than 20g saturated fats a day). Instead, much of their fat is eaten as omega-3 fats via a fish-rich diet.

Add these facts together and it's easy to see it's probably not so much the total amount of fat we have in our diet that affects our health, but the type of fat we eat.

High intakes of saturated fats and trans fats increase blood cholesterol, a key risk factor for heart disease. But research is increasingly showing these fats may also increase the risk of other diseases, including obesity, type 2 diabetes, dementia, and certain cancers, most likely because they trigger inflammation in the body. Unsaturated fats, it seems, either don't increase the risk or seem to help protect us from such diseases.

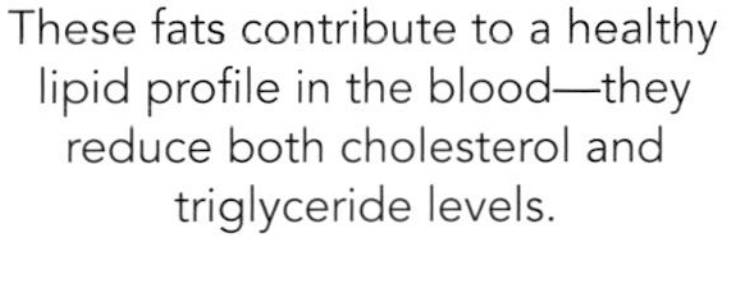

LIKE

Polyunsaturated fats

These fats (omega-3 and -6) promote levels of "good" cholesterol and provide essential fats for a healthy brain and skin.

OILY FISH

SUNFLOWER OIL

SOY

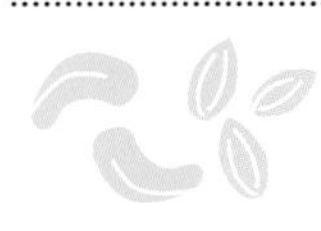

NUTS AND SEEDS

LOVE

Monounsaturated fats

These fats contribute to a healthy lipid profile in the blood—they reduce both cholesterol and triglyceride levels.

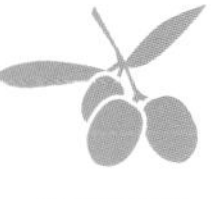

OLIVE OIL

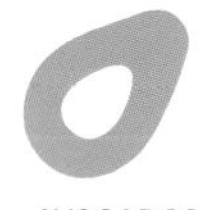

AVOCADOS

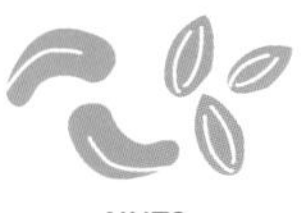

NUTS AND SEEDS

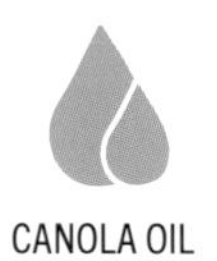

CANOLA OIL

The coconut conundrum

Coconut oil is over 85 percent saturated fat—far higher than butter (52 percent). Advocates say the fat in coconut is different and doesn't raise blood cholesterol. Most studies don't back this up; in fact, some studies show that it does indeed raise "bad" cholesterol.

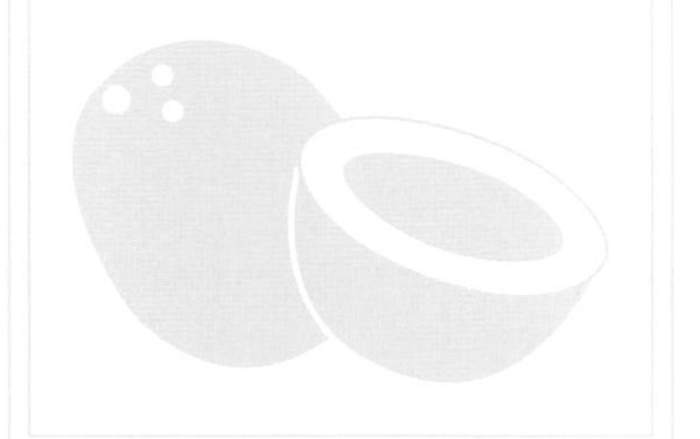

Dose up on the sunshine vitamin

Despite being able to make vitamin D ourselves, a lack of vitamin D is one of the most common nutritional deficiencies in the world. Since it's so vital to health and longevity, it's time to address the situation.

The figures are staggering: more than 4 in 10 adults over the age of 50 in the US and Europe are deficient in vitamin D. The "sunshine vitamin"—it's made in the body when the skin is exposed to sunlight—is best known for its role in keeping bones strong and healthy. Vitamin D helps the body absorb calcium from foods and deposit it in bones, thereby helping to prevent bone conditions, such as osteomalacia in adults and rickets in children.

Naturally well-rounded

But its benefits go way beyond the health of our bones. Vitamin D keeps our muscles functioning properly and is vital for a strong immune system. One 2017 study of about 11,000 people found supplements of vitamin D reduced the risk of acute respiratory tract infections (such as colds, flu, bronchitis, and pneumonia) by 12 percent. The effects were particularly strong for those initially deficient in vitamin D.

Scientific studies also reveal that a deficiency of vitamin D may increase the risk of many conditions, including type 2 diabetes, heart

TOP FOOD SOURCES OF VITAMIN D

We can top up our body's store of vitamin D with foods, including oily fish, mushrooms, and eggs. The World Health Organization recommends a daily vitamin D intake of 5mcg for everyone under 50, 10mcg for 51–65-year-olds, and 15mcg for over-65s. Some health organizations suggest that everyone take a vitamin D supplement in fall and winter to guarantee levels for optimal health.

Vitamin D (mcg) per 3½oz (100g)

CHANTERELLE MUSHROOMS
5.3

FARMED SALMON
4.7

FRESH SARDINES
4

EGGS
3.2

RED SNAPPER
2.3

CANNED TUNA
1.1

disease, certain cancers (especially colon cancer), multiple sclerosis, rheumatoid arthritis, and osteoarthritis. Other research shows a link between low intakes of vitamin D and an increased risk of mental decline, dementia, and Alzheimer's disease.

More research is needed, but with so many potential links to better health, vitamin D is creating a buzz in the nutrition world.

Who's at risk?

Because most vitamin D is made when the skin is exposed to the sun's UVB rays, people who cover up for cultural reasons or who are housebound are at particular risk of vitamin D deficiency, as their skin isn't exposed to sunlight. Using sunscreen has a similar effect since it blocks UVB rays.

The sun's rays need to be of a certain strength to create vitamin D, so where we live, the season, and the time of day can affect how much is made. People with darker skin may also be at risk, even if they live in a sunny climate, since higher pigment levels affect the skin's vitamin D–making ability. Older people are more prone to a deficiency, because age-related skin changes mean less vitamin D is made. So be safe in the sun, but be sure to get enough, and let food play its part.

Getting enough sun

When UVB rays are at the right strength, the skin only needs short periods of direct exposure to make vitamin D. It's vital to follow sun safety advice and make sure skin doesn't burn, as sunburn is linked to an increased risk of skin cancer.

MACKEREL, CANNED IN BRINE **7.4**

RAINBOW TROUT **7.9**

KIPPERS **8**

FRESH MACKEREL **8**

WILD SALMON **8.6**

COLD-SMOKED SALMON **8.9**

RED SALMON, CANNED **10.9**

PINK SALMON, CANNED **13.6**

SARDINES, CANNED IN TOMATO SAUCE **14**

40% of adults in the US and Europe over the age of 50 are deficient in vitamin D.

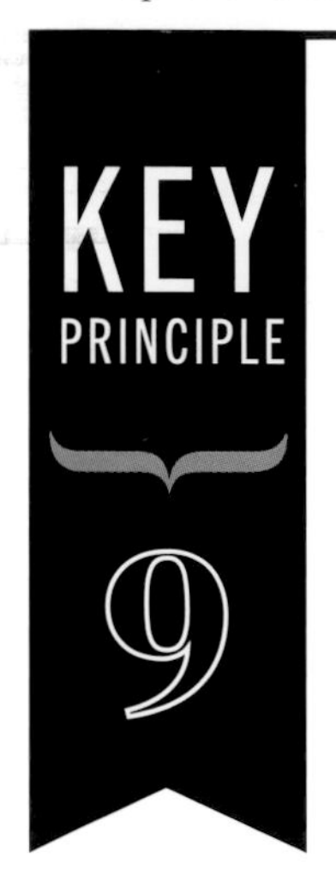

Choose foods across the color spectrum

For a long and healthy life, you need to be eating more than "your greens." The phytochemicals in colorful produce have been linked to protection against heart disease, cancer, and Alzheimer's disease.

Until recently, the health-promoting benefits of plant foods were put down to them containing plenty of fiber, vitamins, and minerals. Those elements do offer benefits, but that's not the whole story. Now research is revealing they naturally contain thousands of other compounds, known as phytochemicals or phytonutrients ("phyto" roughly translates as "plants" in Greek).

Tangible benefits

Phytochemicals evolved to help plants protect themselves (from disease, pests, and UV light). So, often, they reside in the outer layers and are responsible for

EAT A RAINBOW

Phytonutrients are found on or near the surface, so whenever possible, eat the skin—be it the zest of lemons, the peel on cucumbers, or the skin on potatoes. The remainder exist within the interior flesh, so whole fruits and vegetables will give you a complete package of nutritional goodness. Here are just some of the potential health and longevity benefits of "eating the rainbow," as suggested by lab research.

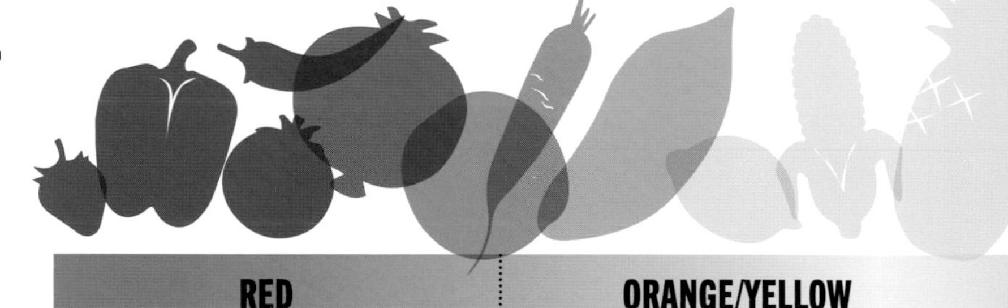

RED

Lycopene—A carotenoid that may protect against some cancers and reduces blood cholesterol levels.

Ellagic acid—An antioxidant chemical that may help counter body-wide free-radical damage and a potential anticancer agent.

Anthocyanins—These also occur but at lower levels in red foods; see Purple/blue (right).

ORANGE/YELLOW

Alpha- and beta-carotene—These carotenoids are precursors to vitamin A. Beta-carotene is the most common and has antioxidant powers. It is beneficial for strong immunity and good vision.

Beta-cryptoxanthin—A chemical that is transformed into vitamin A in the body. It may also reduce the risk of lung cancer.

64x

more antioxidants exist in plant foods than in animal foods.

fruits' and vegetables' colors—such as the dark purple of blackberries (anthocyanins), the redness of tomatoes (lycopene), and the dark green of spinach (lutein); their flavors—for instance, the bitter taste of kale (glucosinolates); and their aromas—like the pungent odor of garlic (allicin). It's not surprising to discover that the more colors you eat, the wider the variety of phytochemicals you'll consume, and the greater the spread of benefits you'll reap.

Now, for the science

Phytochemicals tend to be separated into groups according to their structural make-up. For example, polyphenols (one of the largest and most-studied groups) are further divided into smaller groups, including flavonoids, anthocyanins, flavonols, flavones, isoflavonoids, flavanones, and flavanols. Other groups include carotenoids, such as alpha- and beta-carotene, zeaxanthin, lutein, beta-cryptoxanthin, and lycopene.

The total package

It's difficult to pinpoint the role individual phytochemicals have on our health and longevity, partly because phytochemicals don't exist in isolation—one plant may contain hundreds, along with fiber, vitamins, and minerals. That said, there is much scientific lab-based research that provides good insight into the potential benefits that phytochemicals may have in helping to prevent disease and promote optimum health.

In the meantime, boosting our intake of phytochemicals is key: simply eat a variety of differently colored fruits and vegetables—just think "rainbow."

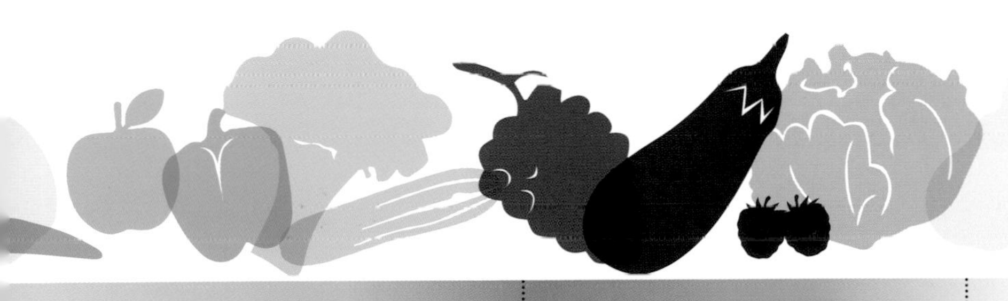

GREEN

Lutein and zeaxanthin—Two antioxidant carotenoids that are linked to a reduction in the risk of age-related macular degeneration.

Glucosinolates—These are broken down into chemicals that may protect against lung cancer.

Chlorophyll—Gives plants their green pigment and has antioxidant and anti-inflammatory benefits.

PURPLE/BLUE

Anthocyanins—Polyphenols that help to dilate blood vessels, so they're good for heart health and are linked to better memory.

Resveratrol—A polyphenol with potent anticancer actions. It's also been linked to better heart health.

Phenolic acids—Chemicals with potent antimicrobial, antiviral, and antioxidant activities.

WHITE/BEIGE

Quercetin—A flavonoid that's good for circulation and for body-wide inflammation.

Allicin—A sulfur-containing compound that may lower blood pressure and cholesterol and reduce the risk of some cancers.

Anthoxanthins—Flavonoids that may reduce stroke risk and promote heart health.

Drink plenty of fluids

Dehydration at any age can make you feel tired, weak, dizzy, and confused; affect your concentration and memory; and increase the risk of low blood pressure and urinary tract infections. But as we get older, staying hydrated becomes harder, so it's vital to know exactly what and how much you should be drinking.

The human body is two-thirds water, so it's no wonder that water is vital for all bodily functions: it transports nutrients in the blood; removes waste products in the urine; helps us regulate our body temperature; and acts as a lubricant and shock absorber in our joints. The brain, in particular, is 77 percent water, so even mild dehydration can wreak havoc on a person's mental function.

Dehydration issues

Unfortunately, we become more susceptible to dehydration as we get older. First, the amount of water in our body decreases with age—at birth, the body is about 75 percent water, but this drops to around 55 percent in elderly people. Next, the kidneys become less efficient at conserving water in the body; this is combined with the fact that the mechanism that triggers thirst becomes less effective, so we're less likely to feel

THE LOWDOWN ON DRINKS

When it comes to fluid intake, surprisingly, almost all fluids count (see right for which to choose). The only exception is alcohol, which promotes dehydration. Follow in the steps of those who live the longest by drinking plentiful amounts of water and green tea.

Water

Experts universally agree on water as the number-one choice for fluids, as it's super-hydrating, doesn't damage teeth, and is calorie free.

Coffee

Moderate amounts of coffee (four cups a day) may confer some health gains. Coffee has beneficial antioxidants and may reduce the risk of Alzheimer's disease.

thirsty and therefore drink less. On top of this, worries about incontinence mean some people limit their fluid intakes. Bottom line: as we get older, it becomes even more important to pay attention to how much we drink so that we stay hydrated.

How much fluid is enough?

Everyone's requirements are different, depending on their weight, age, gender, level of activity, and the climate where they live—hotter temperatures and increased humidity, for example, make us sweat more, so we need more fluid to replenish what's been lost. Added to this, what we eat can affect how much extra fluid we need to get from drinks.

For most of us, about one-fifth of the fluid in our diet comes from foods, such as milk, soup, stews, yogurts, fruits, and vegetables.

Research from the European Food Safety Authority suggests adequate daily intakes of water are about 3½ pints (2 liters) for women and 4¼ pints (2.5 liters) for men. If 20 percent of this comes from food, then women need to drink 2¾ pints (1.6 liters) and men 3½ pints (2 liters) of fluids—that's about six to eight glasses—each day (see The lowdown on drinks, below). Good hydration helps your body operate better for longer.

A Japanese study showed that women drinking the most green tea were 17 percent less likely to die earlier.

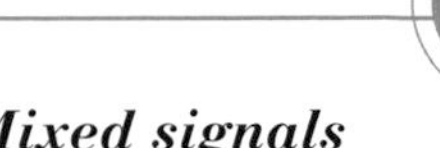

Mixed signals

People can easily mistake thirst for hunger and reach for food instead of fluids. When in doubt, drink a glass of water when you first experience hunger pangs. If they subside, you were dehydrated; if they continue, then you really are hungry.

Tea

Tea—particularly green tea—features in the diets of some of the longest-living groups. Tea drinking has been linked to protection against cancer and cognitive decline. Plus, it's rich in fluoride.

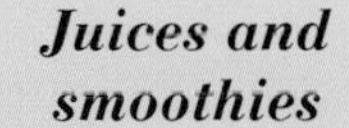

Juices and smoothies

Although they contain some vitamins and minerals, these drinks can damage teeth if drunk often. It's better to eat the whole fruit or vegetable than blend it with milk or water.

Sugary and sports drinks

Avoid these drinks; they contain no nutrients and are packed with sugar (or artificial sweeteners). For most people (who exercise for an hour at a time), sports drinks are just not necessary.

-PART-

3

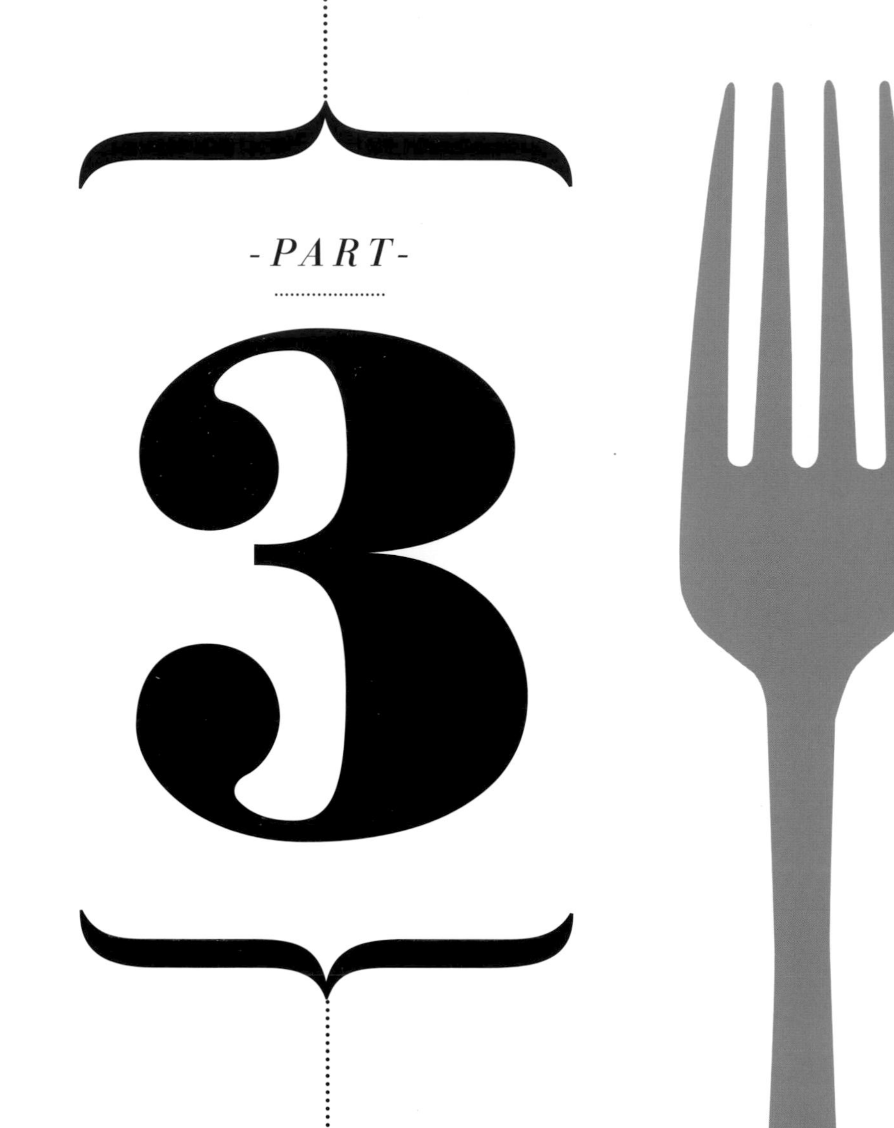

The longevity eating plan

Follow the month-long program of menus with delicious recipes for whole-body health. Discover the longevity "wonderfoods" and "supergroups."

The next four weeks

Follow the longevity eating plan and you'll find yourself digging into delicious meals and snacks that will leave you feeling and looking younger in just 4 weeks. What are you waiting for?

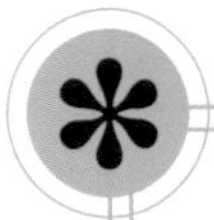

How the icons work

The recipes in the plan have been designed to deliver optimum nutrition for health and longevity. Although all recipes offer health benefits across the board, some ingredients come with even greater bonuses for certain parts of the body or for preventing specific conditions—and these are shown as icons, which correspond to the body sections (see page 155).

Positive benefits—When icons are highlighted, it means the recipe is packed with nutrients that are particularly good for promoting health in this part of the body.

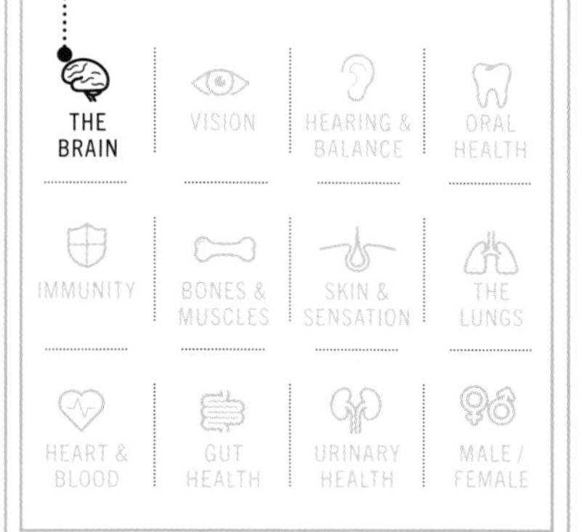

Unlike some anti-aging diets, the longevity eating plan isn't about depriving yourself. After all, who wants to extend their life if every mealtime feels like a penance rather than a pleasure? Although the plan is designed with nutrition in mind, it's so much more than that. The aim is to also provide plentiful meal ideas that are easy to make, look fantastic, taste delicious, and, above all else, are what you really want to eat.

The plan in a nutshell

In essence, over the next 4 weeks, the plan aims to get you eating a predominantly plant-based diet that's packed with fruits; vegetables; and starchy, fiber-rich foods. It helps you significantly reduce the amount of meat in your diet but still encourages you to eat fish. And it's designed to help you shift your calorie intake from evening-heavy to morning-heavy.

Nutritional design

The eating plan across the weeks provides around 2,000 calories a day. But over the course of the plan, we distribute these calories

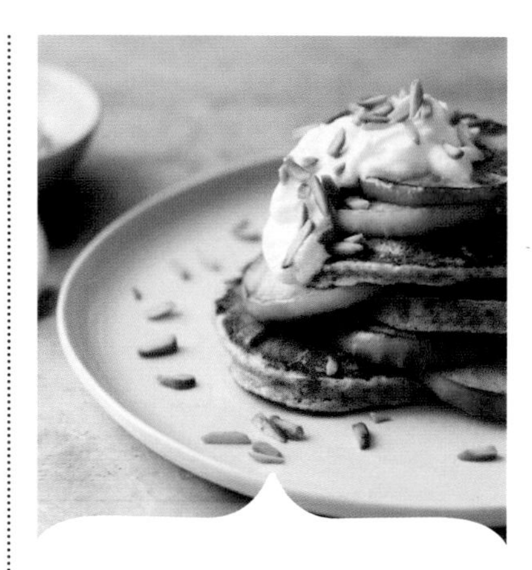

FOCUS ON EATING BREAKFAST EVERY DAY; IT'S EASY WHEN THERE ARE PLENTY OF DELICIOUS EXAMPLES, SUCH AS THESE BANANA PANCAKES WITH SPICED APPLE RINGS (SEE PAGE 67).

between the meals differently to follow Key principle 1 (see page 22). You may well find you're eating more food than you're used to because the meals are packed with fruits and vegetables, which add bulk but few calories. The plan is high in fiber, so be sure to drink plenty of fluids (see page 40). All snacks provide about 250 calories each.

The great news is that from week 1, the plan has the right levels of healthy fats, carbs, and protein for health and longevity.

MAKING THE PLAN WORK

No plan can suit everyone all of the time, so to make things fit with real life, here we cover some of the common questions about adapting the plan.

Q} I'm a big exerciser. Will I need to adjust anything?

A} You may want to slightly increase your portions of starchy carbs and whole grains and of plant proteins, such as beans and tofu, to balance out the extra energy you use. Men may also want to boost portion sizes unless they want to lose weight.

Q} Can I follow the plan if I'm cooking for one?

A} Most of the recipes in this plan are designed for two people. But they're easily adapted to be halved for one or doubled up for four, for example, if you have more mouths to feed. Alternatively, make the recipe as it stands, then cool and store the second portion in a sealed container in the freezer.

Q} I'd like to lose a bit of weight. Can I?

A} If you have a little amount of weight (14lb/6kg) to lose, the easiest option is to omit one or both of the snacks from the plan. If you have more weight to lose, such as 28–41lb (12.7–19kg), you may lose weight just by following the plan as it is (the heavier you are, the more your body burns calories).

Q} What if I don't like some of the options?

A} There is flexibility in swapping meals and snacks around. When it comes to lunches and snacks, feel free to swap one for another from any week; but for breakfasts and dinners, only replace it with another from the same week.

Q} Does the plan work for vegetarians?

A} This plan already contains plenty of vegetarian recipes. However, if you want to replace any meat or fish options, follow the same advice as above on swapping.

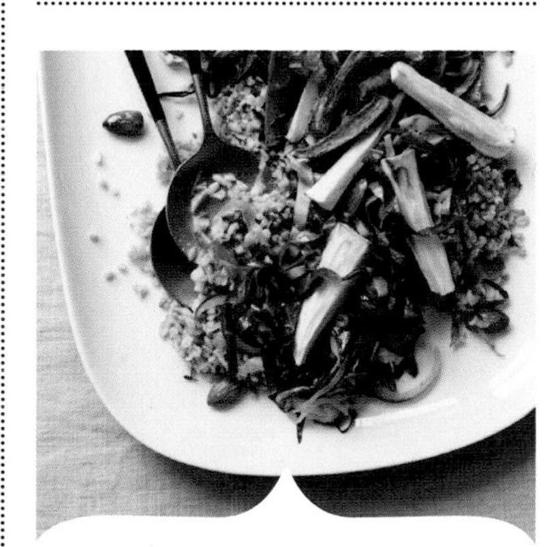

ENJOY A SELECTION OF EASY-TO-COOK MEALS BURSTING WITH NUTRITION AND TASTE, SUCH AS FREEKEH WITH ROASTED VEGGIES AND GREENS (SEE PAGE 93).

THE PATH TO LONGEVITY MEANS...

Tablespoon and teaspoon measurements are level; 1 tsp = 5ml; 1 tbsp = 15ml.

A serving of fruit and veg should be 3oz (80g).

Eggs should be medium, unless otherwise stated.

Cow's milk should be the skim variety.

Nondairy milks, such as soy or almond milk, should be unsweetened and fortified with calcium.

All types of yogurt should be unsweetened and plain. Buy calcium-fortified soy yogurt.

Nut butters should be free from added salt or sugar.

Nuts and seeds should always be unsalted.

Beans and lentils should be canned in water and free from added sugar or salt.

Salt should never be added.

Swap foods to suit the seasons.

Always buy **sustainable fish.**

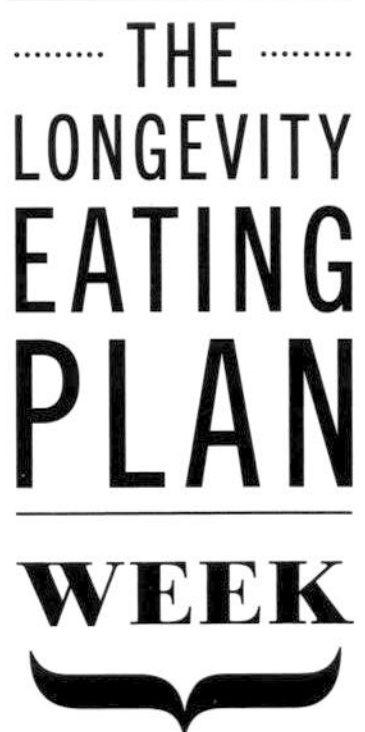

Week 1 is all about getting into the habit of eating regularly and making sure you start each and every day with a healthy and tasty breakfast. At the same time, you'll be getting used to eating more fruits, veggies, beans, and whole grains, while cutting down on (but not totally avoiding) red meat and poultry. Welcome to the first week of eating better to live longer.

	MONDAY	TUESDAY	WEDNESDAY
BREAKFAST	Buckwheat and oat porridge (see page 59)	2 slices rye bread with 3 tbsp low-fat cottage cheese, 2 sliced figs, and 4 crushed walnut halves	2 slices whole-grain toast topped with 2 scrambled eggs, mixed with 2½oz (75g) smoked haddock and 2 grilled tomatoes
SNACK	2 tbsp unsalted peanuts, 1 handful of blueberries, and 1 orange	Shake: blend 1 banana with 1 handful of raspberries, 1 tbsp chia seeds, and ¾ cup (200ml) skim milk	4 tbsp fat-free Greek yogurt with 1 chopped pear and 1 tbsp chopped hazelnuts
LUNCH	Greek salad: based on 2 tomatoes, 1 green bell pepper, 1 small red onion, ¼ cucumber, 1¼oz (40g) reduced-fat feta, 10 olives, and 1 tbsp olive oil; serve with 1 whole-wheat pita, plus 1 pear	Shrimp, pomegranate, and quinoa bowl (see page 80)	Pesto pasta salad with broccoli and tomatoes (see page 79)
SNACK	2 oatcakes topped with ½ small avocado mashed with a little lime juice	2 celery sticks filled with 2 tbsp nut butter, plus 1 pear	2 tbsp unsalted cashew nuts, plus a glass of skim milk
DINNER	Turkey stir-fry (see page 107)	Tasty tofu wraps (see page 107)	Sumac fishcakes with greens (see page 111)

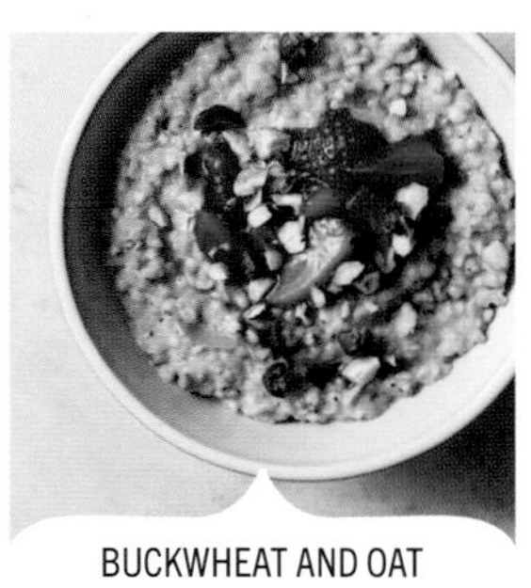

BUCKWHEAT AND OAT PORRIDGE

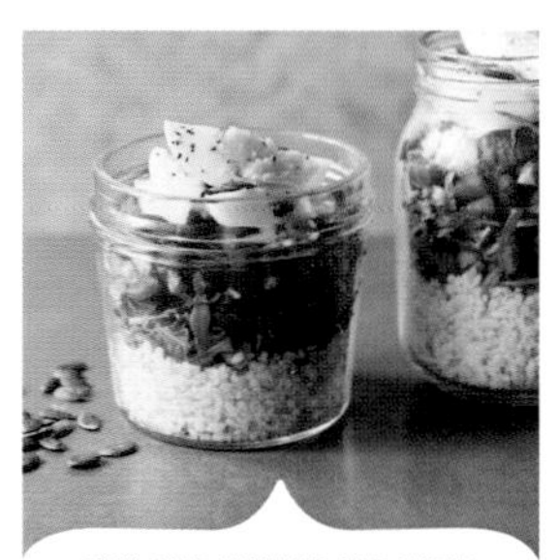

BULGUR WHEAT JAR WITH EGGS AND SALSA

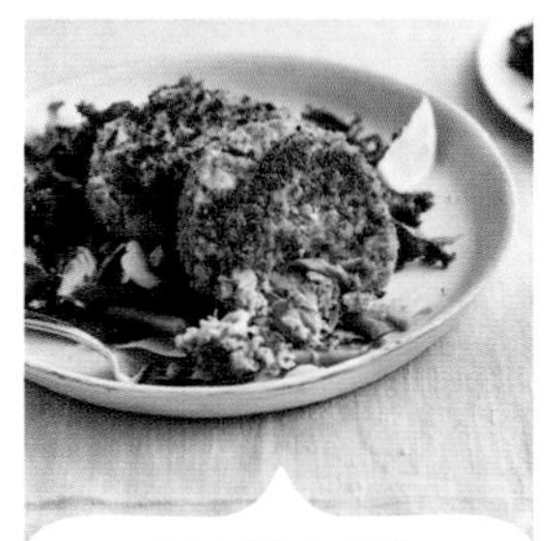

SUMAC FISHCAKES WITH GREENS

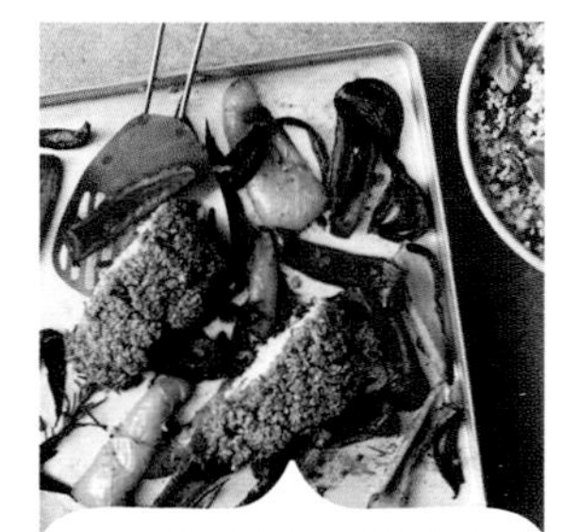

ROASTED HADDOCK WITH A HERBY CRUMB

THURSDAY	FRIDAY	SATURDAY	SUNDAY
Tropical fruit salad (see page 55)	1 whole-wheat wrap filled with ½ small mashed avocado, 2 hard-boiled eggs, and 1 tomato	Breakfast tortilla (see page 55)	1 sliced banana, 1 chopped peach with 4 tbsp fat-free Greek yogurt and topped with 5 tbsp toasted oats
3 oatcakes topped with 3 tbsp low-fat cottage cheese and 1 sliced peach	2 tbsp pumpkin seeds and 1 pear	1 banana, mashed, on 1 slice of whole-grain toast with a sprinkling of cinnamon, plus 1 glass of skim milk	10 walnut halves
Bulgur wheat jar with eggs and salsa (see page 83)	Salad: mix 7oz (200g) cooked whole-wheat pasta with 5¾oz (160g) can tuna in water (drained), 1 handful each of baby spinach and watercress, and 1 tomato; toss with 1 tbsp each olive oil and balsamic	Salad: mix 6 tbsp cooked bulgur wheat with 4oz (120g) canned kidney beans (drained), 1 tomato, 4 scallions, ¼ cucumber, 2 celery sticks, and chopped cilantro; toss with 1 tbsp olive oil and lemon juice	Moroccan-style couscous salad (see page 79)
1 slice rye bread with 1 tbsp peanut butter and 1 banana	Tzatziki: mix 4 tbsp fat-free Greek yogurt with ¼ cucumber (grated), crushed garlic, lemon juice, and freshly chopped mint; serve with 1 whole-wheat pita	2 handfuls of blueberries, 1 kiwi fruit, 1 tbsp skin-on almonds with 4 tbsp fat-free Greek yogurt	Guacamole: mix ½ small avocado, 1 diced tomato, lemon juice, crushed garlic, and chili to taste; serve with 1 whole-wheat pita
Steak and wedges (see page 116)	Roasted haddock with a herby crumb (see page 115), plus 2 handfuls of blackberries	Lemon chicken pasta (see page 116)	Roast pork and veggies (see page 117)

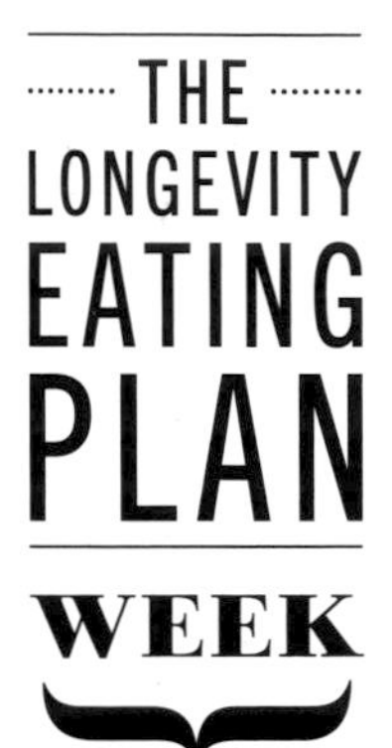

You're most likely already seeing and feeling the benefits of the plan. Eating regularly—and sticking with starchy, high-fiber carbs—should be boosting your energy levels. Plus, you'll be feeling satisfied for longer after eating. This week, you'll see breakfasts get a little bigger and dinners a little smaller as you work toward breakfasting like a king.

	MONDAY	TUESDAY	WEDNESDAY
BREAKFAST	1 whole-wheat wrap filled with 1 mashed banana, 4 sliced dates, and 4 crushed walnut halves	2 eggs scrambled with 1 small (3oz/80g) grilled kipper and 1 tomato, served with 2 slices whole-grain toast	Fruit salad: 2 fresh figs, 1 pomegranate, 1 orange, 1 kiwi fruit, and 2 handfuls of blueberries with 4 tbsp fat-free Greek yogurt, and 2 tbsp pistachio nuts
SNACK	1 slice whole-grain bread topped with 3 tbsp low-fat cottage cheese and 1¾oz (50g) canned pink salmon	1 tbsp each of sunflower seeds, pumpkin seeds, and raisins	3 oatcakes topped with ½ small avocado and 1 tomato
LUNCH	Mixed bean bowl with pita nachos (see page 86)	1 large baked potato with 5 tbsp low-fat cottage cheese mixed with 1 slice chopped fresh pineapple, 1 nectarine, and 1 tbsp skin-on chopped almonds	Freekeh with roasted veggies and greens (see page 93)
SNACK	Fruit salad: 1 apple, 1 nectarine, and 1 orange with 4 tbsp fat-free Greek yogurt	3oz (80g) whole-grain baguette, thinly sliced, toasted, and rubbed with garlic; top with a mix of 2 tomatoes, ½ small red onion, garlic, basil, and 1 tsp olive oil	Shake: blend 1 cup (250ml) skim milk, 1 banana, and 1 tbsp peanut butter
DINNER	Mushroom stew (see page 117)	Barley risotto with roasted squash (see page 120)	Cod with sweet potato wedges (see page 128)

CINNAMON TOAST WITH BLUEBERRY COMPOTE

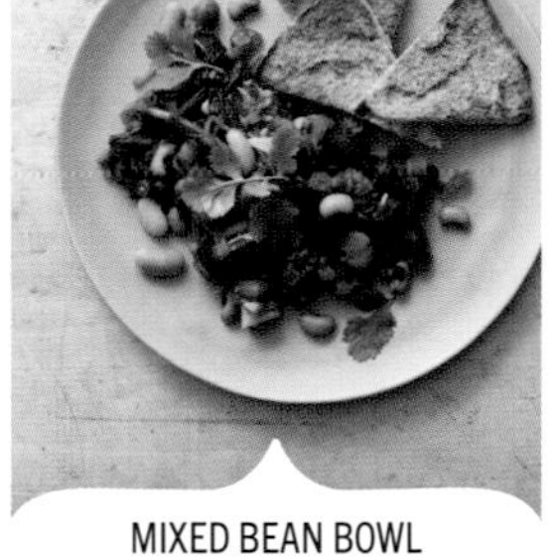

MIXED BEAN BOWL WITH PITA NACHOS

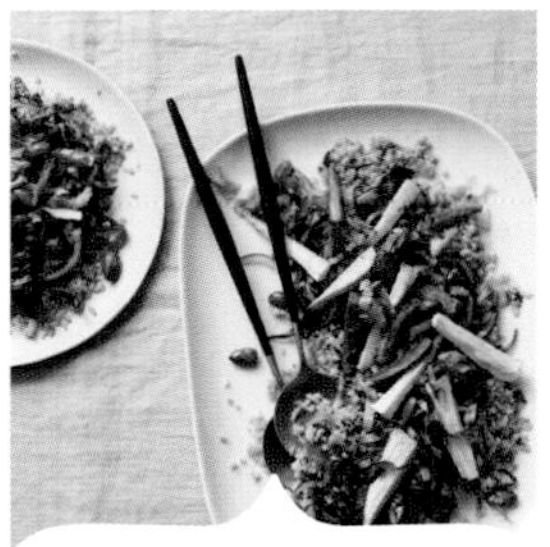

FREEKEH WITH ROASTED VEGGIES AND GREENS

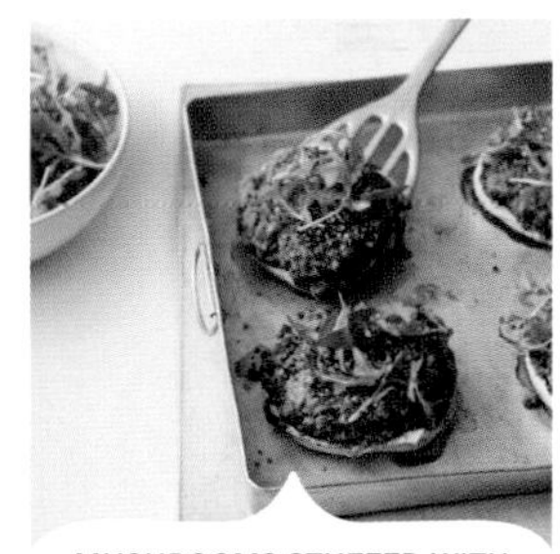

MUSHROOMS STUFFED WITH TOMATO COUSCOUS

THURSDAY	FRIDAY	SATURDAY	SUNDAY
Porridge: 4 tbsp oats and 1¼ cups (275ml) soy milk, with 1 banana and 4 tbsp (30g) chopped pecan nuts	Eggs on toast with roasted tomatoes (see page 72)	Cinnamon toast with blueberry compote (see page 63)	Mango and coconut smoothie bowl (see page 72)
1 slice whole-grain toast with 1 tbsp peanut butter and 1 pear	2 tbsp unsalted pistachio nuts and 1 glass of skim milk	Protein pot: 4 tbsp cooked quinoa, 1 hard-boiled egg, and 1 tbsp edamame	2 tbsp almonds and 1 pear
Salad: 8 tbsp cooked whole-wheat giant couscous, 1 small can tuna in water (drained), 3 scallions, ½ red bell pepper, 5 olives, lemon zest and juice, 2 tsp garlic-flavored olive oil, and basil, plus 1 tangerine	Indian-style chicken wrap (see page 88)	4 oatcakes with 3 celery sticks, 1 apple, 1 handful of seedless grapes, and 6 tbsp low-fat cottage cheese mixed with chives and 4 scallions, plus 1 tangerine	Sandwich: 3 slices whole-grain bread filled with ½ avocado mashed with garlic, lemon juice, and chili to taste, 1 tomato and 1 handful of arugula, plus 1 apple and 1 kiwi fruit
8 strawberries and 2 handfuls of blueberries topped with 4 tbsp fat-free Greek yogurt and 1 tbsp hazelnuts	1 whole-wheat pita filled with cucumber and 3½oz (100g) shrimp cooked and mixed with 1 tbsp soy yogurt and lemon zest and juice	10 walnut halves and 2 handfuls of blackberries	1 whole-wheat wrap cut into triangles, brushed with oil, sprinkled with herbs, and baked with 4½oz (125g) soy yogurt mixed with mint, and lemon juice
Mushrooms stuffed with tomato couscous (see page 125)	Ratatouille (see page 128)	Pasta with tuna and roasted veggies (see page 129)	Rosemary lamb (see page 129)

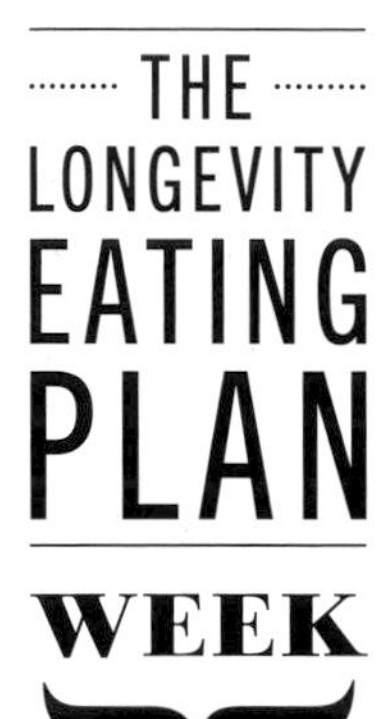

During this week, you consolidate the changes you've made in weeks 1 and 2 and shift even further toward a predominantly plant-based diet. You'll see more soy products, nuts, and seeds taking center stage, and you'll find out how to put an anti-aging twist on classics, such as chili, chicken dinners, kebabs, pasta dishes, and even milkshakes.

	MONDAY	TUESDAY	WEDNESDAY
BREAKFAST	Fruit salad: 1 apple, 1 banana, 1 pear, 1 orange, and 1 handful of raspberries with 4 tbsp fat-free Greek yogurt, and 4 tbsp oats	Porridge: 4 tbsp oats with 1¼ cups (275ml) skim milk, 6 dried apricots, 1 pomegranate, 1 tbsp whole (skin-on) almonds, and cinnamon to taste	Sandwich: 3 slices whole-grain bread filled with ½ avocado, 1 hard-boiled egg, 1 tomato, and 1 handful of arugula, plus 1 handful of blueberries
SNACK	3 tbsp unsalted peanuts	Shake: blend ¾ cup (200ml) soy milk, 4½oz (125g) soy yogurt, 8 strawberries, and 1 banana; top with 1 tsp chia seeds	Fruit salad: 1 orange, 1 banana, 1 handful of grapes, and 1 peach
LUNCH	Beet, pepper, and chunky hummus wrap (see page 96)	Omelet: 1 tsp sunflower oil, ½ small red onion, 1 handful of mushrooms, ½ red bell pepper, ½ zucchini, and 2 eggs with salad and a 3oz (80g) piece of whole-grain baguette, plus 1 pear	1 large baked potato with 1 grilled turkey steak and coleslaw (1 grated carrot, 1 handful of shredded red cabbage, ½ sliced small onion, and 2 tbsp soy yogurt mixed with garlic and lemon zest)
SNACK	3 oatcakes with 3 tbsp low-fat cottage cheese and 1 sliced kiwi fruit	4 dates and 1 tbsp raisins	3 tbsp pumpkin seeds
DINNER	Pasta with chili and garlic shrimp (see page 136)	Tofu skewers (see page 136)	Roasted flounder with sweet potato noodles (see page 132)

BANANA PANCAKES WITH SPICED APPLE RINGS

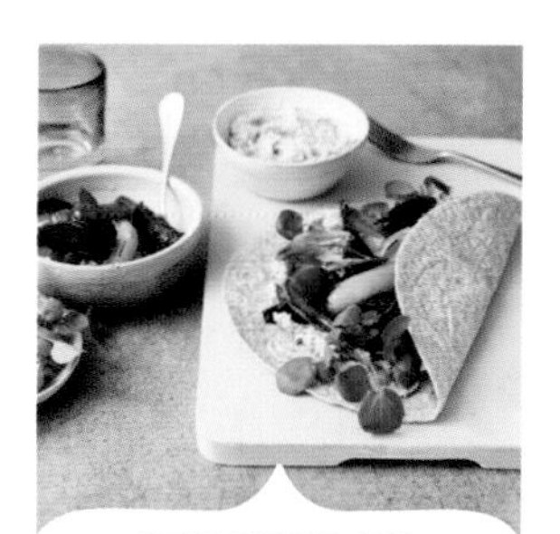

BEET, PEPPER, AND CHUNKY HUMMUS WRAP

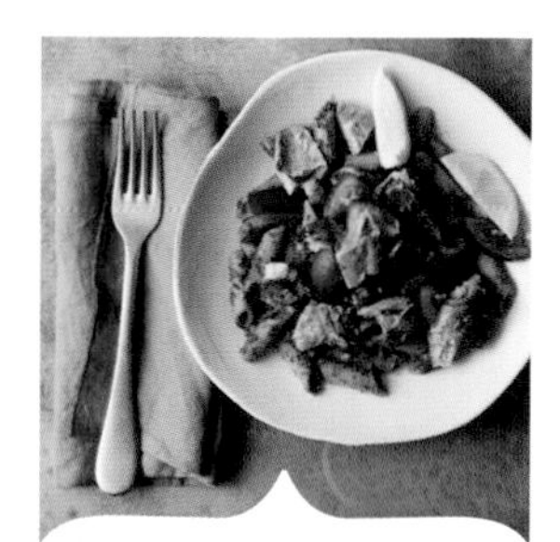

WHOLE-WHEAT PASTA SALAD WITH SARDINES

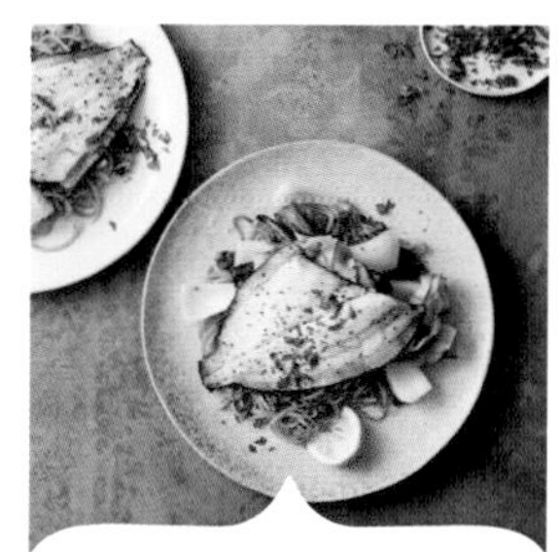

ROASTED FLOUNDER WITH SWEET POTATO NOODLES

THURSDAY	FRIDAY	SATURDAY	SUNDAY
Muesli: 3 tbsp oats, 1 tbsp chopped hazelnuts, 3 dried dates, and 1 tbsp golden raisins with 1 chopped apple and soy milk (use as much or as little as you like)	Veggie breakfast pita pockets (see page 73)	Banana pancakes with spiced apple rings (see page 67)	2 slices whole-grain toast with 2 tbsp nut butter; 1 slice topped with 1 banana and the other with 1 sliced pear
Sandwich: 2 slices whole-wheat bread and 1 tbsp peanut butter	7 walnut halves and 1 tbsp raisins	1 orange and 2 tbsp sunflower seeds	Tropical fruit salad: 1 slice cantaloupe melon, 1 slice pineapple, 1 pomegranate, 1 nectarine, and 1 orange
Asian-style tuna salad (see page 99)	Salad: 6 tbsp cooked brown rice, ½ can chickpeas (drained of water), 1 small red onion, 1 grated carrot, 2 celery sticks, mint, lemon juice and zest, and 2 tsp olive oil	Salad: lettuce, 4 boiled new potatoes (skins on), 3½oz (100g) canned pink salmon, 1 tomato, steamed green beans, 5 olives, 1 hard-boiled egg, 1 tbsp each of olive oil and balsamic, and 1 slice cantaloupe melon	Whole-wheat pasta salad with sardines (see page 103)
Sundae: layer 2 handfuls of raspberries, 1 pear, and 4½oz (125g) soy yogurt; top with 1 tbsp hazelnuts	3 oatcakes topped with ½ small avocado and 1 tomato	1 small pot soy yogurt with grated cucumber, garlic, lemon juice, and mint, served with 1 whole-wheat pita and ½ red and ½ yellow bell peppers	3 celery sticks filled with 3 tbsp low-fat cottage cheese and topped with 7 crushed walnuts
Vegetable chili (see page 137)	Fish and chips with peas (see page 137)	1 large baked potato with 4oz (120g) mixed beans (drained), 3 tbsp sweetcorn, chili to taste, cilantro, lime zest and juice, served with 1 handful of arugula and 2 tbsp soy yogurt, plus 10 strawberries	Oven-roasted chicken and veggies (see page 144)

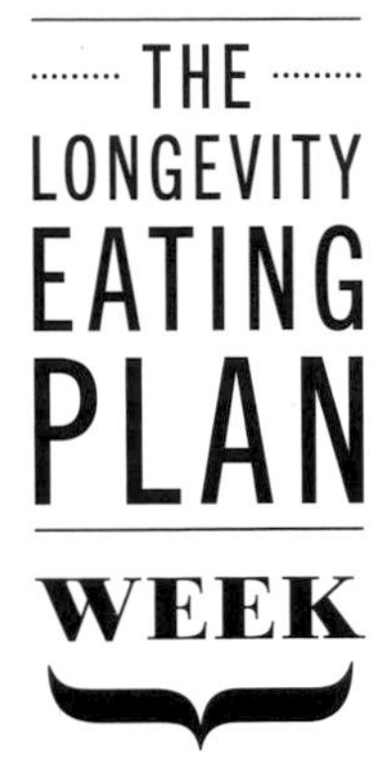

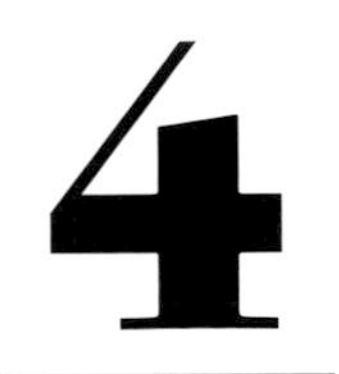

This is the week that puts into practice all the changes you've been making. Breakfast is now your biggest meal of the day and dinner is the smallest. You'll be getting most of your nutrients from plant foods, although you'll still find eggs, fish, small amounts of dairy, and even a serving of turkey. By now, you should be hooked on a new way of eating.

	MONDAY	TUESDAY	WEDNESDAY
BREAKFAST	2 slices whole-grain toast with 2 scrambled eggs mixed with 3½oz (100g) canned pink salmon, 1 handful of baby spinach, and 2 tomatoes, plus 1 pear and 1 nectarine	Porridge: 5 tbsp oats and 1½ cups (350ml) soy milk, topped with 1 banana, 1 nectarine, and 1 tbsp each of chopped almonds and raisins	Homemade muesli with soy yogurt and berries (see page 73)
SNACK	4½oz (125g) soy yogurt with 1 banana, 1 peach, and 1 tbsp pumpkin seeds	2 slices whole-grain bread topped with 2 tbsp low-fat cottage cheese, and 2 handfuls of raspberries	3 oatcakes with 1 sliced banana and 2 handfuls of blueberries
LUNCH	Salad: 8 tbsp cooked bulgur wheat, 3oz (120g) canned green lentils (drained), ½ small red onion, 6 cherry tomatoes, 1 grated carrot, lemon juice and zest, and parsley	Quinoa, tuna, and bean salad (see page 88)	1 large baked potato, with 3½oz (100g) fresh crab mixed with ½ small avocado, lemon juice and zest, and parsley, served with salad, plus 1 apple
SNACK	6 walnut halves and 6 dried apricots	2 tbsp unsalted peanuts and 1 tbsp raisins	2 slices whole-grain bread topped with coleslaw (1 handful of shredded cabbage, ½ small red onion, 1 grated carrot, lemon zest and juice, and 1 tbsp soy yogurt)
DINNER	Japanese-style noodle soup (see page 139)	Wild mushroom pie (see page 143)	Turkey steak with kale and squash (see page 148)

PLANT-BASED COOKED BREAKFAST

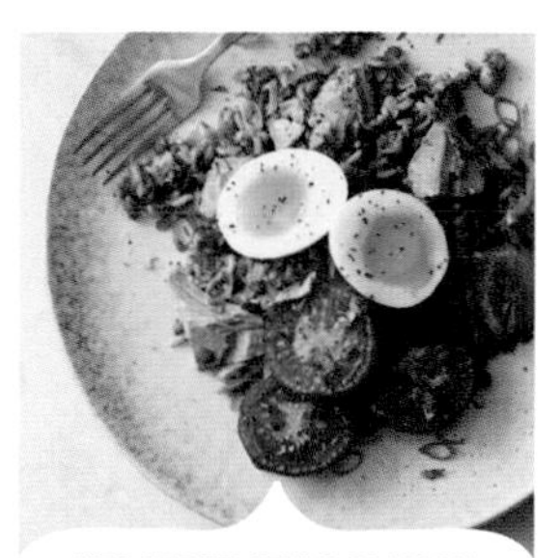

KEDGEREE-STYLE SALMON AND RICE

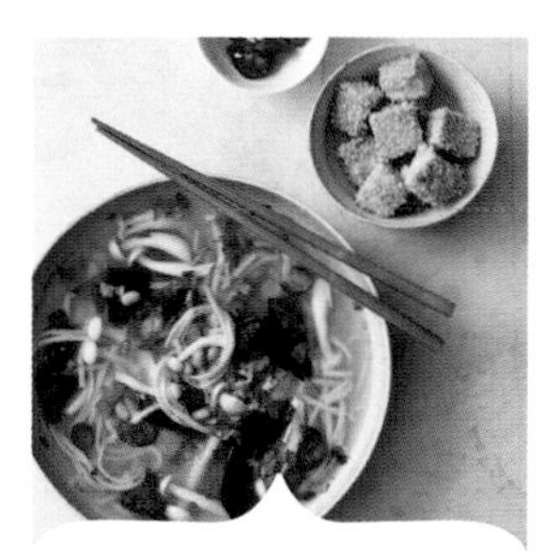

JAPANESE-STYLE NOODLE SOUP

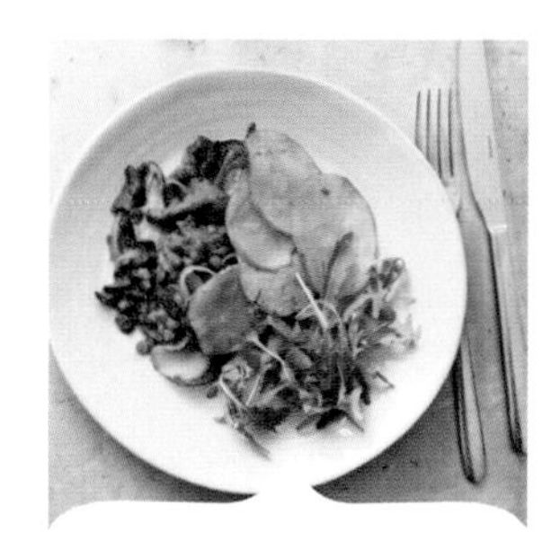

WILD MUSHROOM PIE

THURSDAY	FRIDAY	SATURDAY	SUNDAY
2 slices whole-grain toast topped with 2 tbsp peanut butter, 1 banana, and 3 dried dates, plus 1 peach	3 slices whole-grain toast topped with 3 tbsp low-fat cottage cheese, ½ avocado, and 1 hard-boiled egg, plus 10 strawberries	Plant-based cooked breakfast (see page 68)	Kedgeree-style salmon and rice (see page 77)
1 tbsp pumpkin seeds, 1 pear, 1 handful of grapes, and 1 slice cantaloupe melon	4 tbsp fat-free Greek yogurt with 4 dried dates and 2 handfuls of blackberries	Shake: blend 1 cup (250ml) soy milk with 1 banana, ½ ripe mango, and 2 tsp chia seeds	1 whole-wheat pita filled with 3 tbsp hummus (see recipe, page 96) and cucumber
Sardine bruschetta (see page 89)	Spicy bean and red pepper soup (see page 89)	1 whole-wheat wrap filled with 4oz (120g) canned chickpeas (drained), 1 carrot, ½ red bell pepper, ½ red onion, 3 tbsp soy yogurt mixed with lemon zest and juice, and cilantro, plus 1 nectarine	Salad: 7oz (200g) cooked whole-wheat pasta, 1 tomato, 1¾oz (50g) reduced-fat mozzarella, 5 olives, basil, and 1 tbsp balsamic vinegar; plus 2 handfuls of raspberries with 4 tbsp fat-free Greek yogurt
Sweet potato wedges made from 1 large sweet potato (about 9oz/250g), 1 tsp olive oil, and a sprinkle of paprika	Fruit salad: 1 banana, 1 handful of grapes, 1 apple, and 1 orange	1 tbsp unsalted peanuts, 1 tbsp raisins, and 6 dried apricots	6 dried apricots and 4 dried dates
Roasted Greek veggies with feta (see page 144)	Hot and crispy salmon (see page 145)	Quorn 5-spice stir-fry (see page 145)	1 large baked sweet potato with 4oz (120g) canned kidney beans (drained), salsa (made from 1 tomato, ½ small red onion, and cilantro), and 1 tbsp soy yogurt

BREAKFASTS

Trials have shown that people who start their day with a substantial meal are more likely to be a healthy weight and have better blood sugar levels—both of which contribute to long life. So repeat your new mantra, "I will breakfast like a king."

65%

more weight was lost by people who ate an egg-based breakfast, compared to a bagel breakfast.

TROPICAL FRUIT SALAD

This technicolored breakfast serves up longevity-boosting sprinkles with its "wonderfood" yogurt.

SERVES **2**

Ingredients

1¾oz (50g) oats
2 tbsp skin-on almonds, chopped
3 tbsp desiccated coconut
1 mango, peeled, pit removed, and cut into chunks
1 slice cantaloupe melon, skin removed, and cut into chunks
8oz (227g) can pineapple chunks canned in juice, drained
9oz (250g) fat-free plain yogurt

1 Heat a dry nonstick frying pan over medium heat. Put in the oats, almonds, and coconut and cook, shaking the pan constantly, until the mixture starts to brown. Transfer to a bowl and leave to cool.

2 Divide the mango, melon, and pineapple between two bowls. Top with the yogurt and the toasted oat mix.

NUTRITION PER SERVING Calories **408** Total fat **17.4g** Saturated fat **6.8g** Cholesterol **3mg** Carbohydrates **51.8g** Dietary fiber **9.8g** Sugars **33.2g** Protein **14.4g** Sodium **102mg**

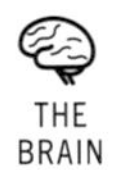
THE BRAIN
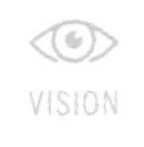
VISION
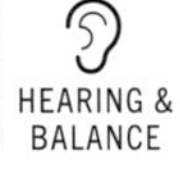
HEARING & BALANCE
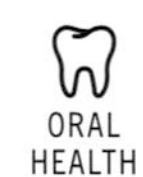
ORAL HEALTH
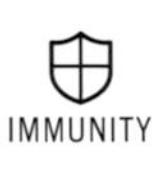
IMMUNITY
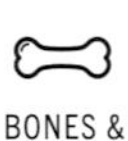
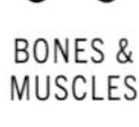
BONES & MUSCLES
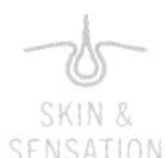
SKIN & SENSATION
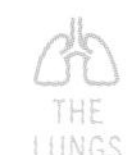
THE LUNGS
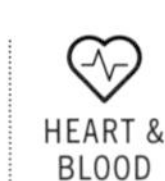
HEART & BLOOD
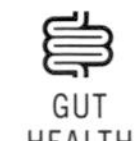
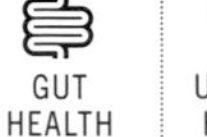
GUT HEALTH
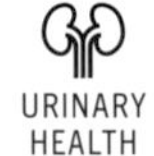
URINARY HEALTH
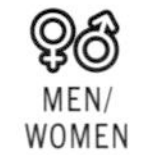
MEN/ WOMEN

BREAKFAST TORTILLA

Start your day with this protein-packed plateful: use leftovers for breakfast-on-the-go another day.

SERVES **2**

Ingredients

1 tbsp canola oil
5½oz (150g) mushrooms, sliced
freshly ground black pepper
10oz (300g) boiled potatoes (skins on), sliced
2 handfuls of baby spinach
5¾oz (160g) can tuna in water, drained
4 large eggs, beaten
1¼oz (40g) reduced-fat feta cheese, crumbled

1 Heat the oil in a 8in (20cm) nonstick frying pan over medium heat. Add the mushrooms and black pepper and fry gently for 5–7 minutes until browned.

2 Add the sliced potato, baby spinach, and tuna; cover; and leave to wilt and heat through for 2–3 minutes.

3 Remove the lid and pour over the beaten eggs, making sure they cover the bottom of the pan evenly. Cook until the tortilla is almost set. Preheat the grill to medium.

4 Top with the feta and more black pepper, then grill until the egg is fully set. Cut into wedges and serve.

NUTRITION PER SERVING Calories **404** Total fat **18.1g** Saturated fat **5.3g** Cholesterol **394mg** Carbohydrates **26.7g** Dietary fiber **3.2g** Sugars **1.4g** Protein **35.3g** Sodium **706mg**

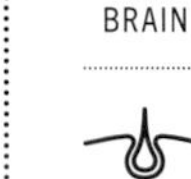
THE BRAIN
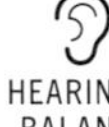
VISION
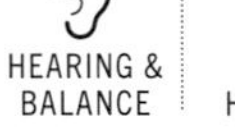
HEARING & BALANCE
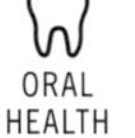
ORAL HEALTH
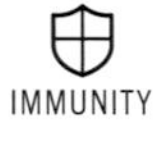
IMMUNITY
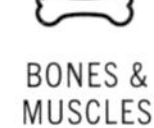
BONES & MUSCLES
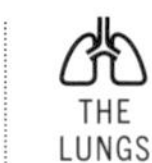
SKIN & SENSATION
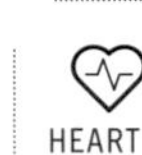
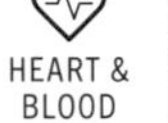
THE LUNGS
HEART & BLOOD
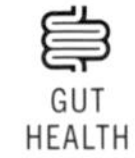
GUT HEALTH
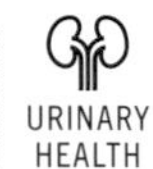
URINARY HEALTH
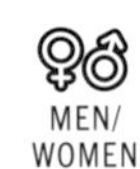
MEN/ WOMEN

-WONDERFOOD-

YOGURT

Packed with gut-friendly probiotics as well as protein, calcium, and phosphorus, yogurt's longevity benefits lie in its protective powers. Studies have shown that yogurt can help counter many of the health problems associated with getting older, such as high blood pressure, osteoporosis, and unwanted weight gain.

WHICH YOGURTS?

All yogurts are a great source of protein and calcium. Here are the various benefits offered by the most popular kinds of plain yogurts.

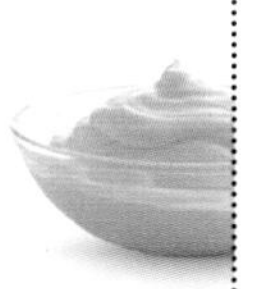

Regular

- Is made from whole milk and usually contains the most nutrients
- Has good levels of calcium, vital for strong bones and helping prevent osteoporosis

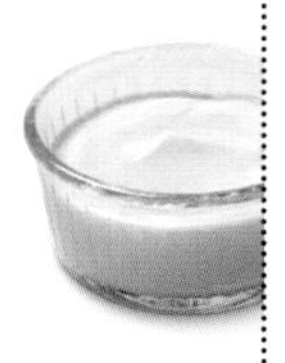

Fat-free/low-fat

- Are the lowest in calories, fat, and saturated fat, so are the best choice for weight management and heart health

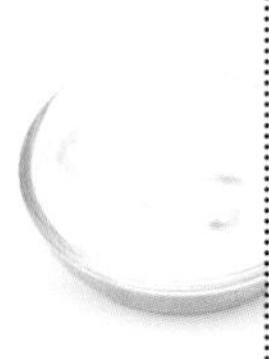

Greek

- Has fewer natural sugars, but is much higher in fat (unless a fat-free version)
- Is a good source of vitamin A, an immune-boosting antioxidant

HOW MUCH?

Studies suggest one small pot (3 to 4 tablespoons) a day offers the greatest health benefits.

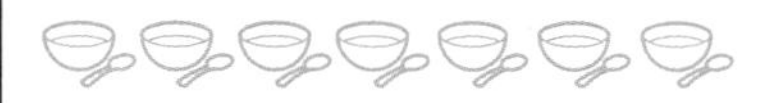

BEST BOUGHT

Choose probiotic or live and active culture yogurts, which have friendly bacteria added to them. Select unsweetened, plain, or natural varieties of yogurt.

HOW TO STORE

Keep refrigerated, or freeze for a homemade frozen yogurt.

RAW OR COOKED?

Eat raw, as cooking kills the probiotics.

Blood pressure lowering

In the late 1990s, a landmark study found that adding low-fat dairy to a diet rich in fruits and vegetables lowered blood pressure more than fruits and vegetables alone. Further research has backed up this link and shown that yogurt in particular has impressive results.

20%

drop in risk of developing high blood pressure when yogurt is eaten five times a week rather than once a month.

Diet helpers

Numerous studies show that people who eat yogurt gain less weight over time and are more likely to have a lower body mass index, a smaller waist, and less body fat. The newest research suggests that "friendly" probiotic bacteria in yogurt "crowd out" bad bacteria that may affect satiety or the absorption of nutrients, meaning that we limit our calorie intake.

Brilliant bone strengthener

From our mid-30s, we start to lose bone mass, with an increased loss around the time of menopause for women. Calcium is vital for strong bones, and yogurt is rich in calcium, along with protein and phosphorus. Several studies have linked good intake of yogurt to stronger bones. This is important, as osteoporosis affects around 200 million women worldwide, according to the International Osteoporosis Foundation.

Women

39%

drop in risk of developing osteoporosis from eating one serving of yogurt a day.

Men

52%

drop in risk of developing osteoporosis from eating one serving of yogurt a day.

The combination of protein and calcium in yogurt boosts its bone-building power.

Osteoporosis can cause bones to break more easily, particularly the hip, femur, spine, wrist, radius, and ulna.

Eating yogurt boosts calcium levels, supplying ingredients for making bones.

Many yogurts are fortified with vitamin D, which helps the body to absorb calcium, promoting the growth of strong bones.

Gut friendly

Fermented foods such as live and active culture yogurt are packed with probiotic bacteria, which help to boost friendly bacteria in the gut. This in turn has been linked to many health benefits, including improving digestion-related problems, such as diarrhea, irritable bowel syndrome (IBS), and lactose intolerance, as well as boosting immunity and protecting against some cancers.

Diabetes protection

Many studies have shown how yogurt helps to protect against type 2 diabetes. In one of the largest studies, adults who ate 1lb 2oz (500g) of yogurt a week were 28 percent less likely to develop the disease over the study period of 11 years.

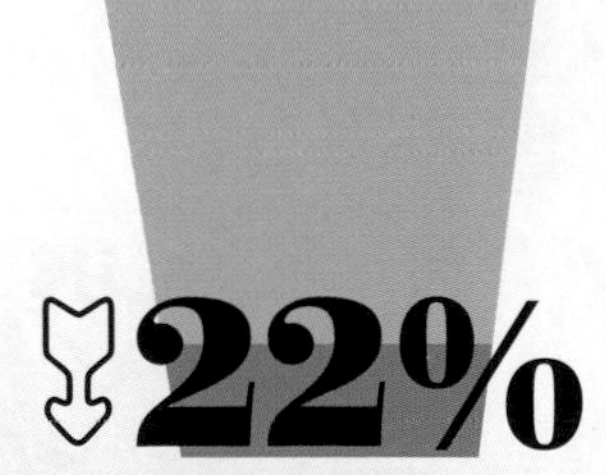

22%

In a review of 17 studies, eating 7oz (200g) of yogurt each day was linked to a 22 percent reduction in the risk of diabetes.

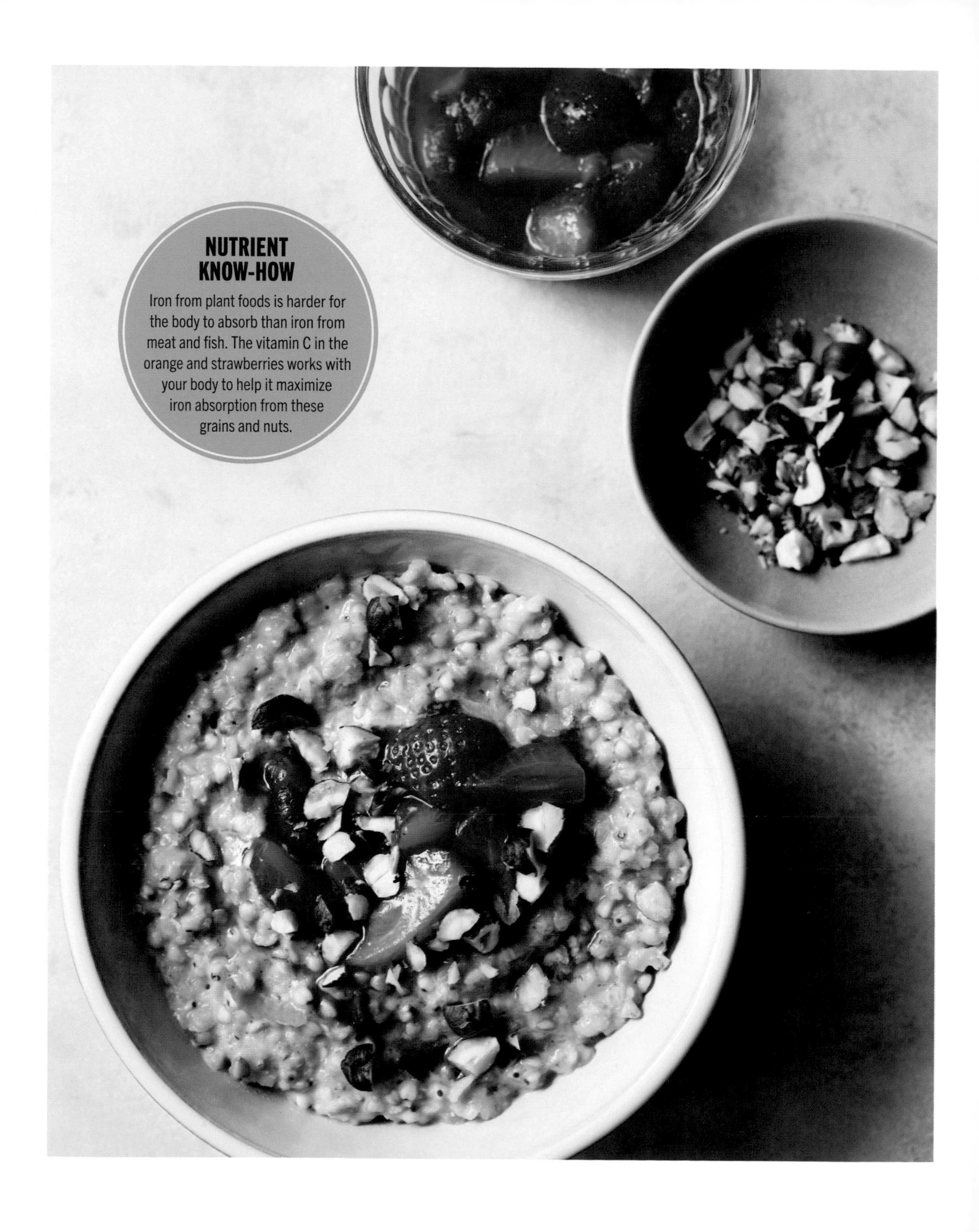
NUTRIENT KNOW-HOW
Iron from plant foods is harder for the body to absorb than iron from meat and fish. The vitamin C in the orange and strawberries works with your body to help it maximize iron absorption from these grains and nuts.

THE BRAIN | VISION | HEARING & BALANCE | ORAL HEALTH | IMMUNITY | BONES & MUSCLES | SKIN & SENSATION | THE LUNGS | HEART & BLOOD | GUT HEALTH | URINARY HEALTH | MEN/WOMEN

BUCKWHEAT AND OAT PORRIDGE

Buckwheat adds a nutty taste and texture to regular rolled oats, while the no-added-sugar compote provides vitamin-rich and immune-boosting sweetness.

SERVES **2**

Ingredients

3oz (85g) buckwheat groats

1½ cups (350ml) skim milk

7oz (200g) strawberries

finely grated zest and juice of 1 orange

1¾oz (50g) rolled oats

¼ cup (30g) unblanched (skin-on) hazelnuts, roughly chopped

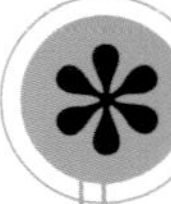

Smart swaps

- Replace the dairy milk with unsweetened **soy milk** or **almond milk** for an entirely vegan breakfast.
- Short on time? Simply replace the strawberry compote with **fresh berries**; a handful of **blueberries** comes with memory-boosting anthocyanins, too.
- Swap the hazelnuts for **pistachios** to get more eye-friendly lutein and zeaxanthin.

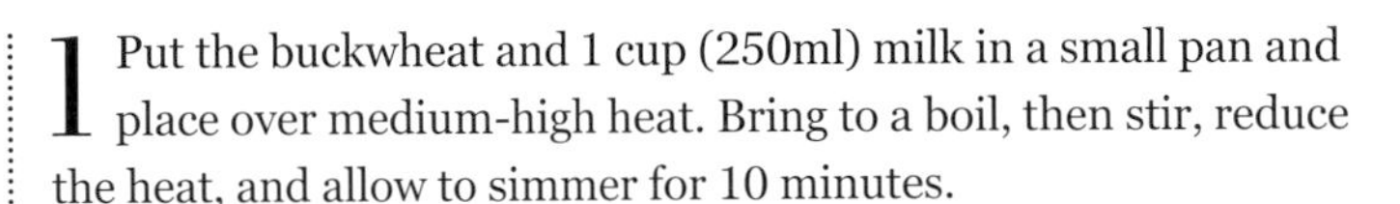

1 Put the buckwheat and 1 cup (250ml) milk in a small pan and place over medium-high heat. Bring to a boil, then stir, reduce the heat, and allow to simmer for 10 minutes.

2 Meanwhile, make the strawberry compote. Hull and quarter the strawberries and place in a second small pan, with 1 tablespoon of the orange juice. Put on very low heat and allow the strawberries to warm for about 10 minutes, so that they release their juices. Stir occasionally, using a rubber spatula so that the berries are not broken down too much.

3 When the buckwheat has simmered for 10 minutes, stir in the oats. Add some or all of the remaining milk if the porridge is getting too thick. Return the porridge to a simmer and leave it to cook for another 5 minutes.

4 Once the porridge is cooked, remove it from the heat and stir in the orange zest and remaining juice.

5 Divide the porridge between two bowls, sprinkle on the hazelnuts, and top with a good spoonful of strawberry compote. Add more of the strawberry juice if you prefer a runny porridge.

NUTRITION PER SERVING Calories **446** Total fat **13.2g** Saturated fat **1.3g** Cholesterol **7mg** Carbohydrates **71.4g** Dietary fiber **8g** Sugars **17.6g** Protein **15.2g** Sodium **80mg**

-SUPERGROUP-

BERRIES

All berries are good for you—the vibrant blues, purples, and reds of this supergroup are an indication that they are packed with damage-fighting antioxidants. But not all berries are created equal—some are better than others when it comes to longevity. Discover which protect against memory loss, cancer, and heart disease.

WHICH BERRIES?

These berries—ones commonly eaten—benefit health and longevity differently.

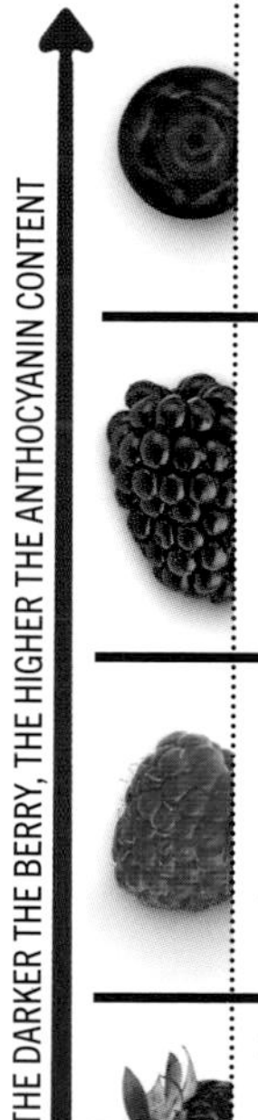

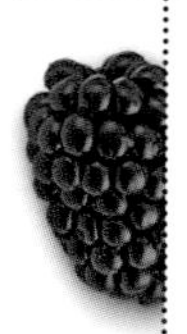

Blueberries
- Help boost memory
- Improve blood flow and also protect against high blood pressure

Blackberries
- Rank top in terms of antioxidant power
- Offer diverse anti-inflammatory actions via their tannins

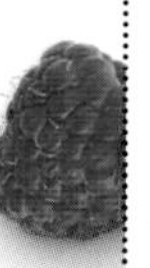

Raspberries
- Contain ellagic acid, a polyphenol with anticancer properties
- May help us burn fat better

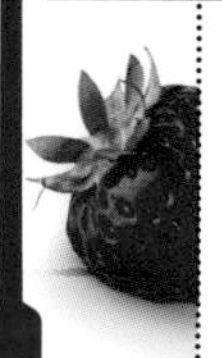

Strawberries
- Are rich in immune-boosting vitamin C
- Are packed with folate, which helps to reduce tiredness and fatigue

HOW MUCH?

Eat a couple of handfuls (one serving) three to four times a week.

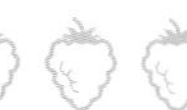

BEST BOUGHT

Fresh and frozen are both nutrient rich, but frozen fruit is cheaper.

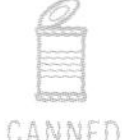

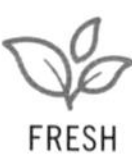

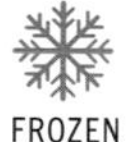

HOW TO STORE

Refrigerate fresh berries for optimum levels of vitamin C. It's handy to have frozen berries, too, as freezing has little impact on anthocyanin levels.

RAW OR COOKED?

Cooking degrades certain nutrients, so berries are best eaten raw.

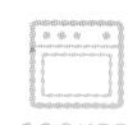

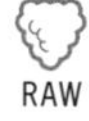

Leveling out blood sugar

Despite berries containing the sugar fructose, studies show that they help to improve insulin sensitivity, as well as regulate blood sugar levels. Berries are high in fiber and have a low glycemic index. So a regular dose of any type of berries could help reduce the risk of type 2 diabetes.

A mental boost

Adding to a wealth of lab-based research, studies of elderly adults confirm that berries improve memory and slow down age-related loss in cognitive function. Blueberries have gained the most attention, but other berries are also linked to delays in cognitive aging. One study showed that eating just two servings of strawberries a week (about 16 strawberries) reduced memory decline in people over 70.

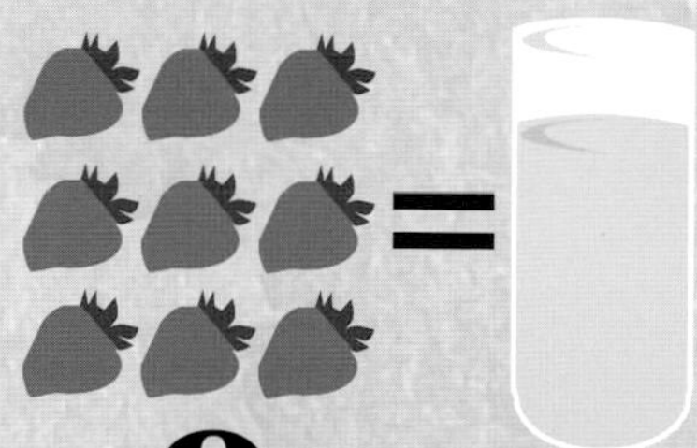

9 strawberries give you the same amount of vitamin C as one small glass of orange juice.

Heart health benefits

All berries have been linked to cardiovascular improvements. (It's the winning combination of antioxidants and fiber.) Research shows that eating at least three servings of blueberries or strawberries a week can reduce the risk of a heart attack. The high levels of polyphenols in berries have also been shown to lower high blood pressure.

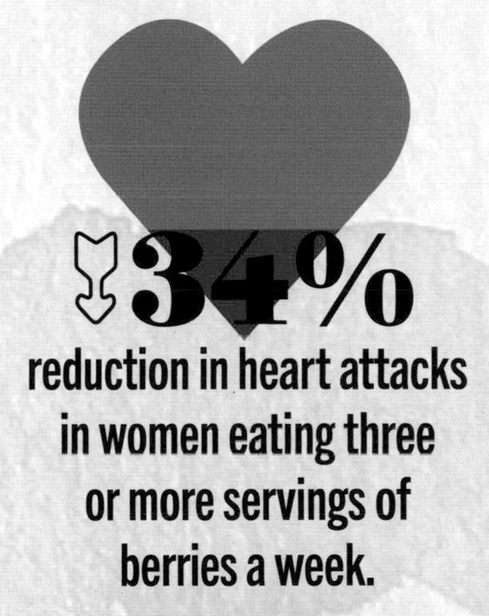

Cancer protection

Good intakes of berries may help to lower the risk of certain cancers. Berries are jam-packed with phytochemicals (such as ellagic acid and anthocyanins; see also page 38), many of which have cancer-fighting properties. The research evidence is currently strongest for berries' anticancer effects in cancers of the breast, esophagus, and colon.

Protective powerhouses

Berries come naturally packaged with a host of plant-based antioxidants, including anthocyanins, quercetin, and vitamins C and E. These berry-based compounds can confer a diverse array of benefits all over the body by helping to counteract damage caused by free radicals (see also page 11).

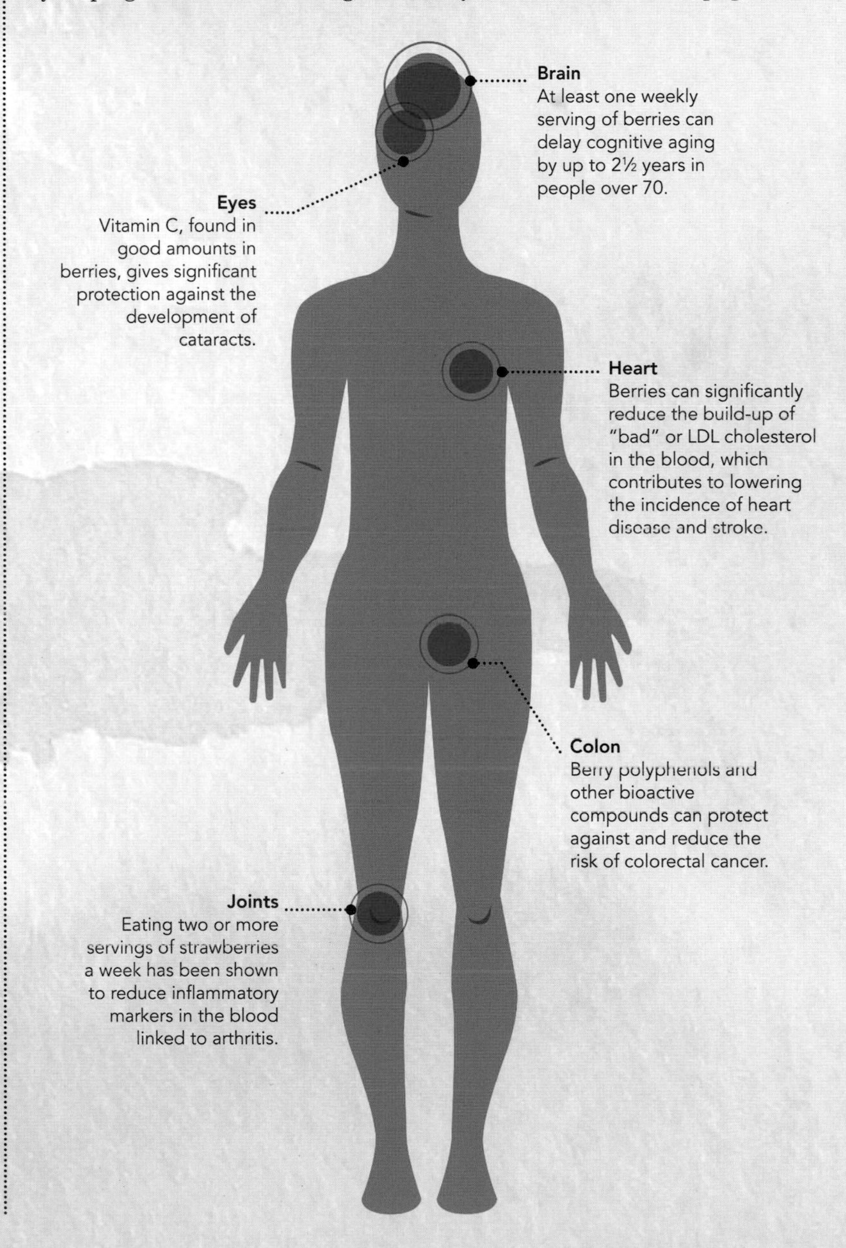

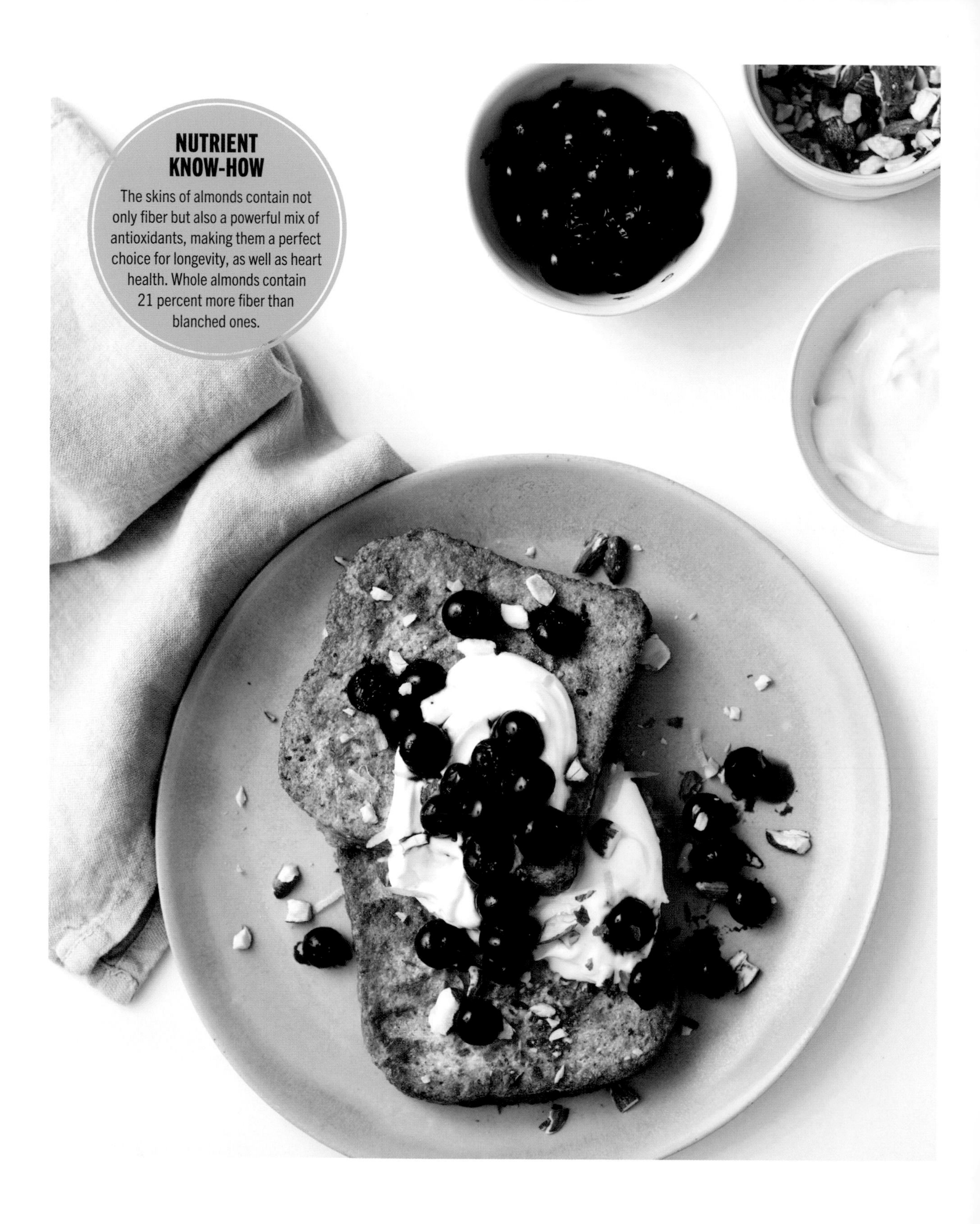

NUTRIENT KNOW-HOW

The skins of almonds contain not only fiber but also a powerful mix of antioxidants, making them a perfect choice for longevity, as well as heart health. Whole almonds contain 21 percent more fiber than blanched ones.

CINNAMON TOAST WITH BLUEBERRY COMPOTE

Love French toast? This recipe uses wholesome bread for its digestion-friendly fiber and olive oil (great for a healthy heart), plus tasty nutrient-packed toppings.

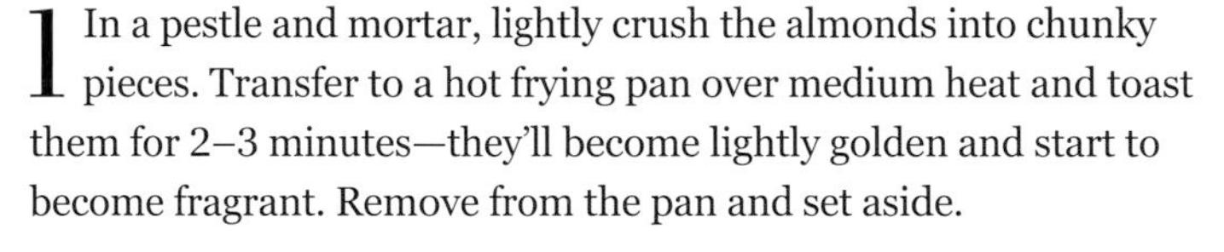

SERVES **2**

Ingredients

- ¼ cup (30g) whole, unblanched (skin-on) almonds
- 3 eggs
- ½ tsp ground cinnamon
- 4 thick slices whole-wheat bread
- 5¾oz (160g) blueberries
- ½ tsp vanilla extract
- 1 tbsp olive oil, canola oil, or other mild oil
- 2 heaped tbsp low-fat yogurt
- zest of ½ lemon, plus extra to garnish (optional)

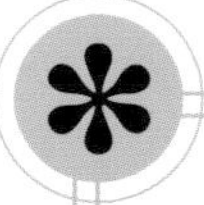

Smart swaps

- For a savory dish packed with lycopene (an antioxidant thought to reduce the risk of some cancers), swap the blueberries for **cherry tomatoes** roasted with a drizzle of olive oil, and use cayenne, not cinnamon.
- Replace the almonds with toasted **walnuts** for some alpha-linolenic acid, a plant form of omega-3 fat.

1 In a pestle and mortar, lightly crush the almonds into chunky pieces. Transfer to a hot frying pan over medium heat and toast them for 2–3 minutes—they'll become lightly golden and start to become fragrant. Remove from the pan and set aside.

2 Beat the eggs in a shallow bowl and mix in the ground cinnamon. Dip the bread into the egg, turning the slices so that they absorb egg on both sides. Leave the bread sitting in the egg mixture while you make the blueberry compote.

3 Steam the blueberries in a steamer, or place a metal colander over a pan of simmering water and cover with a lid. Steam for 2–3 minutes until the berries start to drip colored juice, then take them off the heat. Place the berries in a small bowl and stir in the vanilla extract. The berries will start to break down a little and release their juices; set aside.

4 Return the frying pan to medium heat and add the oil. When the oil is hot, carefully place the egg-soaked bread into the pan so the slices sit flat. Cook for 2–3 minutes, until the underside is golden and the egg has "sealed" and set. Flip the bread and cook it for another 2–3 minutes on the other side. Remove from the heat.

5 Put the yogurt in a bowl and stir in the lemon zest. Serve the slices of toast in pairs, topped with the lemon yogurt, warm blueberry compote, and a sprinkle of almonds, and zest (if using).

NUTRITION PER SERVING Calories **495** Total fat **23.6g** Saturated fat **4.1g** Cholesterol **268mg** Carbohydrates **49.4g** Dietary fiber **7.9g** Sugars **13.6g** Protein **23.9g** Sodium **507mg**

-WONDERFOOD-

BANANAS

Whether you like your bananas slightly green or spotted, they all come with triple levels of mood-boosting powers. They are good sources of carbohydrates (fuel for the brain and muscles), and of tryptophan and vitamin B6 (both of which are needed for production of feel-good chemicals). What's more, bananas improve digestion and may help regulate blood pressure.

WHICH BANANAS?

All bananas contain mood-boosting and longevity nutrients. But the degree of ripeness affects their level of natural sugars, antioxidants, and resistant starch (see opposite).

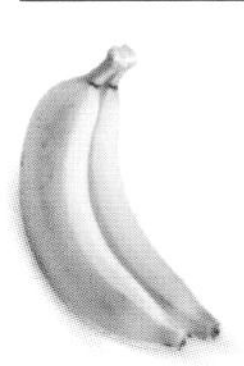

Bananas

- Are rich in carbs that provide a source of energy for the body
- Provide fiber to help keep us satisified
- Are a good source of potassium, which benefits the heart and blood pressure
- Are one of the best fruits for vitamin B6, which is important for the nervous system and well-being

HOW MUCH?

Enjoy three to four bananas a week.

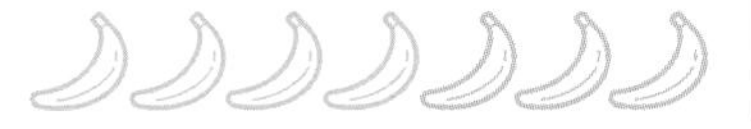

BEST BOUGHT

However you like to eat your bananas is a personal preference, but their benefits do vary with their ripeness.

FRESH

HOW TO STORE

Bananas will ripen at home—if you want to speed up the process, keep them in a bunch or with other fruits. Once ripe, they can be refrigerated to stop them ripening further. Bananas freeze well, so chop up very ripe ones and freeze for later use.

RAW OR COOKED?

Best enjoyed raw for maximum nutrient benefits.

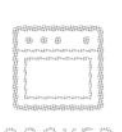

COOKED

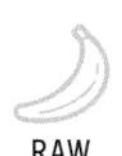

RAW

Mood boosters

Bananas contain small amounts of an amino acid called tryptophan, which is converted into a feel-good chemical called serotonin in the brain. They also provide vitamin B6, which helps this conversion take place. Low levels of serotonin and vitamin B6 have been linked to depression, while higher levels may be protective.

↓43%

In one study, elderly women with the highest intakes of vitamin B6 from food were 43 percent less likely to become depressed.

Blood pressure helpers

Studies confirm that increasing your potassium intake (for instance, from bananas) while reducing your sodium intake can help maintain a healthy blood pressure. This is important, because the World Health Organization estimates high blood pressure causes around 51 percent of deaths from stroke.

Reducing the risk of kidney cancer

Bananas may help protect against kidney cancer. In a 13-year study of Swedish women, higher intakes of all fruits reduced the risk of renal cancer, but bananas seemed to offer the best protection. An earlier study also found eating at least four bananas a week (rather than less than three a month) resulted in a 50 percent reduction in the risk of kidney cancer.

Fuel for good bacteria

Bananas are rich in a soluble fiber called fructooligosaccharides. This passes undigested into the large intestine, where it becomes food for probiotics or good bacteria, which flourish and "crowd out" bad bacteria. This increased number of good bacteria is linked to better digestive health and immunity.

In one small study, women had increased levels of beneficial bacteria after eating two bananas a day for 2 months.

Filling factor

Bananas are rich in a fiber called pectin, and unripe bananas also contain good amounts of resistant starch (starch that isn't digested). Both pectin and resistant starch help to slow down stomach emptying, which in turn causes smaller and slower rises in blood sugar and can help us to feel fuller for longer, so may aid weight management.

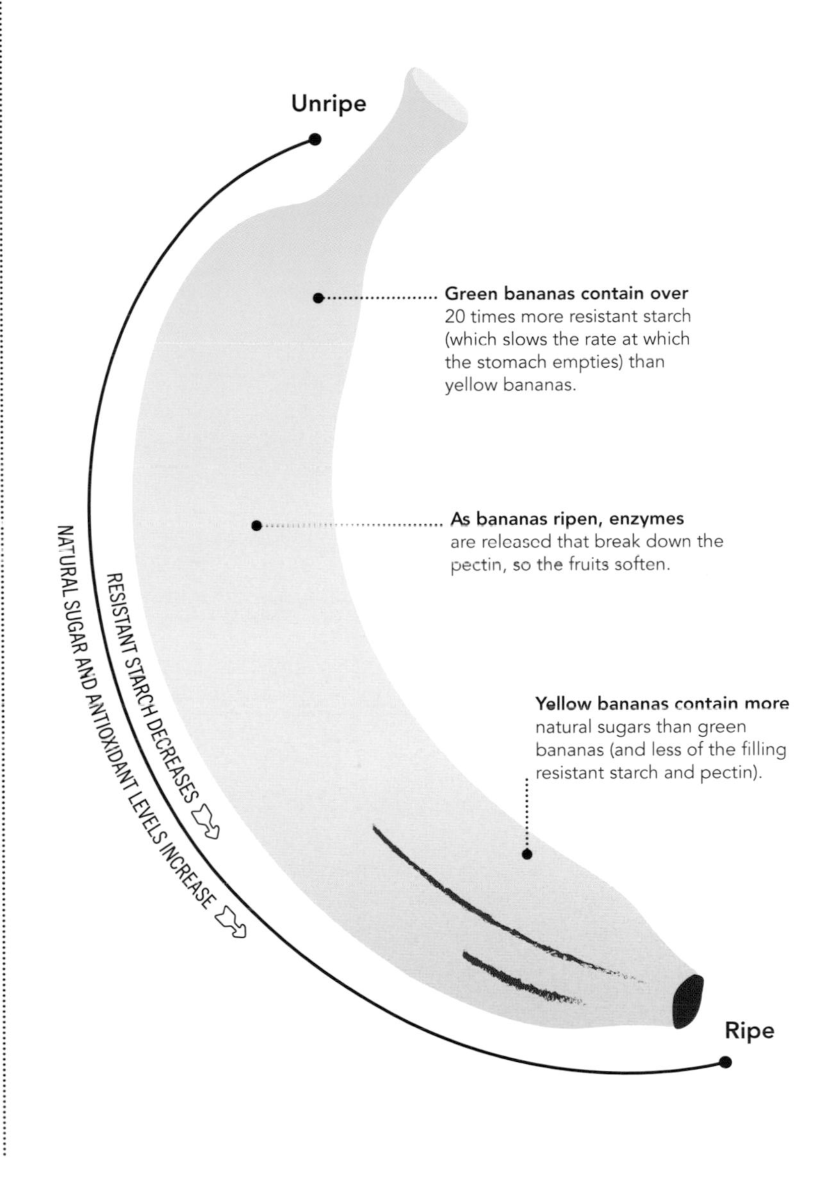

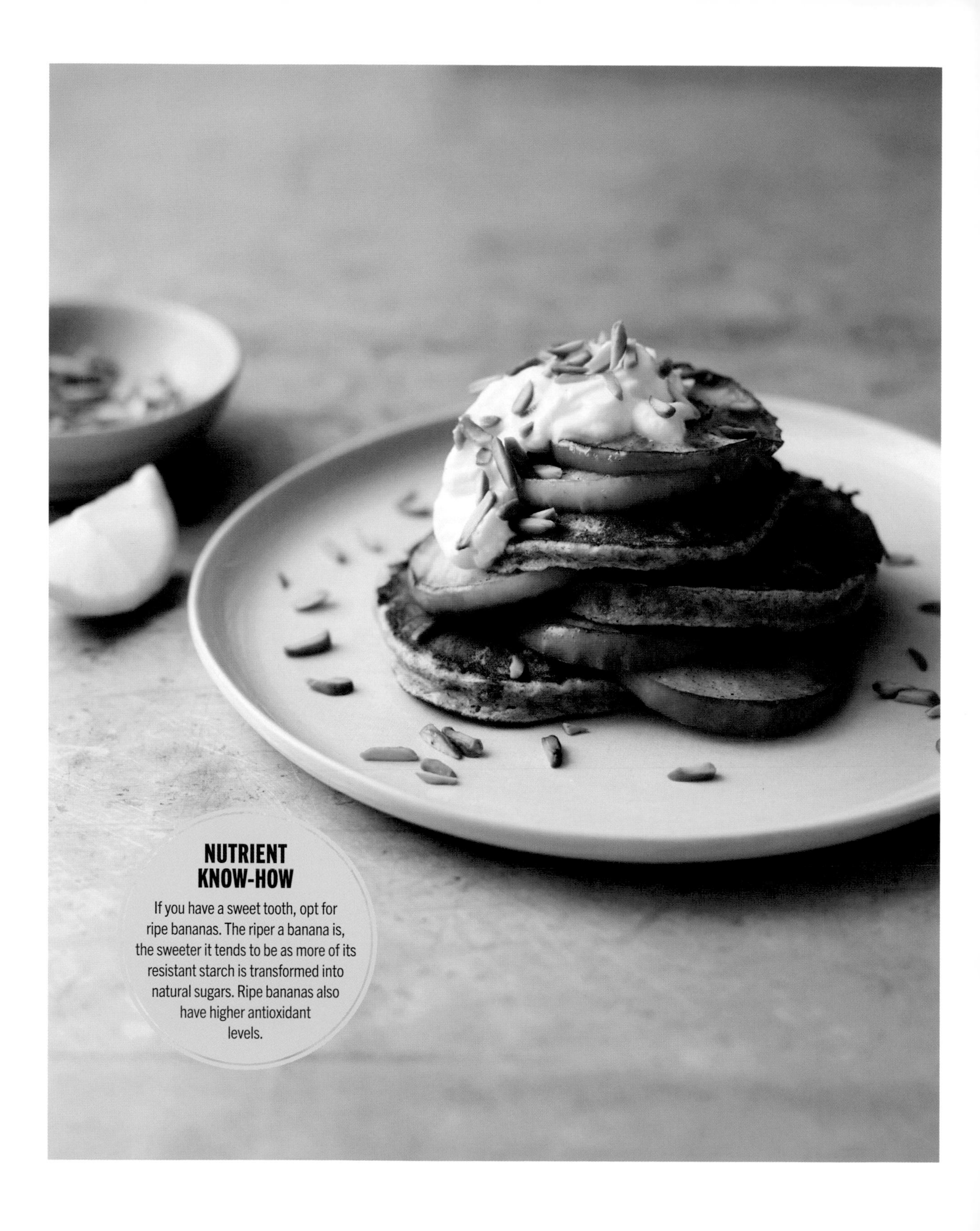

NUTRIENT KNOW-HOW

If you have a sweet tooth, opt for ripe bananas. The riper a banana is, the sweeter it tends to be as more of its resistant starch is transformed into natural sugars. Ripe bananas also have higher antioxidant levels.

BANANA PANCAKES WITH SPICED APPLE RINGS

Adding mashed banana to this pancake batter adds a glorious sweetness, as well as blood-pressure-lowering potassium. Make the pancakes small so they stay moist.

THE BRAIN | VISION | HEARING & BALANCE | ORAL HEALTH
IMMUNITY | BONES & MUSCLES | SKIN & SENSATION | THE LUNGS
HEART & BLOOD | GUT HEALTH | URINARY HEALTH | MEN/WOMEN

MAKES 6 PANCAKES

Ingredients

½ cup (50g) whole-wheat flour

1 tsp baking powder

½ tsp vanilla extract

1 ripe banana

1 egg, beaten

4 tbsp (60ml) skim milk

2 sweet apples

1–2 tsp ground nutmeg

2 tbsp mild olive oil

7oz (200g) fat-free plain yogurt, to serve

⅓ cup (40g) unsalted pistachio nuts, roughly chopped, to serve

lemon wedges, to serve

1 In a large bowl, mix together the flour, baking powder, and vanilla extract. Use a fork to mash the banana to a pulp, before adding it into the bowl along with the egg. Mix together everything in the bowl and then incorporate the milk gradually, whisking well to give a smooth and lump-free batter. Set aside.

2 Core the apples and, leaving the skins on, slice them into rings ½in (1cm) thick. Dust each ring with a little ground nutmeg.

3 Heat 1 tablespoon of oil in a nonstick frying pan over medium heat. When hot, add the apple rings, laying them flat on the base of the pan so that they brown evenly. Cook them for 1–2 minutes, and then use a spatula to flip them and cook the other sides. When done, transfer them to a plate and keep them warm.

4 Add another 1 tablespoon of oil to the pan. When the oil is hot, add one ladleful of batter into the pan to make a small thick pancake 3–4in (7.5–10cm) in diameter. Cook two or three pancakes at a time in batches—whatever fits easily. Lift and swirl the pan to distribute the oil evenly, then leave it to cook for 2 minutes until bubbles appear on top and it is golden brown underneath. Flip over and cook for another 1–2 minutes until the second side is cooked. Keep warm while you cook the rest.

5 Pile three pancakes onto each serving plate with the warm apple rings stacked between them. Serve warm, with a good dollop of yogurt, a sprinkling of pistachios, and lemon wedges.

NUTRITION PER SERVING Calories **489** Total fat **24.2g** Saturated fat **4.1g** Cholesterol **90mg** Carbohydrates **55.2g** Dietary fiber **6.9g** Sugars **32.5g** Protein **18.1g** Sodium **361mg**

Smart swaps

- Swap the skim milk for unsweetened **almond milk**—choose one that's fortified with calcium to ensure it remains a bone-friendly choice.
- For a boost in vitamin C, swap the apple rings for **raspberries**, scattering a few onto the pancakes as the first side is cooking in the pan. When the pancakes are golden on one side, flip them over and lightly cook on the second side.

PLANT-BASED COOKED BREAKFAST

THE BRAIN | VISION | HEARING & BALANCE | ORAL HEALTH | IMMUNITY | BONES & MUSCLES | SKIN & SENSATION | THE LUNGS | HEART & BLOOD | GUT HEALTH | URINARY HEALTH | MEN/WOMEN

From the sweet potatoes' beta-carotene for healthy eyes to the fiber-filled beans for controlling blood cholesterol levels, every bite of this satisfying dish is beneficial.

SERVES **2**

Ingredients

- 3 tbsp olive oil, plus extra for drizzling
- 1 small red onion, finely chopped
- 1 garlic clove, sliced
- ½ tsp smoked paprika
- ¼ tsp cayenne pepper, plus a pinch for the tomatoes
- 14oz (400g) can navy beans, rinsed and drained
- 9oz (250g) crushed and sieved tomatoes
- freshly ground black pepper
- 5½oz (150g) chestnut mushrooms
- 1 baby eggplant (3½oz/100g), cut into small cubes
- 1 tsp dried mixed herbs
- 3 ripe medium tomatoes, halved
- 1 large sweet potato (about 7oz/200g), scrubbed not peeled
- 1 tbsp cider vinegar
- 2 eggs
- 2 tbsp (15g) sunflower seeds
- parsley, to serve

Smart swaps

- Swap the sunflower seeds for **pumpkin seeds** to get extra iron, potassium, phosphorus, and zinc.
- Replace the navy beans with **soy beans** to boost intakes of phyto-estrogens. Dried varieties will need to soak for 8–10 hours or overnight before use.

1 Preheat the oven to 400°F (200°C). Heat 1 tablespoon of oil in a pan and fry the onion for 2–3 minutes until soft. Add the garlic and fry for another minute. Then, add the spices, beans, and tomatoes, stirring well. Season the mixture with black pepper, bring it to a simmer, cover, and let it cook gently, stirring occasionally.

2 Place the mushrooms on a large baking sheet and drizzle them with a little oil. Put the eggplant cubes at the other end of the sheet and season them with the dried herbs and black pepper, then drizzle on a little more oil. Roast for 10 minutes, before adding the tomatoes, seasoning the tops with a pinch of cayenne. Return to the oven for another 5–10 minutes until the eggplant is cooked.

3 Put a pan of water on to boil and grate the sweet potatoes. Heat 2 tablespoons of oil in a frying pan over medium-high heat, then press the grated potato into 3in (7.5cm) cooking rings to shape the hash browns. Fry for 3 minutes on one side, pressing the potato down (to compact into a "cake"), and 2 minutes on the other.

4 Add the vinegar to the boiling water and break one egg into a small bowl. Reduce the heat to a simmer and carefully drop the egg into the simmering water; repeat for the second egg. Poach the eggs for 3–4 minutes; lift the eggs out with a slotted spoon.

5 Serve a hash brown per plate with a poached egg, a spoonful of beans, roasted vegetables, and a sprinkle of the seeds and parsley.

NUTRITION PER SERVING Calories **608** Total fat **32.1g** Saturated fat **5.3g** Cholesterol **179mg** Carbohydrates **56.7g** Dietary fiber **17.7g** Sugars **19.3g** Protein **21.4g** Sodium **355mg**

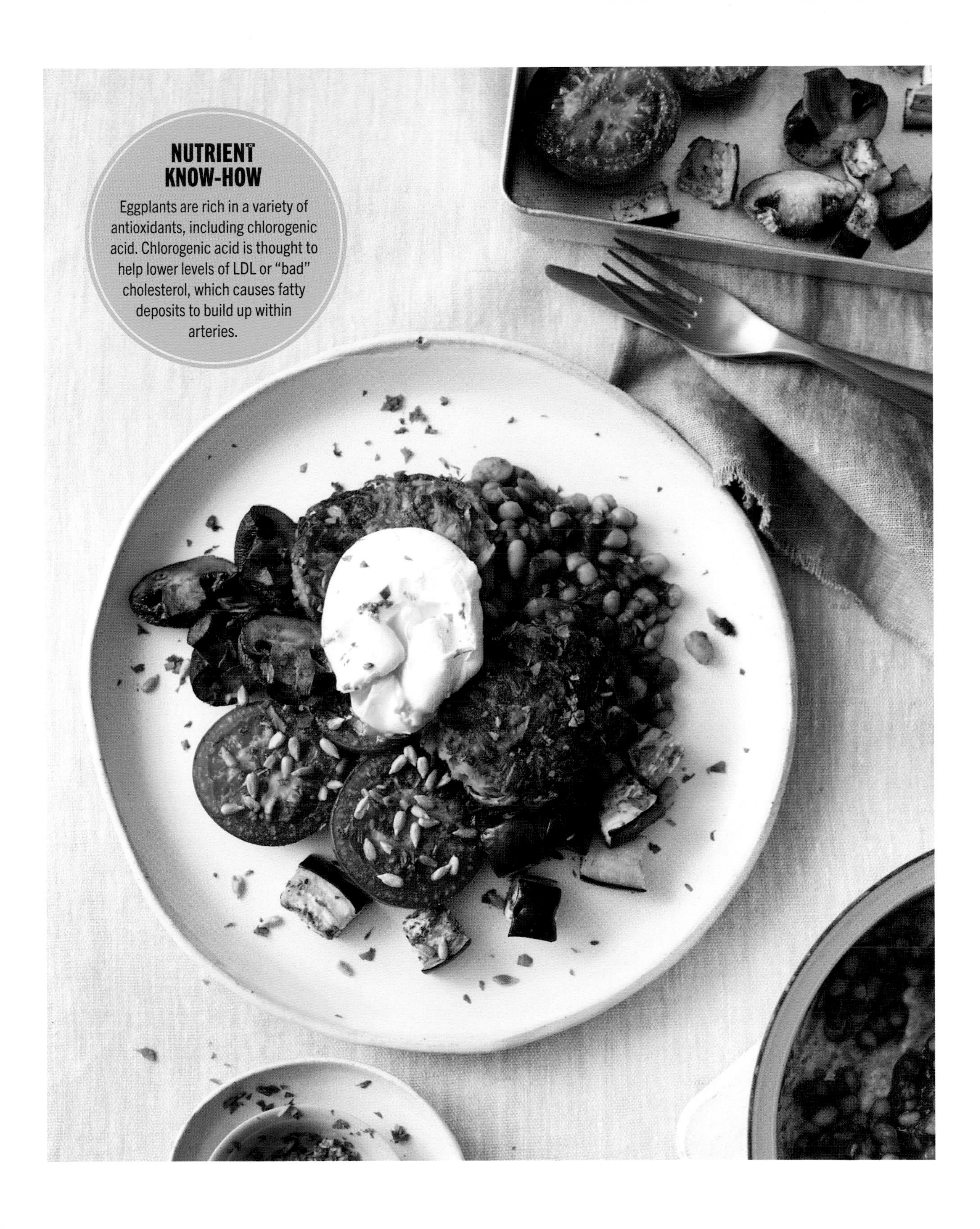

NUTRIENT KNOW-HOW

Eggplants are rich in a variety of antioxidants, including chlorogenic acid. Chlorogenic acid is thought to help lower levels of LDL or "bad" cholesterol, which causes fatty deposits to build up within arteries.

-WONDERFOOD-

EGGS

These powerhouses are packed with nutrients linked to good health and the prevention of many age-related diseases. Their positive effects on weight loss, memory, and eye and bone health mean that eggs are a great protein food to put on your menu.

WHICH EGGS?

Whether you enjoy a quail egg in a salad or you choose omega-3-enriched eggs, there are small but noteworthy nutritional differences between different types of eggs.

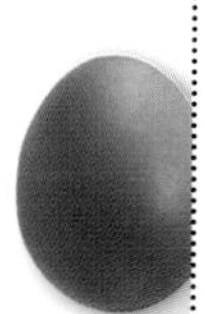

Hen eggs

- Provide good-quality protein, important for healthy muscles
- Contain a range of B vitamins and choline, essential for brain function
- Vary depending on the type; for example, there are omega-3-enriched and organic eggs. An organic egg yolk may contain more protein and potassium than a regular egg yolk

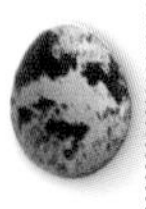

Quail eggs

- Are rich in iron—eat just three quail eggs to get the same amount of iron as from one hen egg

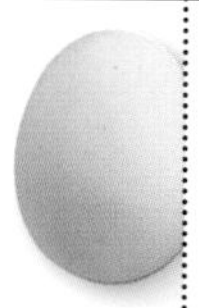

Duck eggs

- Contain five times more vitamin A than regular hen eggs (which is important for eye health), but they also contain more fat

HOW MUCH?

About six eggs a week seems to be the optimum amount for good health.

BEST BOUGHT

Buy fresh eggs, and check that the shells are intact.

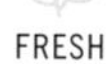

FRESH

HOW TO STORE

Eggs are best kept at a constant temperature of 68°F (20°C) or below. If in doubt, keep them in the refrigerator.

RAW OR COOKED?

If you are in good health, cook hen eggs according to your preference; other eggs, however, should be cooked until the white and yolk are solid.

COOKED

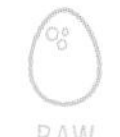

RAW

Great for eyes

Eggs contain vitamin A, which is vital for healthy vision. In addition, they contain lutein and zeaxanthin, antioxidants known as carotenoids, which are concentrated in the macula and are critical for healthy eyes. A good intake of these nutrients is linked to a lower risk of age-related macular degeneration and cataracts, both of which can lead to blindness.

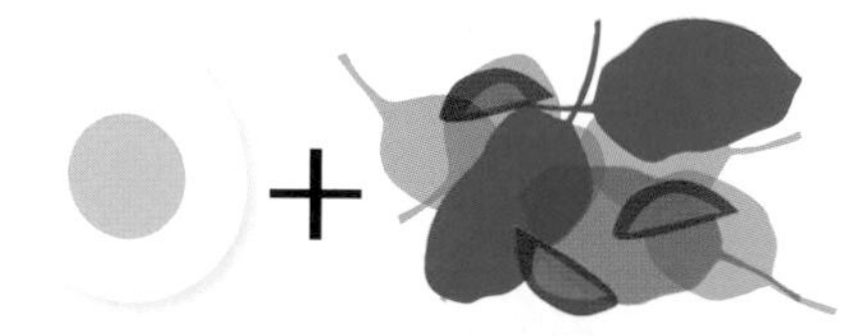

Add eggs to your salad—the fat in eggs helps the body absorb eye-friendly antioxidants.

Heart friendly

Eggs may have a high cholesterol content, but current research shows that cholesterol in food generally has little impact on blood cholesterol levels or heart disease risk (except for people with a genetic condition called familial hypercholesterolemia). Instead, it's saturated and trans fats that raise blood cholesterol (see page 34); yet only 28 percent of the fat in an egg is saturated fat.

Strong muscles

Protein influences muscle mass, strength, and function, all of which can decline with age. Eggs are a complete protein, containing all the essential amino acids, for good muscle health and repair after working out.

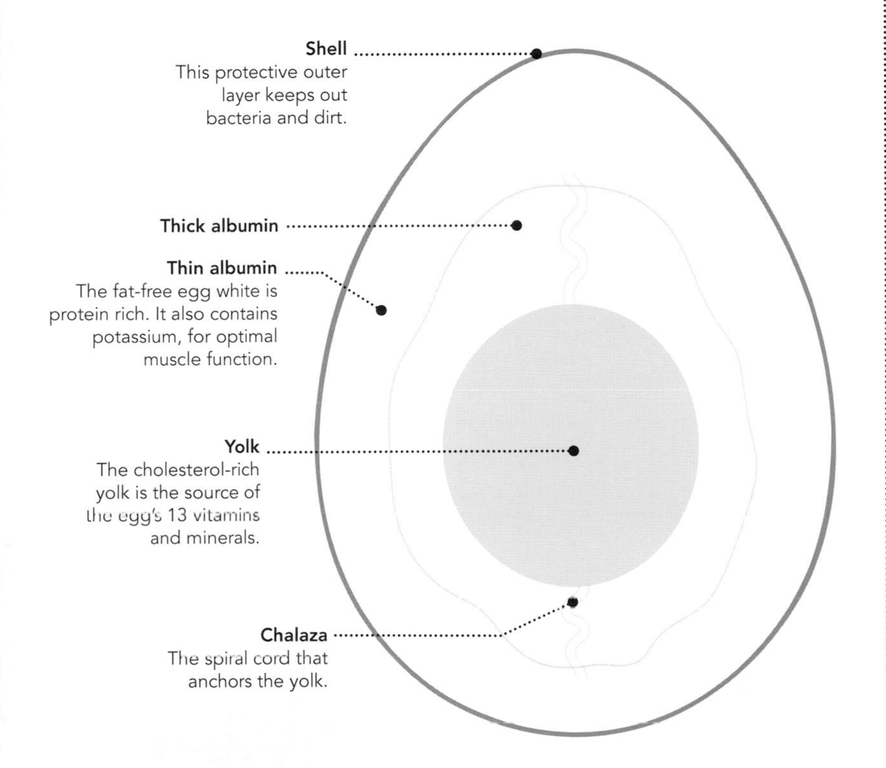

Fracture protector

Eggs are one of the few foods that are naturally rich in vitamin D, which is important, as it helps the body to absorb calcium. It is therefore vital for keeping bones strong and healthy and protecting against osteoporosis and fractures.

Calorie cutter

Research shows eggs keep us fuller for longer, so we take in fewer calories after eating them, which in turn helps with weight loss. In one study, normal-weight men who ate two poached eggs on toast for breakfast consumed 123 fewer calories at lunch and 315 fewer calories at dinner than those who ate cornflakes and toast for breakfast.

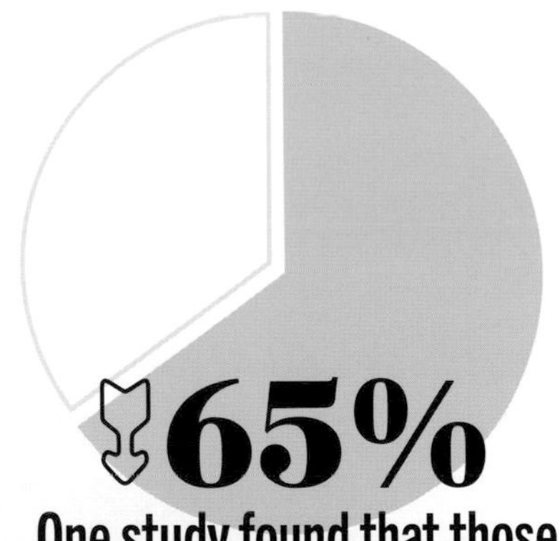

65%

One study found that those who ate an egg-based breakfast lost 65 percent more weight than those who had a bagel breakfast.

Mental well-being

Eggs contain many B vitamins, including B12, folate, pantothenic acid, and biotin, all of which are important for mental well-being. Eggs are also rich in choline, a nutrient crucial to the production of the neurotransmitter acetylcholine in the brain, which aids brain function and memory.

Vegetarian nutrient boost

As well as being a great source of protein and providing vitamins A and D, a range of B vitamins, phosphorus, selenium, and iodine, eggs also contain useful amounts of iron and zinc, which are especially important for those following vegetarian diets.

EGGS ON TOAST WITH ROASTED TOMATOES

Cooking the tomatoes enhances their nutritional goodness in this easy-to-make breakfast.

SERVES **2**

Ingredients

10oz (300g) cherry tomatoes
2 tbsp olive oil
2 tbsp balsamic vinegar
1 tbsp torn basil
1 sprig thyme
freshly ground black pepper
4 eggs
4 slices whole-grain bread
2 handfuls of baby spinach

1 Preheat the oven to 400°F (200°C). Toss the tomatoes with the oil, balsamic, and herbs in a small roasting pan and season with black pepper. Roast for around 10–15 minutes until the tomatoes have softened.

2 While the tomatoes are cooking, poach the eggs and toast the bread.

3 Mix the baby spinach leaves into the hot tomatoes to wilt a little (remove the thyme), then pile onto the toast and top with the eggs and a little more black pepper.

NUTRITION PER SERVING Calories **483** Total fat **24.8g** Saturated fat **5.2g** Cholesterol **432mg** Carbohydrates **43.6g** Dietary fiber **8.2g** Sugars **11.5g** Protein **24g** Sodium **459mg**

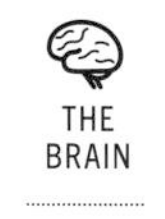
THE BRAIN
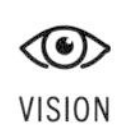
VISION
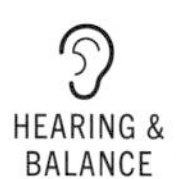
HEARING & BALANCE
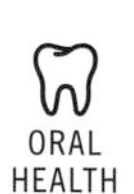
ORAL HEALTH
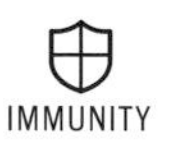
IMMUNITY
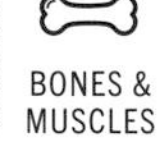
BONES & MUSCLES
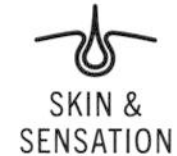
SKIN & SENSATION
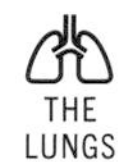
THE LUNGS
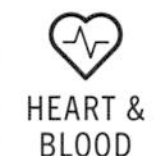
HEART & BLOOD
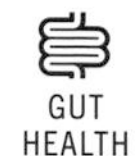
GUT HEALTH
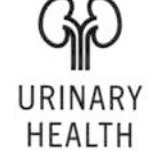
URINARY HEALTH
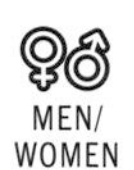
MEN/ WOMEN

MANGO AND COCONUT SMOOTHIE BOWL

Using frozen fruit means you can make this nutritious breakfast even when pressed for time.

SERVES **2**

Ingredients

3oz (90g) oats, any type
1¼ cups (300ml) unsweetened coconut milk drink
2 frozen bananas, in chunks
7oz (200g) frozen mango chunks
1 tsp vanilla extract
¼ cup (30g) skin-on almonds, chopped
¼oz (10g) desiccated coconut
2 handfuls of blueberries

1 Heat a nonstick frying pan over medium heat. Add the oats and cook, shaking the pan constantly, until the oats start to brown. Transfer to a bowl and leave to cool.

2 Blend the coconut milk drink, bananas, mango, and vanilla extract until smooth and creamy.

3 Divide the smoothie between two bowls and top with the toasted oats, almonds, coconut, and blueberries.

NUTRITION PER SERVING Calories **485** Total fat **16.8g** Saturated fat **5.4g** Cholesterol **0mg** Carbohydrates **75.6g** Dietary fiber **11.4g** Sugars **39.8g** Protein **10.8g** Sodium **85mg**

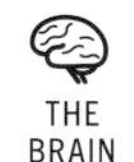
THE BRAIN
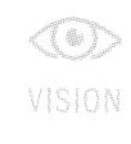
VISION
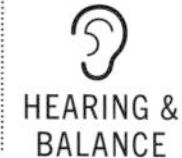
HEARING & BALANCE
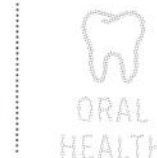
ORAL HEALTH
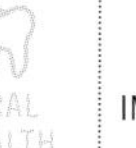
IMMUNITY
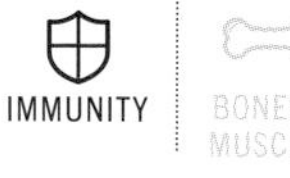
BONES & MUSCLES
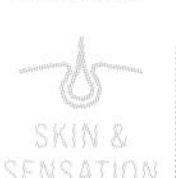
SKIN & SENSATION
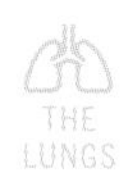
THE LUNGS
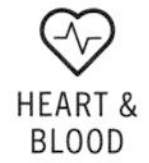
HEART & BLOOD
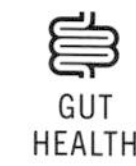
GUT HEALTH
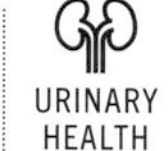
URINARY HEALTH
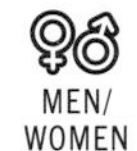
MEN/ WOMEN

VEGGIE BREAKFAST PITA POCKETS

This vitamin- and protein-rich combo comes in its own little parcel and makes for a super-satisfying breakfast.

SERVES **2**

Ingredients

1 tbsp canola oil
5½oz (150g) mushrooms, sliced
5½oz (150g) cherry tomatoes, halved
2 handfuls of baby spinach
4 eggs, beaten
freshly ground black pepper
4 whole-wheat pitas, warmed

1 Heat the oil in a nonstick frying pan over medium heat. Add the mushrooms and fry for 2 minutes until they start to brown. Next, add the tomatoes and cook for 2 minutes until they've started to split. Then, throw in the spinach and cook for 1 minute until it starts to wilt.

2 Season the eggs with black pepper, then pour them into the pan as well. Stir the mixture continuously and cook until the eggs have scrambled.

3 Fill the pita breads with the egg and vegetable mixture to serve.

NUTRITION PER SERVING Calories **494** Total fat **17.2g** Saturated fat **3.4g** Cholesterol **357mg** Carbohydrates **58.1g** Dietary fiber **8.2g** Sugars **6.1g** Protein **27.1g** Sodium **652mg**

THE BRAIN | VISION | HEARING & BALANCE | ORAL HEALTH | IMMUNITY | BONES & MUSCLES
SKIN & SENSATION | THE LUNGS | HEART & BLOOD | GUT HEALTH | URINARY HEALTH | MEN/WOMEN

HOMEMADE MUESLI WITH SOY YOGURT AND BERRIES

This no-nonsense breakfast offers maximum nutrition for minimal effort. In fact, why not make double and keep in an airtight container?

SERVES **2**

Ingredients

3½oz (100g) oats, any type
¼ cup (30g) mixed nuts
¼ cup (30g) sunflower seeds
1¾oz (50g) raisins
3½oz (100g) dried apricots, chopped
9oz (250g) plain soy yogurt
2 handfuls of raspberries

1 Combine the oats, nuts, seeds, raisins, and apricots in a bowl. Divide between two serving bowls.

2 Top each of the mueslis with the yogurt and scatter over the raspberries.

NUTRITION PER SERVING Calories **594** Total fat **22g** Saturated fat **3.3g** Cholesterol **0mg** Carbohydrates **83.4g** Dietary fiber **14.7g** Sugars **44.7g** Protein **20.5g** Sodium **96mg**

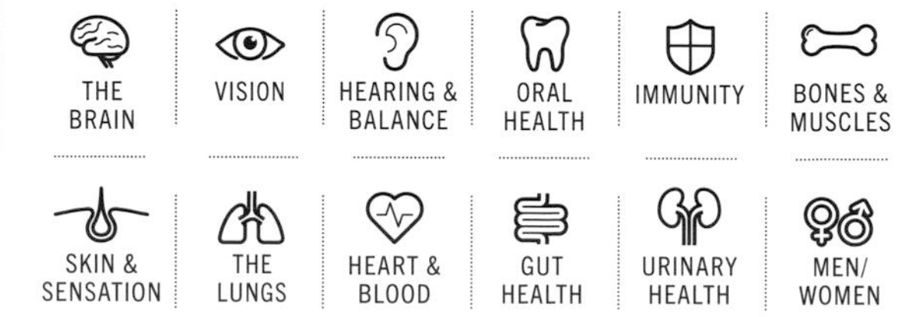

-SUPERGROUP-

WHOLE GRAINS

Whole grains are truly well-rounded when it comes to their health benefits, having a positive effect on the circulatory, digestive, and immune systems and reducing age-related diseases. Switching from refined grains to whole grains is a simple but powerful step to better health and a longer life.

WHICH WHOLE GRAINS?

Whole grains contain more nutrients than refined grains. These commonly eaten whole grains and whole-grain products have many benefits for longevity.

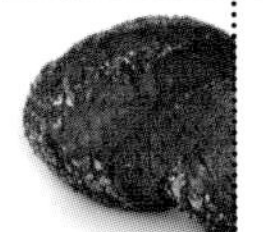

Whole-grain bread

- Has more potassium, iron, magnesium, and zinc than white bread

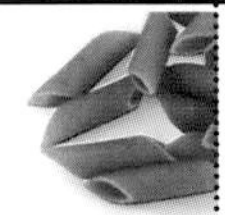

Whole-wheat pasta

- Is higher in fibre, so keeps you fuller for longer.

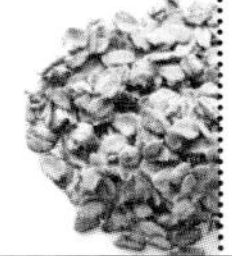

Oats

- Are rich in soluble fiber, so help control blood sugar levels

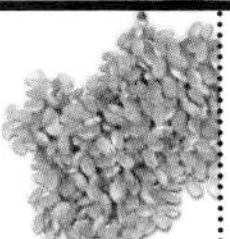

Brown rice

- Is particularly rich in magnesium, manganese, and the B vitamins

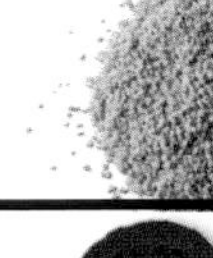

Whole-wheat couscous

- Is rich in the antioxidant selenium and a good source of potassium

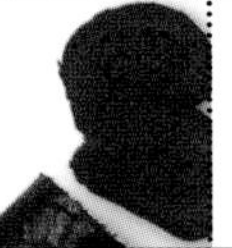

Rye bread

- Is a great source of vitamin E: it contains 15 times more than white bread

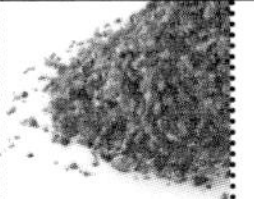

Barley (whole, not pearl)

- Is high in soluble fiber, so helps with weight

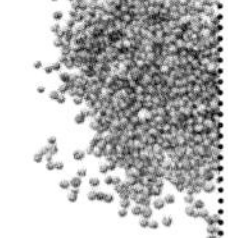

Quinoa

- Is the nutrient winner—extremely rich in iron, potassium, and zinc

HOW MUCH?

Whole grains are so vital to the body, it's important to eat them every day. Eat three servings daily for the best health and longevity benefits.

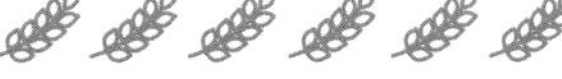
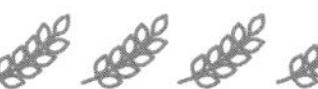
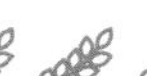

1 serving equals

- 1 medium slice of whole-grain bread such as whole-wheat, brown, or rye
- 1 small whole-wheat tortilla
- 2 oatcakes or rye crisp breads
- 3 tablespoons of whole-grain breakfast cereal
- 1 heaped tablespoon of uncooked oats
- 2 heaped tablespoons of barley, quinoa, or whole-wheat couscous
- 2 heaped tablespoons of cooked brown or wild rice
- 3 heaped tablespoons of cooked whole-wheat pasta

HOW TO STORE

Store whole grains and whole-grain products in their packages or in airtight containers in a cool, dark place, such as a cabinet or pantry.

RAW OR COOKED?

Most grains should be cooked before eating, although oats and bread don't need cooking.

COOKED

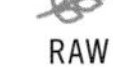
RAW

BEST BOUGHT

Look for the word "whole" on labels and ingredients, except for oats and brown or wild rice, which are always whole.

FRESH

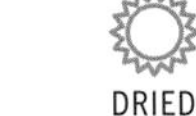
DRIED

Smart swaps for longevity

Changing from refined grains to whole grains has numerous body-wide health and longevity benefits, as whole grains can contain up to 75 percent more nutrients than refined grains. Whole-grain foods offer the complete package and contain all parts of the grain, but when grains are refined, the outer bran layer and germ are stripped away, so the grain loses many of its nutrients and much of its fiber.

Whole grain

Refined grain

Bran
Fiber-filled outer layer, which is rich in B vitamins and minerals. It takes time to digest, so we feel full for longer.

Endosperm
Starchy carbohydrate energy-providing layer. Has some vitamins and minerals.

Germ
Nutrient-rich core packed with B vitamins, vitamin E, essential fatty acids, and phytochemicals.

Health promoter

It's the total whole-grain package that gives whole-grain foods their diverse health benefits. A 2016 review of studies found three servings of whole grains a day were linked to a 12 percent reduction in the risk of stroke, a 15 percent reduction in cancer, and a 22 percent reduction for respiratory disease.

Reducing colon cancer risk

Good intakes of fiber are proven to help protect against colorectal (colon) cancer, and whole grains play an important role in boosting our intakes of fiber. A review of 25 studies found that three servings of whole grains a day reduced the risk of colon cancer by 17 percent.

Cutting the risk of diabetes

A review of 16 studies found that eating three daily servings of whole grains reduced the risk of type 2 diabetes by 32 percent. Interestingly, a small number of studies confirm that while brown rice protects against the disease, high intakes of white rice seem to increase the risk of developing type 2 diabetes.

Weight control

Studies show people who eat more whole-grain foods have a lower body mass index, less body fat, and are less likely to gain weight over time, mainly due to the good fiber content. As the fiber in whole-grain foods takes longer to digest, it helps us to feel fuller for longer and can help to reduce calorie intake.

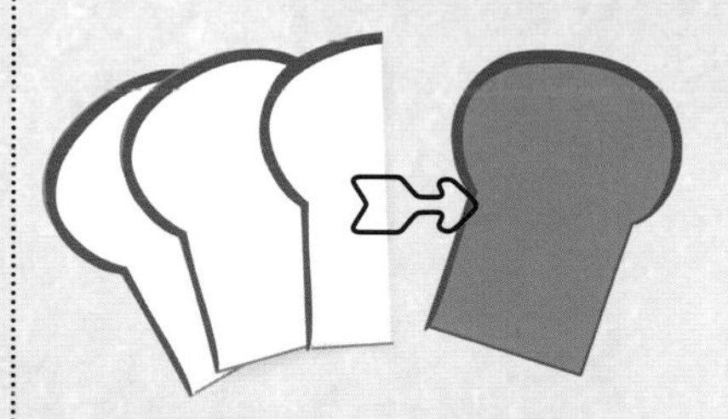

One slice of whole-grain bread provides the same fiber content as 2½ slices of white bread.

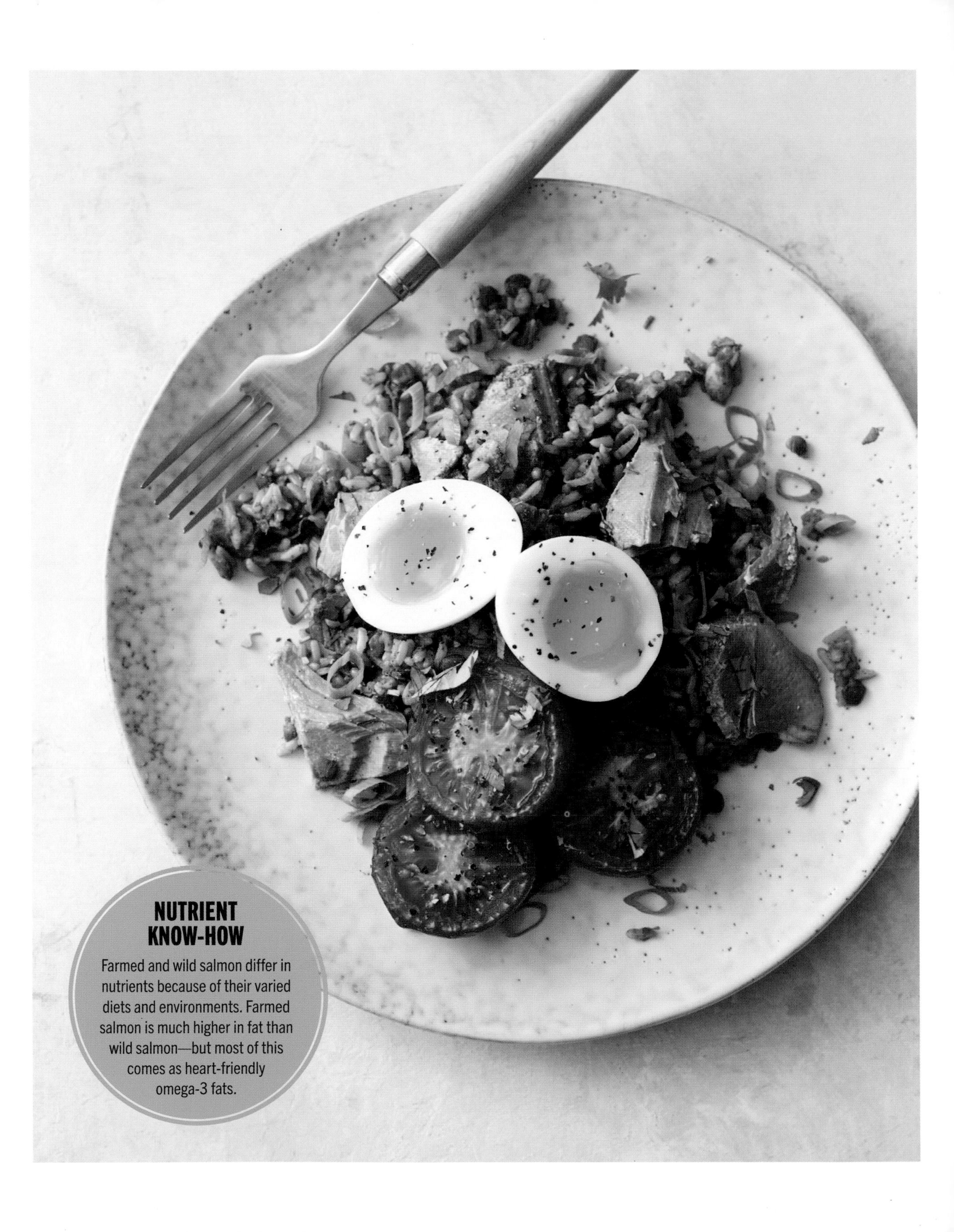

NUTRIENT KNOW-HOW

Farmed and wild salmon differ in nutrients because of their varied diets and environments. Farmed salmon is much higher in fat than wild salmon—but most of this comes as heart-friendly omega-3 fats.

THE BRAIN | VISION | HEARING & BALANCE | ORAL HEALTH
IMMUNITY | BONES & MUSCLES | SKIN & SENSATION | THE LUNGS
HEART & BLOOD | GUT HEALTH | URINARY HEALTH | MEN/ WOMEN

KEDGEREE-STYLE SALMON AND RICE

Rich in omega-3 fats from the salmon and memory-friendly choline from the eggs, this cooked breakfast gives your brain a great start to the day.

SERVES **2**

Ingredients

4½oz (125g) salmon fillet

2 tsp garam masala

2 tsp mustard seeds

1 bay leaf

2 cardamom pods, crushed

1 tbsp olive oil

4 scallions, roughly chopped

¼ tsp turmeric

4½oz (125g) brown rice

3 tbsp lemon juice

14oz (400g) can green lentils, rinsed and drained

3 ripe vine tomatoes, halved

freshly ground black pepper

2 eggs, hard-boiled

cilantro, roughly shredded

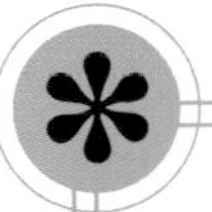

Smart swaps

- For convenience, use **canned salmon** instead of fresh—it's lower in omega-3 fats, but makes up for this by containing good amounts of other nutrients. It's also lower in calories, so it's a good option for those mindful of weight loss.
- Swap the lentils for a can of your favorite **beans**. Each type of bean has its own particular benefits; just be sure to choose varieties without any added sugar or salt.

1 Put the salmon into a medium pan with 1½ cups (350ml) water. Add 1 teaspoon of garam masala, 1 teaspoon of mustard seeds, the bay leaf, and the crushed cardamom pods. Place the pan over medium heat, bring to a gentle boil, and let simmer for 5 minutes until the fish is cooked through (opaque throughout). Use a turner to transfer the salmon to a plate to cool. Keep the cooking water for later, but remove the bay leaf and cardamom.

2 Heat the oil in a medium pan. Add most of the scallions, leaving a few for garnishing, and cook for 1 minute. Add the turmeric and the remaining garam masala and mustard seeds. Let them sizzle for 30 seconds, stirring continuously, then add the rice. Stir to coat the grains, then pour in the salmon cooking water along with the lemon juice and the lentils. Bring to a boil, reduce the heat to the lowest setting, cover, and cook for 25 minutes until the rice is tender. Meanwhile, preheat the grill to medium.

3 While the rice is cooking, place the tomatoes on a baking sheet (cut side up), season them with black pepper, and warm them on the grill for 5 minutes.

4 When the rice is cooked, use a fork to flake the salmon into large pieces and stir it into the rice. Roughly chop the hard-boiled eggs and stir them into the rice with the remaining scallions, cilantro, and plenty of ground black pepper. Serve the "kedgeree" with the grilled tomatoes.

NUTRITION PER SERVING Calories **622** Total fat **22.9g** Saturated fat **4.2g** Cholesterol **221mg** Carbohydrates **74.6g** Dietary fiber **9.9g** Sugars **5.7g** Protein **37.1g** Sodium **119mg**

LUNCHES

Eating a meal midway through your day ensures you don't overeat, allows you to digest your food completely, and gives lunch the emphasis it deserves. All these options refuel your body with all the nutrients you need for a productive afternoon.

92%

more cookies were eaten half an hour after enjoying lunch if people ate while playing games on their phones.

PESTO PASTA SALAD WITH BROCCOLI AND TOMATOES

This classic Italian-style lunch releases its energy slowly and allows you to follow the Mediterranean way of eating for longevity.

SERVES **2**

Ingredients

4½oz (120g) whole-wheat penne
5¾oz (160g) tenderstem broccoli, cut into chunks
1¼oz (40g) basil
2 tbsp olive oil
¼ cup (30g) pine nuts
1–2 garlic cloves
squeeze of lemon juice
freshly ground black pepper
7oz (200g) cherry tomatoes, halved
¾oz (20g) Parmesan cheese, grated, to serve

1 Cook the pasta according to the package instructions, adding the broccoli for the last few minutes of the cooking time. Drain and set aside.

2 Meanwhile, make the pesto: blend the basil, oil, pine nuts, and garlic. Stir in the lemon juice and pepper.

3 Add the tomatoes, along with the pesto, to the pasta and broccoli. Stir well to mix and serve with Parmesan.

NUTRITION PER SERVING Calories **500** Total fat **26.6g** Saturated fat **4.6g** Cholesterol **9mg** Carbohydrates **48.7g** Dietary fiber **11.7g** Sugars **8.3g** Protein **18.1g** Sodium **80mg**

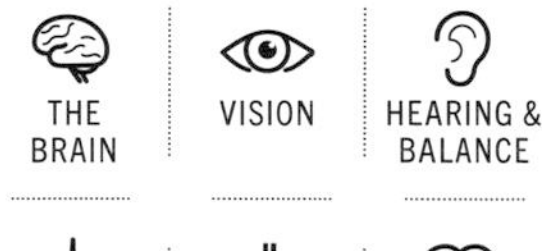
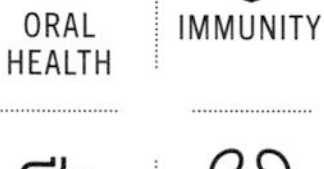

THE BRAIN | VISION | HEARING & BALANCE | ORAL HEALTH | IMMUNITY | BONES & MUSCLES

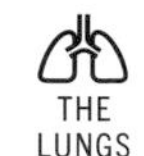
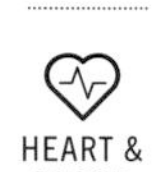
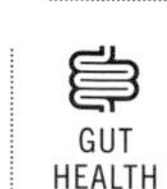
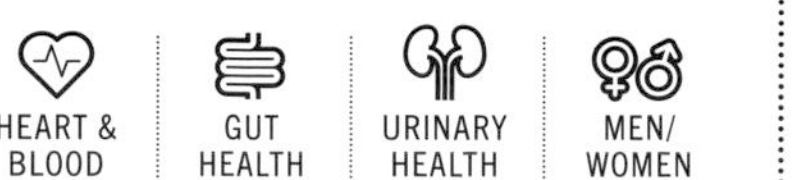
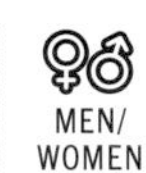

SKIN & SENSATION | THE LUNGS | HEART & BLOOD | GUT HEALTH | URINARY HEALTH | MEN/ WOMEN

MOROCCAN-STYLE COUSCOUS SALAD

A multicolored meal perfectly suited for packed lunches. Even the salad dressing is good for you!

SERVES **2**

Ingredients

3oz (80g) whole-wheat couscous
1 tbsp raisins
14oz (400g) can chickpeas in water, rinsed and drained
1 carrot, grated
1 small red onion, diced
1 orange, segmented and its juice
1 red bell pepper, diced
handful each of cilantro and mint, roughly torn
zest and juice of ½ lemon
2 tbsp olive oil
½ tsp each of ground cumin and ground coriander
1 garlic clove, crushed

1 Mix the couscous and raisins together in a bowl. Prepare according to the couscous package instructions.

2 Mix in the chickpeas, carrot, onion, orange and juice, and bell pepper. Stir through the herbs and lemon zest.

3 Combine the lemon juice, oil, spices, and garlic in a screw-top jar, shake together, and pour over the salad. Season and toss until well combined.

NUTRITION PER SERVING Calories **494** Total fat **16.3g** Saturated fat **2.2g** Cholesterol **0mg** Carbohydrates **73.8g** Dietary fiber **15.5g** Sugars **27.9g** Protein **16.8g** Sodium **31mg**

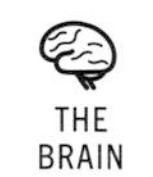
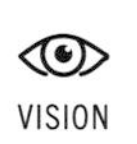
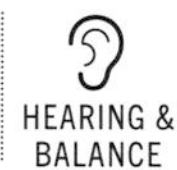
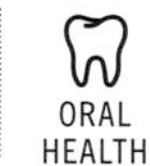
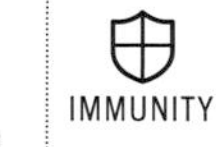
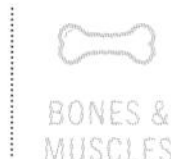

THE BRAIN | VISION | HEARING & BALANCE | ORAL HEALTH | IMMUNITY | BONES & MUSCLES

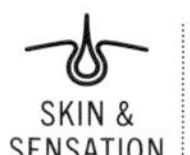
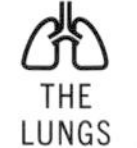
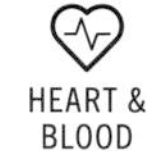
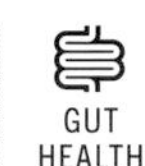
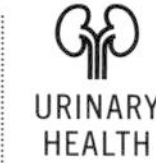
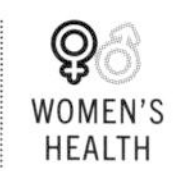

SKIN & SENSATION | THE LUNGS | HEART & BLOOD | GUT HEALTH | URINARY HEALTH | WOMEN'S HEALTH

SHRIMP, POMEGRANATE, AND QUINOA BOWL

Rich in selenium and copper, shrimp offer antioxidant support to muscles and nerves. Make this nourishing packed lunch the night before to let the flavors mingle.

THE BRAIN | VISION | HEARING & BALANCE | ORAL HEALTH | IMMUNITY | BONES & MUSCLES | SKIN & SENSATION | THE LUNGS | HEART & BLOOD | GUT HEALTH | URINARY HEALTH | MEN'S HEALTH

SERVES **2**

Ingredients

- 5½oz (150g) quinoa
- 1 tbsp canola oil
- 5½oz (150g) peeled raw shrimp, deveined
- 1 red chili, finely chopped
- 4 scallions, finely sliced
- zest and juice of 1 lime
- 3½oz (100g) pomegranate seeds (or seeds of 1 large pomegranate)
- handful of cilantro, roughly chopped
- 1 avocado, sliced
- lime wedges, to serve

1 Put the quinoa in a small pan with 1¼ cups (300ml) water. Place on medium heat and bring to a boil. Stir and leave to simmer for 10 minutes or until the water has been absorbed.

2 Heat the oil in a frying pan over medium-high heat. When hot, add the shrimp and cook them for 2–3 minutes until they are dark pink all over. Stir in the chili and half of the scallions, then remove the pan from the heat and allow the flavors to infuse.

3 When the quinoa is cooked, remove the pan from the heat. Add the lime juice, mixing gently and fluffing the grains with a fork. Transfer the quinoa to a large bowl and allow it to cool a little before adding the rest of the scallions, lime zest, pomegranate seeds, and half of the cilantro. Stir to mix.

4 Divide the fruity quinoa between two bowls (or transportable containers). Top with the sliced avocado, chili shrimp, and any cooking juices from the pan. Garnish with the remaining cilantro and serve with lime wedges. If you're taking it for a packed lunch, drizzling lime juice on top will slow the avocado's browning, or take the avocado and slice just before eating.

NUTRITION PER SERVING Calories **509** Total fat **24.2g** Saturated fat **3.9g** Cholesterol **113mg** Carbohydrates **50g** Dietary fiber **11.3g** Sugars **11.7g** Protein **26.2g** Sodium **217mg**

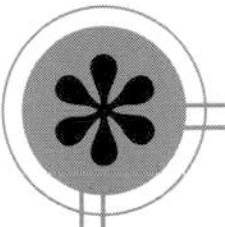

Smart swaps

- Replace the shrimp with **tofu** for a mineral-rich boost of copper, phosphorus, and potassium. Copper is essential for making new red blood cells and has bonus antioxidant activity.
- Swap the pomegranate for **sun-dried tomatoes** to boost your intake of the antioxidant lycopene—sun-dried tomatoes contain the most lycopene of any form of tomatoes.

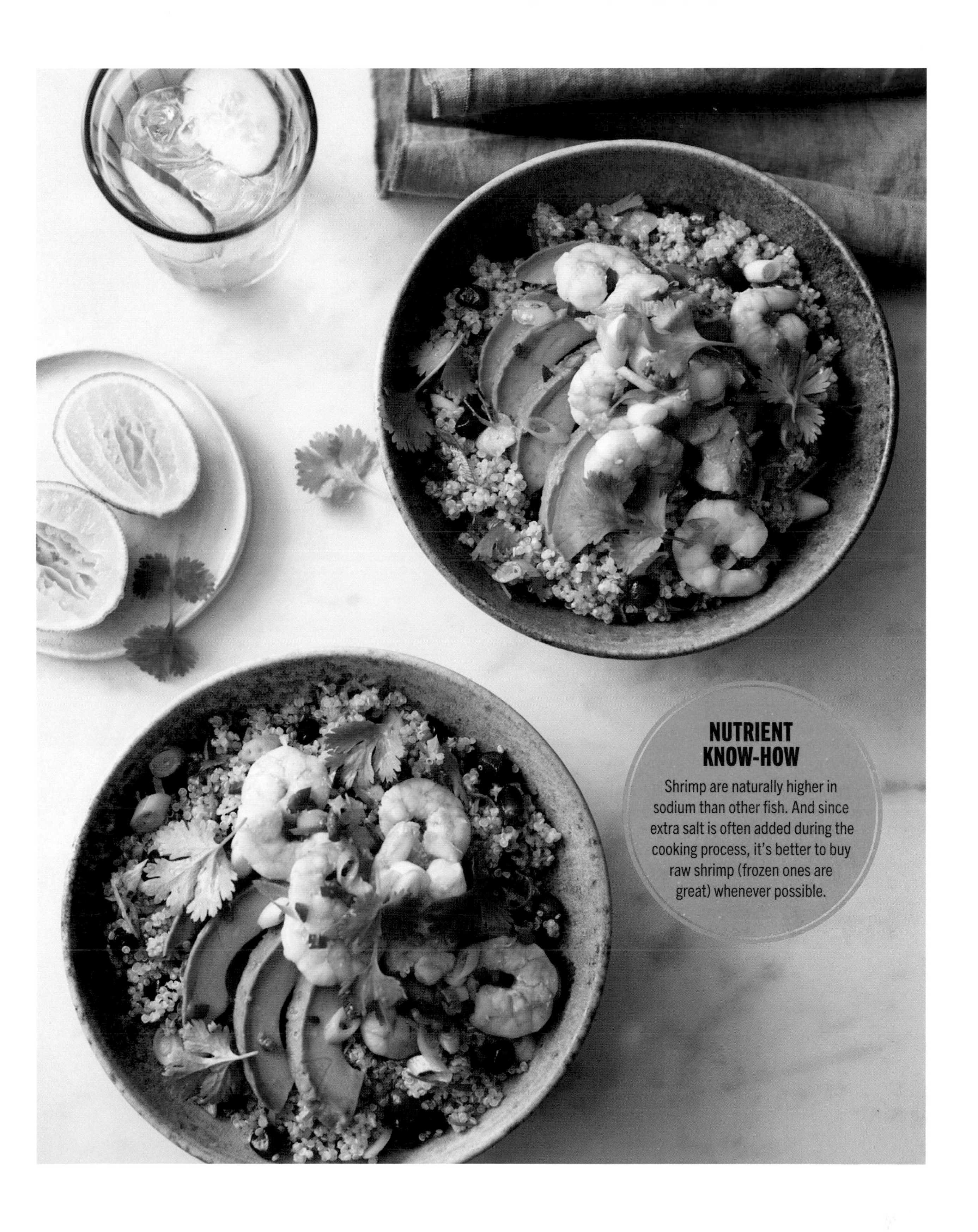

NUTRIENT KNOW-HOW

Shrimp are naturally higher in sodium than other fish. And since extra salt is often added during the cooking process, it's better to buy raw shrimp (frozen ones are great) whenever possible.

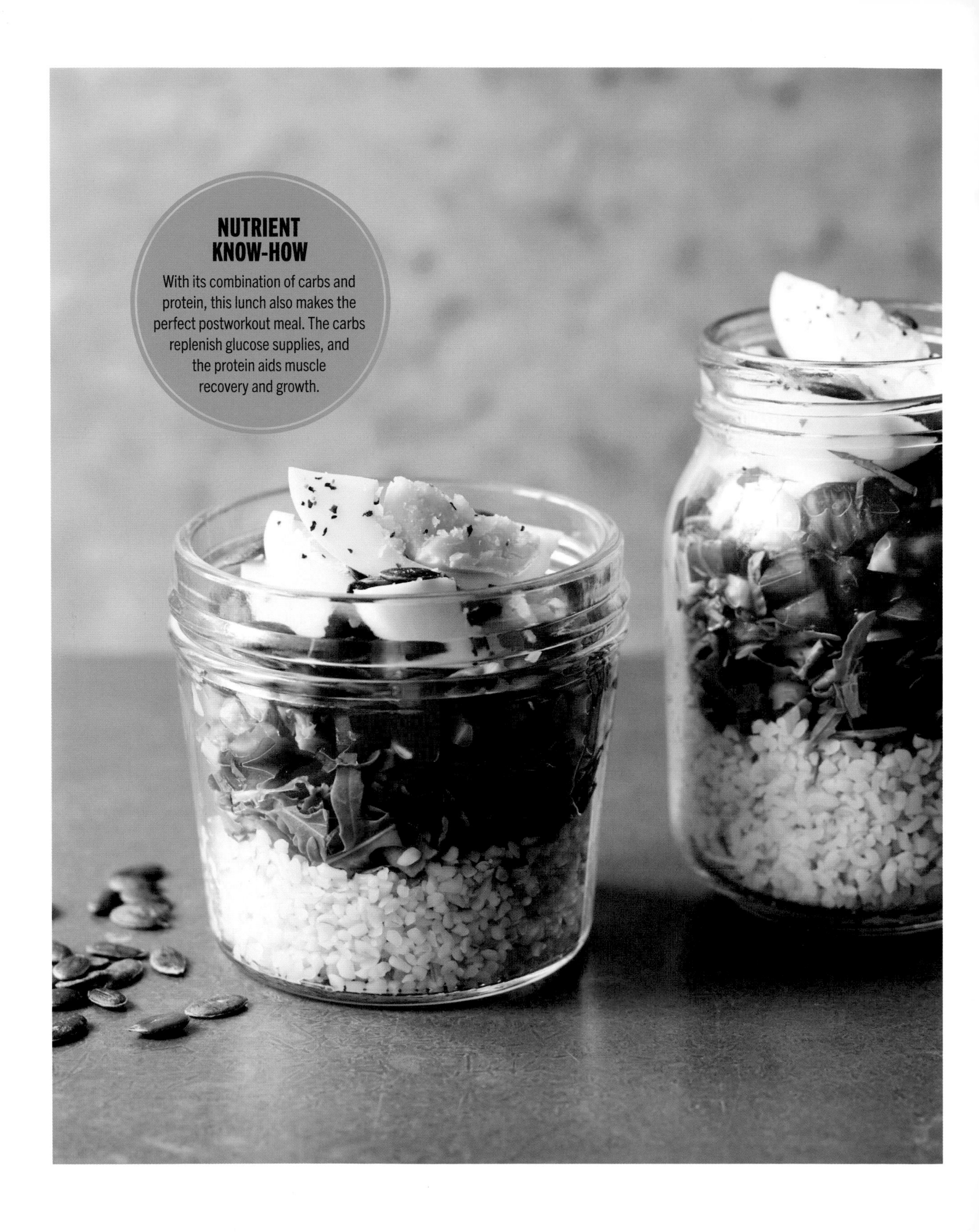
NUTRIENT
KNOW-HOW
With its combination of carbs and protein, this lunch also makes the perfect postworkout meal. The carbs replenish glucose supplies, and the protein aids muscle recovery and growth.

BULGUR WHEAT JAR WITH EGGS AND SALSA

This vibrant, fiber-packed lunch is a great choice for a healthy heart and digestive system. And the whole-grain bulgur wheat helps to keep hunger pangs at bay.

THE BRAIN | VISION | HEARING & BALANCE | ORAL HEALTH | IMMUNITY | BONES & MUSCLES | SKIN & SENSATION | THE LUNGS | HEART & BLOOD | GUT HEALTH | URINARY HEALTH | MEN/WOMEN

SERVES **2**

Ingredients

4½oz (125g) bulgur wheat

3 eggs, hard-boiled

1¾oz (50g) arugula leaves

3 tbsp (30g) pumpkin seeds

For the salsa

2 large vine-ripened tomatoes

1oz (30g) large green olives, pitted

1 mild red chili

1 small garlic clove

handful of basil leaves

2 tbsp olive oil, canola oil, or other mild oil

freshly ground black pepper

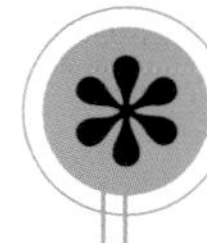

Smart swaps

- Replace the hard-boiled eggs with a can of **crabmeat** and you'll get a boost of omega-3 fats, as well as three times more zinc, which boosts the immune system.
- Swap the chili for chopped **scallion** if you prefer your lunch with less heat.
- Use **barley** instead of bulgur wheat for a boost of soluble fiber—great news if you want to lower cholesterol and keep blood sugar levels steady.

1 Put the bulgur wheat in a small pan with 2 cups (500ml) water. Place the pan on medium heat and bring the water to a boil. Stir and let the water simmer for 8–10 minutes until the bulgur wheat is soft. If the water has not all been absorbed, drain off the excess and set the grains aside to cool.

2 Make the tomato salsa while the bulgur wheat is cooking. Chop the tomatoes into ¼in (5mm) pieces, roughly chop the olives, finely dice the red chili, and lightly crush the garlic clove, placing everything into a small bowl. Shred the basil (both the stalks and the leaves) and stir it into the salsa with the oil and some freshly ground black pepper. Leave to sit for a few minutes.

3 Peel the hard-boiled eggs, then chop and set aside. Roughly shred the arugula leaves.

4 To assemble, divide the cooked bulgur wheat between two jars or bowls. Add a layer of shredded arugula, then spoon over the chunky tomato salsa (remove the garlic clove). Finish with the chopped eggs, a sprinkle of pumpkin seeds, and some black pepper.

NUTRITION PER SERVING Calories **551** Total fat **28.3g** Saturated fat **5.2g** Cholesterol **275mg** Carbohydrates **54.5g** Dietary fiber **7.3g** Sugars **4.1g** Protein **22.9g** Sodium **331mg**

-SUPERGROUP-

LEGUMES

Good intakes of legumes—such as beans, chickpeas, lentils, and dried peas—are linked to a host of health benefits, reducing the risk of many common age-related problems such as heart disease, digestive disorders, and type 2 diabetes. They're also a great weight-loss food, and an excellent source of nutrients for all, but are particularly useful for vegans and vegetarians.

WHICH LEGUMES?

Legumes are in the unique position of counting as both a protein-rich food and a vegetable. All these popular legumes are good sources of fiber, protein, iron, and calcium.

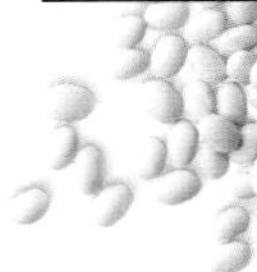

Navy beans

- Have one of the highest amounts of calcium—a nutrient vital for strong bones and protecting against osteoporosis—of all the legumes

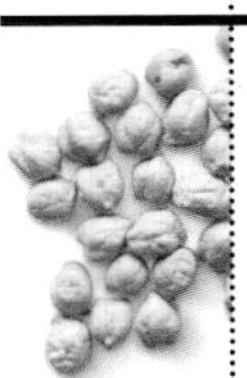

Chickpeas

- Contain good amounts of vitamin E, an antioxidant that protects cells from free radical damage and is needed for healthy skin

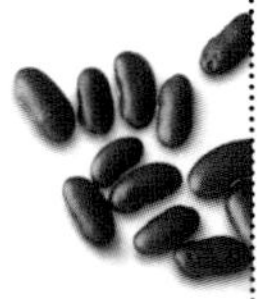

Kidney beans

- Are the star of the legume world for their high fiber content, which is important for weight management and those with type 2 diabetes, and are rich in antioxidants
- Include different types, such as red kidney and cannellini

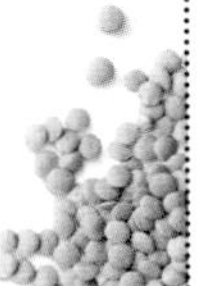

Lentils

- Are a good source of iron
- Come in various colors: choose green or brown for 20 times more selenium and 42 percent more copper

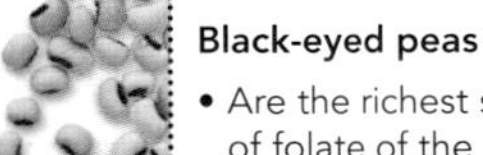

Black-eyed peas

- Are the richest source of folate of the legumes; folate is very important for immunity and for healthy blood

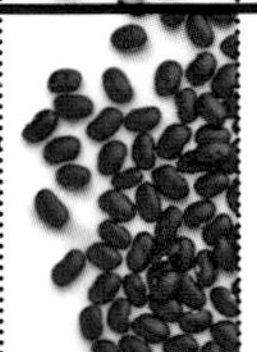

Black beans

- Get their dark color from anthocyanins—antioxidants with many protective and beneficial properties

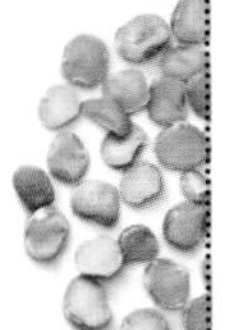

Split peas

- Are a great nutrient that is well-rounded and provides fiber
- Don't need soaking before cooking

HOW MUCH?

Studies show a daily serving of 3oz (80g) offers the best health benefits—choose a variety to ensure a range of nutrients.

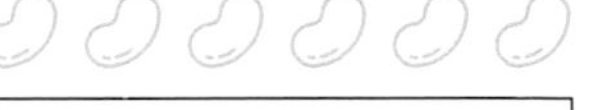

BEST BOUGHT

All beans are nutrient rich, but canned varieties are a little less so than dried versions. If using canned, choose legumes in water without added sugar or salt.

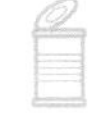

HOW TO STORE

Store legumes in a cool, dry place.

RAW OR COOKED

You need to cook legumes before eating. Soak most dried legumes first to rehydrate, then discard the soaking water and cook.

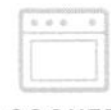

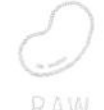

Better heart health

Legumes have many heart-healthy benefits. A landmark study that compared diets and heart health in seven diverse countries found a strong link between good amounts of legumes in people's diets and fewer deaths from heart disease.

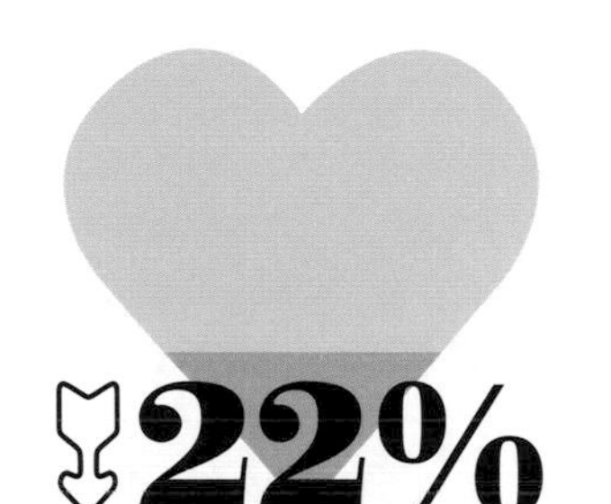

22%

reduction in risk of heart disease when eating legumes four or more times a week, rather than less than once a week.

Drop in diabetes risk

One study found that regularly consuming large portions of legumes (7oz/200g five times a week) improved blood sugar control, making them great foods for people with insulin resistance or type 2 diabetes. Plus, a large study found that women who ate the highest (compared with the lowest) amounts of legumes reduced their risk of developing type 2 diabetes by nearly a quarter.

Digestion benefits

Legumes help to keep the digestive system healthy in various ways (see below). Their undigested oligosaccharides (a form of carbohydrate) and resistant starch (starch that isn't digested) provide food for good bacteria in the large intestine, which helps them flourish. Legumes also contain insoluble fiber, making stools softer and easier to pass, and protecting against diverticular disease, colon cancer, and hemorrhoids (piles).

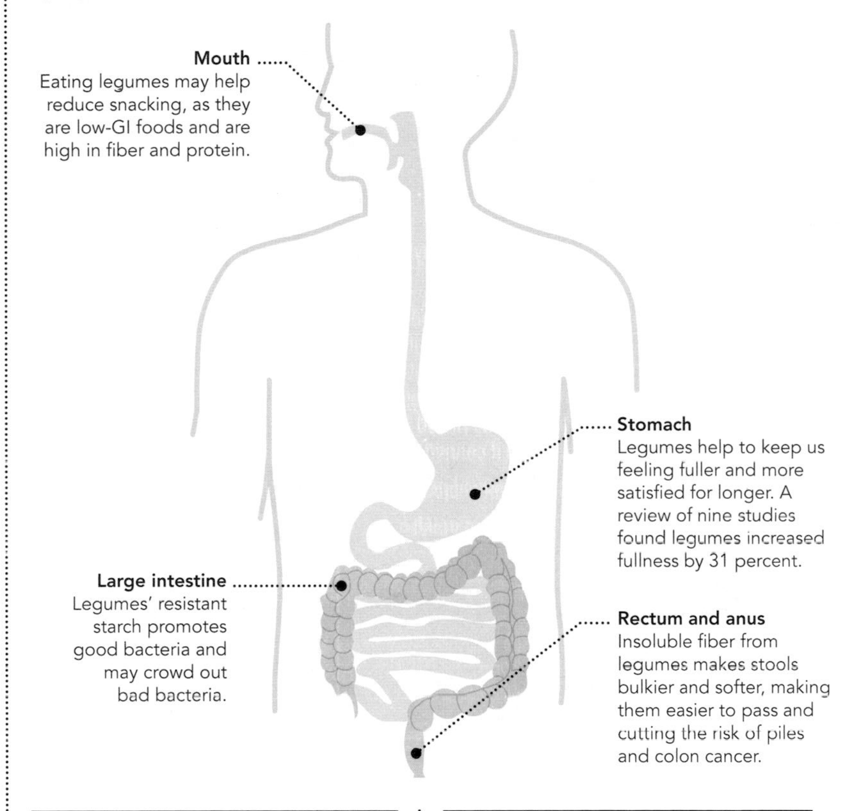

Weight control

Legumes can help us to manage our weight. They have a low glycemic index (GI), so keep blood sugar steady and prevent energy slumps that lead to snacking. They're also packed with protein and fiber—a magic combination for improving fullness so you eat less overall.

Cholesterol reducer

A review of 26 studies found a daily 4¾oz (130g) serving of legumes lowered LDL (or bad) cholesterol. This may be partly because legumes are rich in soluble fiber, which binds with cholesterol in the digestive system and stops it being absorbed into the bloodstream.

MIXED BEAN BOWL WITH PITA NACHOS

When hunger strikes, dive into this delicious and spiced lunch. As well as being a top fiber provider, the beans offer a great source of plant protein and phytonutrients.

THE BRAIN | VISION | HEARING & BALANCE | ORAL HEALTH | IMMUNITY | BONES & MUSCLES | SKIN & SENSATION | THE LUNGS | HEART & BLOOD | GUT HEALTH | URINARY HEALTH | MEN/WOMEN

SERVES **2**

Ingredients

1 tsp cumin seeds

1 tsp caraway seeds

1 tbsp olive oil

1 tsp ground coriander

1 red onion, chopped

1 garlic clove, chopped

4 ripe medium tomatoes, chopped

1 tsp cider or white wine vinegar

4½oz (125g) baby spinach leaves

14oz (400g) mixed beans (any mix of adzuki, cannellini, or borlotti to make the total weight; beans to be rinsed and drained if canned)

3 whole-wheat pita breads

cilantro, to garnish

Smart swaps

- Replace the beans with **chickpeas or lentils**. All legumes are rich in fiber, protein, vitamins, and minerals, and are beneficial for weight control. A review of 21 studies found that eating one serving of legumes a day for six weeks resulted in significant weight loss.
- For a portable packed lunch, swap the pita bread for a large **whole-wheat wrap**. Let the bean mixture cool, then fill the wrap with beans, sprinkle over the cilantro, and wrap up.

1 Put the cumin and caraway seeds in a large frying pan over medium heat and toast them for 1–2 minutes. When they start to "pop" and become fragrant, quickly add the oil and ground coriander and stir. Cook them for another 30 seconds, then add the chopped onion. Stir to coat it in the fragrant spices and leave everything to cook for another 2–3 minutes, without burning.

2 Next, add in the garlic and cook for another minute, before adding the chopped tomatoes (with their seeds) and the vinegar. Stir, reduce to low heat, then cover and cook gently for 4–5 minutes so that the tomatoes break down and release their juices. Toss in the spinach and stir well, letting the leaves cook for 1–2 minutes so they wilt.

3 Put the beans in a large bowl. Spoon the cooked tomato and spinach mixture over them and stir together gently so that the beans don't break up.

4 Preheat the grill to a high setting. With a sharp knife, slice the pita breads in half through the center, opening them out to make thin ovals. Cut each slice into triangular pieces or strips, and place them on a baking sheet. Slide the baking sheet on the hot grill for 2–3 minutes, turning the pitas once during cooking so that they crisp on both sides.

5 Divide the bean mix between two serving bowls, garnish with cilantro, and serve a handful of crisped pita nachos on the side.

NUTRITION PER SERVING Calories **510** Total fat **9.2g** Saturated fat **1.3g** Cholesterol **0mg** Carbohydrates **89.7g** Dietary fiber **24.9g** Sugars **14.2g** Protein **25.1g** Sodium **388mg**

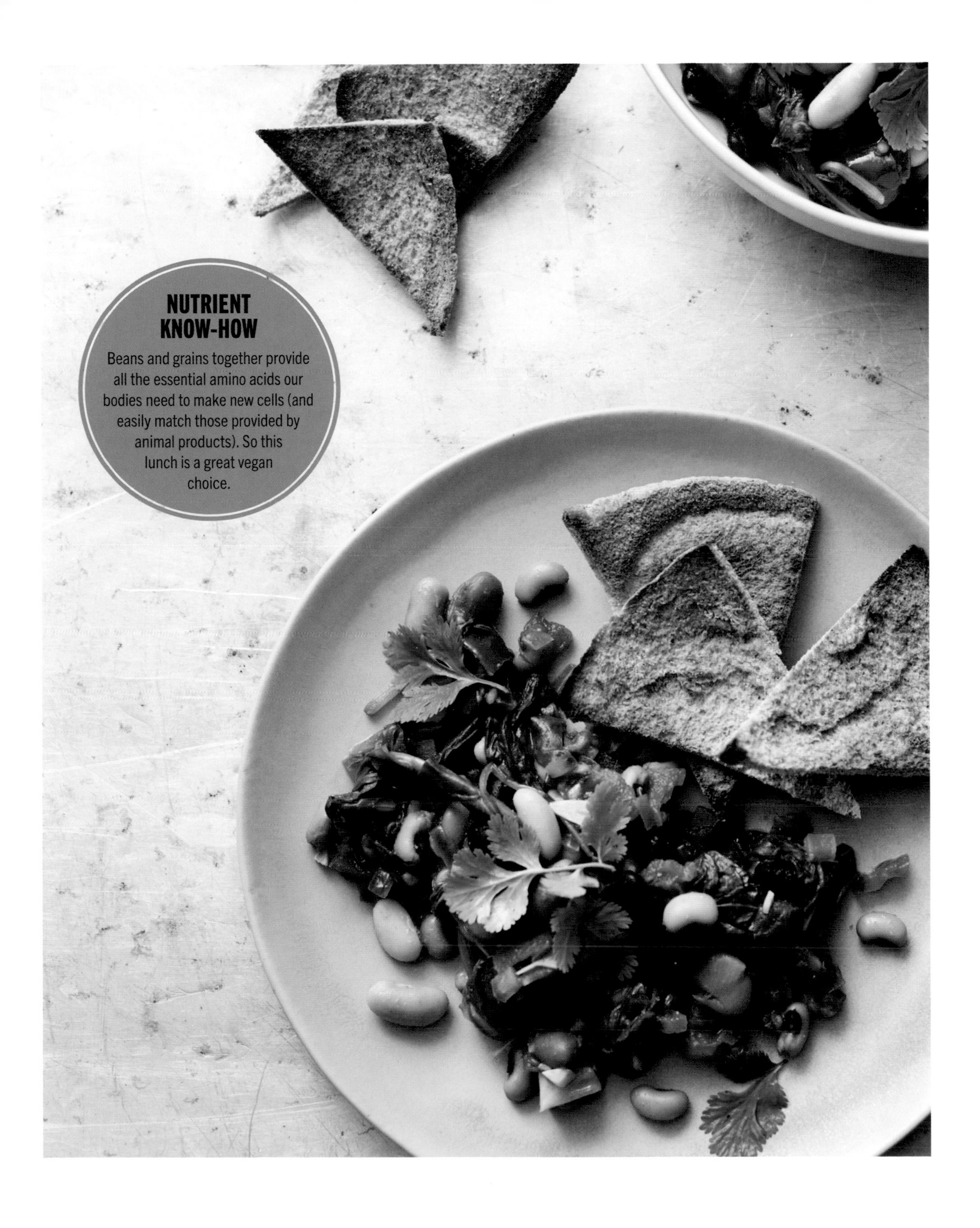

NUTRIENT KNOW-HOW

Beans and grains together provide all the essential amino acids our bodies need to make new cells (and easily match those provided by animal products). So this lunch is a great vegan choice.

INDIAN-STYLE CHICKEN WRAP

Mouth-watering flavors marry with eye-watering benefits from the beta-carotene-rich spinach, whole-grain wraps, and yogurt marinade.

SERVES **2**

Ingredients

5½oz (150g) container fat-free plain yogurt
2 tsp curry powder
1 garlic clove, crushed
1 tsp grated fresh ginger
juice ½ lemon
2 skinless chicken breasts, cut into strips
3 whole-wheat wraps, warmed
1 ripe mango, peeled, pit removed, and sliced
2 handfuls of baby spinach
handful of cilantro

1 Mix together the yogurt, curry powder, garlic, ginger, and lemon juice in a nonmetallic bowl. Add the strips of chicken, toss to coat well, and marinate for 30 minutes.

2 Preheat the grill to high. When ready, grill the chicken, turning midway, until it's cooked through.

3 Warm the wraps, then fill with the grilled chicken, slices of mango, baby spinach leaves, and cilantro. Roll up, cut in half, and serve.

NUTRITION PER SERVING Calories **512** Total fat **8.3g** Saturated fat **3.1g** Cholesterol **109mg** Carbohydrates **58g** Dietary fiber **10.6g** Sugars **18.5g** Protein **50.2g** Sodium **517mg**

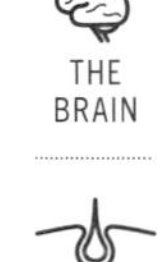
THE BRAIN
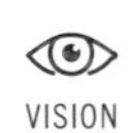
VISION
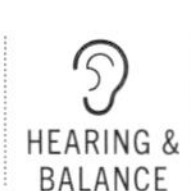
HEARING & BALANCE
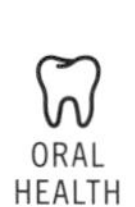
ORAL HEALTH
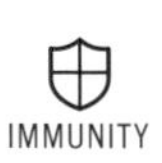
IMMUNITY
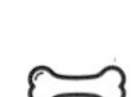
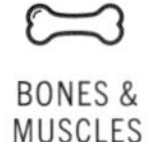
BONES & MUSCLES
SKIN & SENSATION
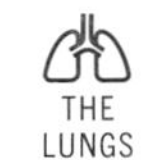
THE LUNGS
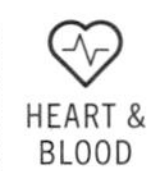
HEART & BLOOD
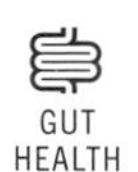
GUT HEALTH
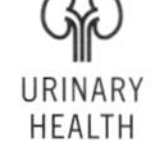
URINARY HEALTH
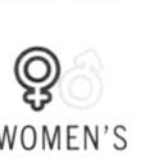
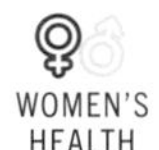
WOMEN'S HEALTH

QUINOA, TUNA, AND BEAN SALAD

A protein-packed lunch that fills you up and keeps blood cholesterol levels down.

SERVES **2**

Ingredients

¾ cup (115g) quinoa
3oz (80g) broccoli, broken into small florets
2 handfuls of chopped kale
5¾oz (160g) can tuna in olive oil, drained
1 small red onion, diced
14oz (400g) can black-eyed peas, rinsed and drained
zest and juice of 1 lime, plus lime wedges to serve
1 tbsp sesame oil
coriander, to taste
freshly ground black pepper

1 In a large lidded pan, cook the quinoa according to the package instructions. Once the water has almost gone, turn down the heat and place the broccoli florets on top of the quinoa. Cover to steam the broccoli, then remove from the heat, stir in the kale, and cover. Add to a bowl to cool.

2 Mix the tuna, onion, and peas into the quinoa and vegetables and stir well. Add the lime zest and juice, sesame oil, and coriander, and season with black pepper. Toss together and serve with lime wedges.

NUTRITION PER SERVING Calories **496** Total fat **13.8g** Saturated fat **1.9g** Cholesterol **28mg** Carbohydrates **60.1g** Dietary fiber **13.1g** Sugars **7.9g** Protein **36.8g** Sodium **279mg**

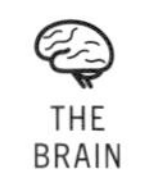
THE BRAIN
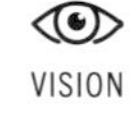
VISION
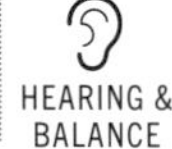
HEARING & BALANCE
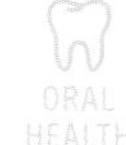
ORAL HEALTH
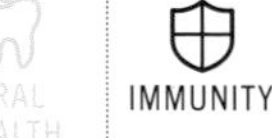
IMMUNITY
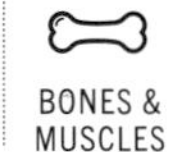
BONES & MUSCLES
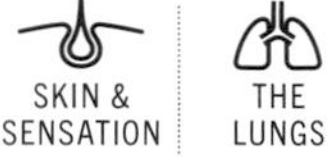
SKIN & SENSATION
THE LUNGS
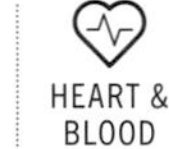
HEART & BLOOD
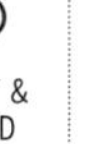
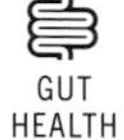
GUT HEALTH
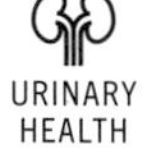
URINARY HEALTH
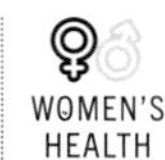
WOMEN'S HEALTH

SARDINE BRUSCHETTA

Since the bones in canned sardines are soft enough to eat, you can boost your own bone-building calcium levels alongside omega-3 fats.

SERVES **2**

Ingredients

1 fat garlic clove
7oz (200g) granary baguette, thinly sliced
3 medium tomatoes, finely chopped
1 small red onion, finely diced
handful of chopped parsley
1 tbsp balsamic vinegar
2 x 4oz (120g) cans sardines in olive oil, drained (reserve 1 tbsp of oil)

1 Preheat the grill to medium. Meanwhile, cut the garlic clove in half and rub one half on one side of each slice of bread. Put the bread onto a baking sheet, garlic side up, and put on the grill until lightly toasted.

2 Crush the remaining garlic and mix with the tomatoes, onion, parsley, balsamic vinegar, and the reserved olive oil from the sardines.

3 Flake the sardines into the tomato mixture and divide between and pile on to the toast slices.

NUTRITION PER SERVING Calories **505** Total fat **20.9g** Saturated fat **4.3g** Cholesterol **59mg** Carbohydrates **50.7g** Dietary fiber **9.4g** Sugars **10.6g** Protein **31.7g** Sodium **765mg**

THE BRAIN | VISION | HEARING & BALANCE | ORAL HEALTH | IMMUNITY | BONES & MUSCLES
SKIN & SENSATION | THE LUNGS | HEART & BLOOD | GUT HEALTH | URINARY HEALTH | MEN/ WOMEN

SPICY BEAN AND RED PEPPER SOUP

This soup offers all the vegetable goodness without a salty stock.

SERVES **2**

Ingredients

1 tbsp canola oil
1 onion, finely chopped
2 garlic cloves, crushed
½ tsp each of ground cumin, chili powder, and paprika
1 red bell pepper, chopped
14oz (400g) can chopped tomatoes
1¾ cups (400ml) homemade vegetable stock (see page 120)
14oz (400g) can mixed beans in water, rinsed and drained
freshly ground black pepper
chopped cilantro, to garnish
4 whole-grain rolls, to serve

1 Heat the oil in a pan over medium heat. Fry the onion gently until softened. Add the garlic and spices, cook for 1 minute, then add the bell pepper and cook for 5 minutes.

2 Add the tomatoes, vegetable stock, and mixed beans; season with black pepper; bring to a boil; then simmer for about 30 minutes until the vegetables are soft.

3 Divide between two bowls and top with the cilantro and a grind of black pepper. Serve with the rolls.

NUTRITION PER SERVING Calories **497** Total fat **12.1g** Saturated fat **1.7g** Cholesterol **0mg** Carbohydrates **77.8g** Dietary fiber **16.5g** Sugars **19.1g** Protein **24.4g** Sodium **530mg**

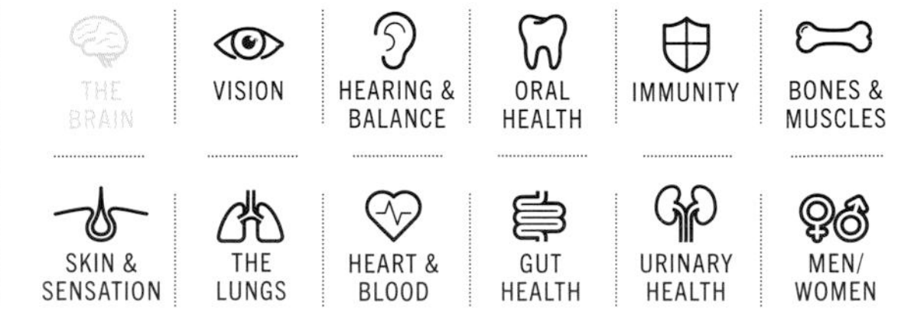

-SUPERGROUP-

BELL PEPPERS AND CHILIES

Bell peppers boost our intake of health-promoting carotenoids and vitamin C, while chilies have been linked to weight loss and better heart health.

WHICH BELL PEPPERS/ CHILIES?

All peppers are packed with similar good amounts of vitamin C, but red bell peppers win for extra nutrients.

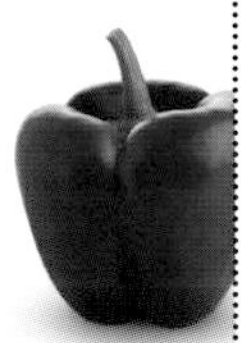

Red bell peppers

- Contain good levels (double that of green bell peppers) of the antioxidant beta-carotene
- Are rich in folate and vitamins A and E

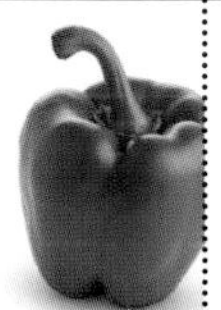

Green bell peppers

- Are the best source of lutein and zeaxanthin, two carotenoids that are important for good eye health

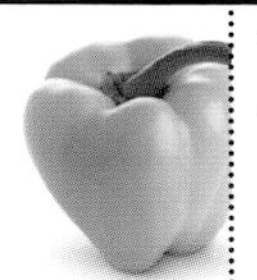

Yellow bell peppers

- Are richer in vitamins B1 and B3, which help release energy from food

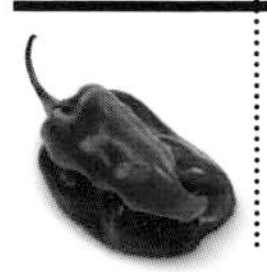

Chilies

- Contain capsaicin—a heart-friendly chemical that aids weight loss

HOW MUCH?

Have three to four bell peppers a week, and small amounts of chilies.

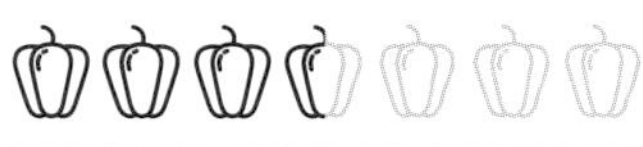

BEST BOUGHT

Choose fresh bell peppers or chilies that are firm, or buy good-quality jarred bell peppers, dried chilies, or chili powder.

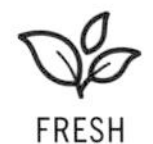

HOW TO STORE

Keep in the refrigerator if fresh, and in a pantry if dried.

RAW OR COOKED?

Enjoy raw or cooked—adding a little fat will help absorb all the carotenoids.

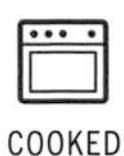

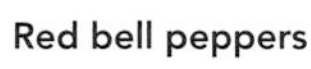

Heart-friendly spice

Studies reveal that capsaicin, the compound present in the flesh and membranes of chilies, has many heart-friendly effects. One of these is that it blocks the action of a gene that makes the arteries constrict. This stops the vessels narrowing, allowing more blood to flow through them. It also helps to stop platelets clumping together, a process that's involved in forming blood clots. In addition, capsaicin helps to reduce cholesterol.

Artery helpers

Bell peppers are also very good for the heart, as they are rich in vitamin C and carotenoids. These nutrients act as powerful antioxidants, helping to mop up free radicals, which can damage cells and start the process that leads to atherosclerosis, or narrowing of the arteries.

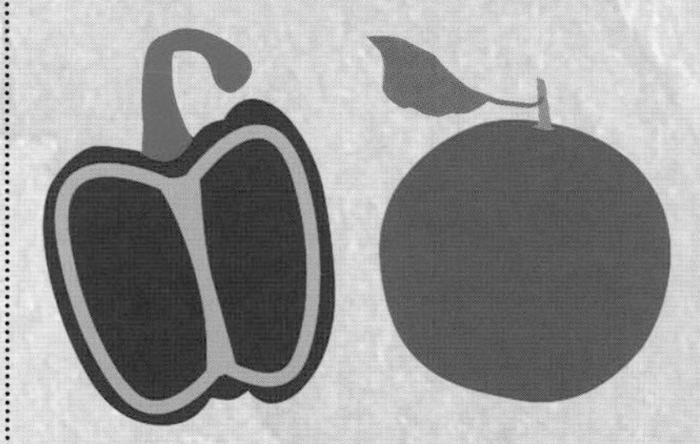

Bell peppers are a great source of vitamin C—half a red pepper has a fifth more vitamin C than an orange.

Weight loss

Much research has focused on how capsaicin, the chemical compound in chilies that gives them their spiciness, can have a positive effect on weight loss. Studies show it may boost the number of calories we burn—one review found about 50 more calories were burned in a day when capsaicin was included in the diet. Capsaicin also seems to temper appetite, so we eat less.

74 fewer calories were eaten if chilies were consumed first.

Cancer protectors

A 2017 study found the risk of lung cancer was 26 percent lower in adults with the highest intakes of vitamin C compared with the lowest, while for beta-carotene it was 34 percent lower. Men who smoked heavily seemed to benefit most from the carotenoids, while women who smoked seemed to benefit most from vitamin C.

Respiratory system helpers

Bell peppers are loaded with vitamin C and carotenoids; see below how they benefit respiratory health. These nutrients are important for healthy lungs and are linked to an improvement in respiratory diseases, such as asthma and chronic obstructive pulmonary disease (COPD). COPD is most common in smokers and, according to the World Health Organization, affects 65 million people around the world.

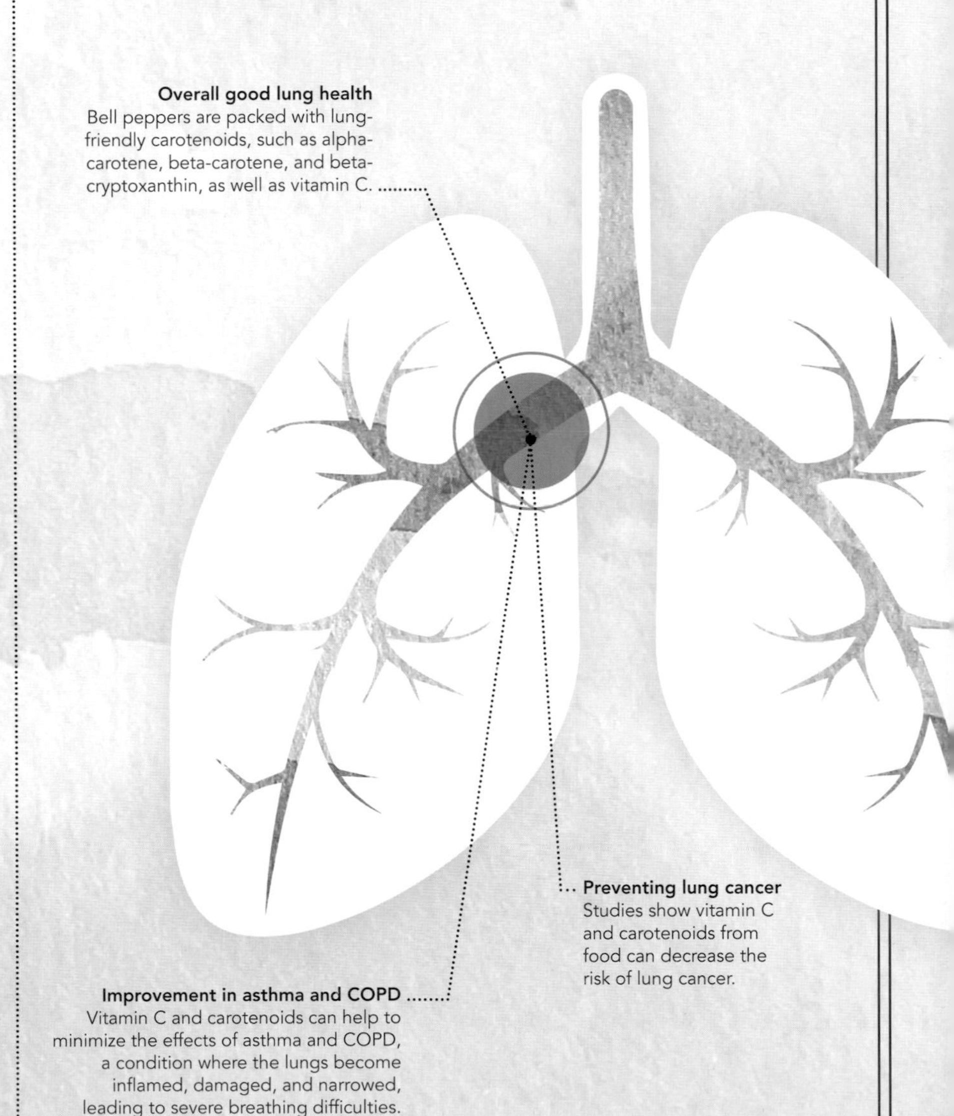

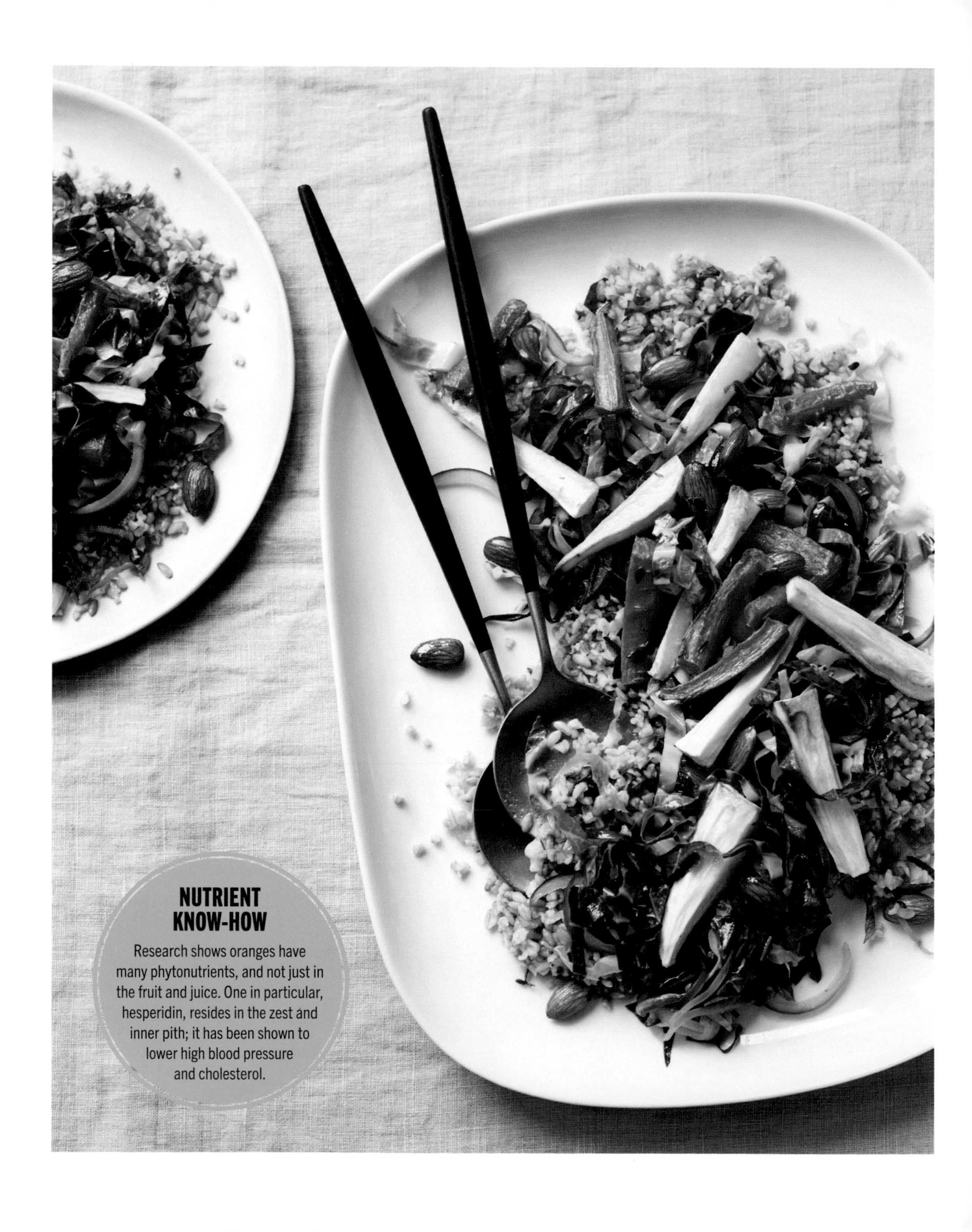

NUTRIENT KNOW-HOW

Research shows oranges have many phytonutrients, and not just in the fruit and juice. One in particular, hesperidin, resides in the zest and inner pith; it has been shown to lower high blood pressure and cholesterol.

THE BRAIN | VISION | HEARING & BALANCE | ORAL HEALTH
IMMUNITY | BONES & MUSCLES | SKIN & SENSATION | THE LUNGS
HEART & BLOOD | GUT HEALTH | URINARY HEALTH | MEN/ WOMEN

FREEKEH WITH ROASTED VEGGIES AND GREENS

As a whole grain, freekeh comes with a long list of longevity credentials, and the combination of vegetables offers better eye health and slows cognitive decline.

SERVES **2**

Ingredients

- 1 medium carrot, peeled
- 1 parsnip, peeled
- olive oil spray
- few sprigs of thyme
- 4 tbsp (40g) whole unblanched (skin-on) almonds
- 3½oz (100g) freekeh grains
- 1 red onion, chopped
- 2 garlic cloves, chopped
- 7oz (200g) spring greens, shredded

For the dressing

- 1 heaped tbsp mint leaves, chopped
- 1 tbsp olive oil
- zest of 1 orange
- 3 tbsp orange juice, plus extra to taste
- 1 tsp white balsamic vinegar, plus extra to taste
- freshly ground black pepper

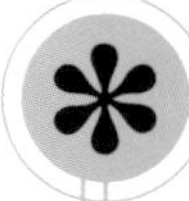

Smart swaps

- Replace the freekeh grains with **brown rice** for a boost of manganese, which is vital for energy production in cells, as well as for the synthesis of fatty acids, which are essential for a healthy nervous system.
- Swap the spring greens for **kale** to get extra immunity-boosting vitamin A, blood-pressure-lowering potassium, and fatigue-busting folate.

1 Preheat the oven to 400°F (200°C). Halve the carrots lengthwise, then divide each into finger-sized batons and put into a roasting pan. Cut the parsnip in the same way and add to the pan. Cover the batons with 3 or 4 spritzes of olive oil spray and toss well to coat. Tuck the thyme sprigs underneath and put the pan into the oven.

2 After 20 minutes, add the almonds to the pan, scattering them over the root vegetables, and roast for another 5 minutes. The vegetables should now be soft and starting to color; take the pan out of the oven and remove and discard the woody thyme. Set aside.

3 Meanwhile, put 2 cups (500ml) water in a medium pan over high heat. Add the freekeh and bring to a boil. Stir the grains, then reduce the heat and simmer for 15–20 minutes until they are tender. Drain any excess water and set the freekeh aside.

4 Put 2–3 spritzes of olive oil spray into a frying pan over medium heat. Fry the onion for 2–3 minutes, then add the garlic. Stir and cook for 1 minute, then add in the greens. Add plenty of black pepper and stir, cooking the greens for 2–3 minutes.

5 In a small bowl, mix all the dressing ingredients. Taste, adding a little more orange juice or vinegar as required. Pour the dressing over the freekeh grains, season with black pepper, and mix well.

6 To serve, spoon the grains on to a large platter and top with the wilted greens, roasted roots, and almonds; works hot or cold.

NUTRITION PER SERVING Calories **482** Total fat **21.3g** Saturated fat **2.4g** Cholesterol **0mg** Carbohydrates **57.3g** Dietary fiber **18.9g** Sugars **19.4g** Protein **19.1g** Sodium **46mg**

-SUPERGROUP-

ROOT VEGETABLES

Root vegetables regularly feature in the diets of communities well-known for their above-average life expectancies. They are especially rich in blood pressure-controlling potassium and digestion-friendly fiber.

WHICH TO CHOOSE?

These popular vegetables are good sources of nutrients.

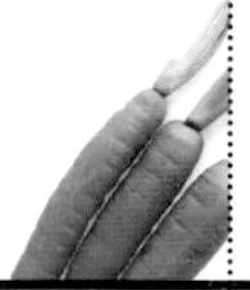

Carrots

- Are one of the richest sources of beta-carotene, essential for good eye health

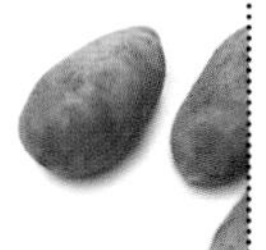

Potatoes

- Are an excellent source of potassium, which helps regulate blood pressure

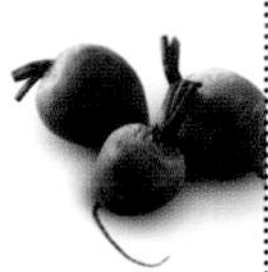

Beets

- Are rich in the B vitamin folate, which is needed for a strong immune system

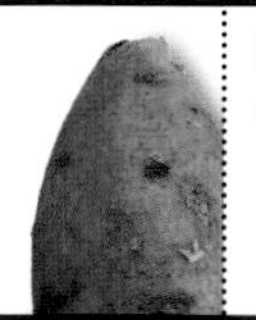

Sweet potatoes

- Come in two varieties: orange contain beta-carotene; purple have anthocyanins

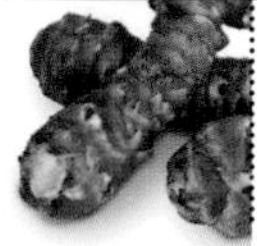

Sunchokes

- Are packed with inulin, a prebiotic that aids digestion

HOW MUCH?

Enjoy root vegetables daily.

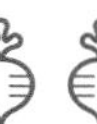
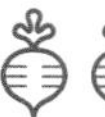

BEST BOUGHT

Choose firm, brightly colored vegetables—the deeper the color, the more antioxidants they contain.

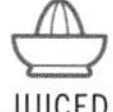
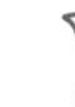

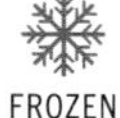

JUICED FRESH FROZEN

HOW TO STORE

Keep beets and carrots in the refrigerator; store other root vegetables in a cool, dark place (not the refrigerator).

RAW OR COOKED?

Some, such as carrots, can be eaten raw, but most need to be cooked first.

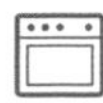

COOKED RAW

Fiber fillers

All root vegetables are rich in fiber, so they can help with blood sugar and weight control and lower cholesterol. They also contain insoluble fiber, which keeps the digestive system healthy, protecting against constipation, hemorrhoids (piles), diverticular disease, and colon cancer. Good fiber intakes are also linked to a lower risk of type 2 diabetes—one large study found high intakes of root vegetables reduced the risk of type 2 diabetes by 13 percent.

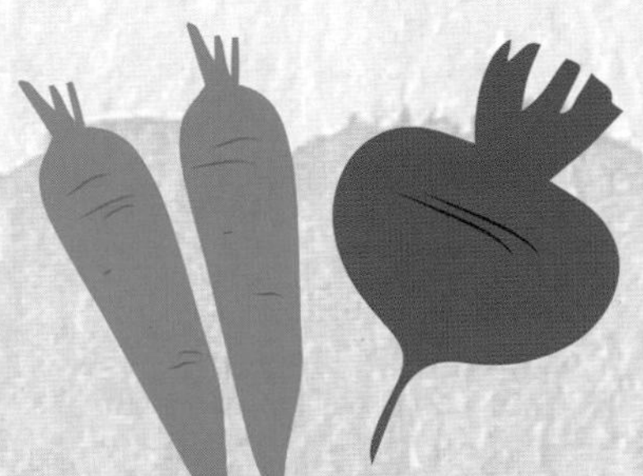

Scrub rather than peel root vegetables, as many of the nutrients and insoluble fiber are found in or just below the skin.

Heart health

Good intakes of root vegetables have been found to protect against cardiovascular disease. One study found higher intakes of carrots lowered the risk of coronary heart disease by 32 percent.

Cancer protector

Orange-fleshed root vegetables are rich in carotenoids, such as beta-carotene. Good intakes of this nutrient have been shown to protect against some cancers. One review of studies found the odds of having esophageal cancer were reduced by 42 percent when comparing the highest and lowest intakes of beta-carotene.

Blood pressure aid

Most root vegetables are rich in potassium, which can lower blood pressure when combined with a lowered intake of sodium. All root vegetables are also rich in nitrates, which are converted into nitric oxide in the blood. This helps to relax the blood vessels, reducing blood pressure. One review of 16 studies found having beet juice every day significantly reduced systolic blood pressure.

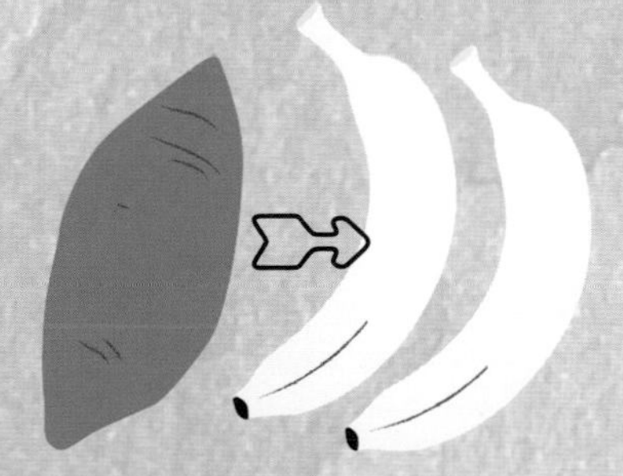

A 7oz (200g) baked sweet potato has more potassium than two medium bananas.

Nutrient-rich energy boosters

Root vegetables provide starchy carbohydrates that come packaged with fiber, vitamins, and antioxidants, making them a nutritious energy source. Potatoes are also reasonably low in calories—just 130 calories in 6¼oz (175g) of boiled potato. Compared with eating just the flesh of a baked potato, eating a baked potato with its skin provides 39 percent more fiber, 66 percent more potassium, 83 percent more vitamin B6, and 80 percent more folate. Discover how cooking can affect a potato's nutrition below.

Peeled and boiled potatoes contain 50 percent more vitamin C than baked, as this vitamin is destroyed by heat.
Baked potatoes are richer in fiber and most nutrients, as these are concentrated in or near the skin.

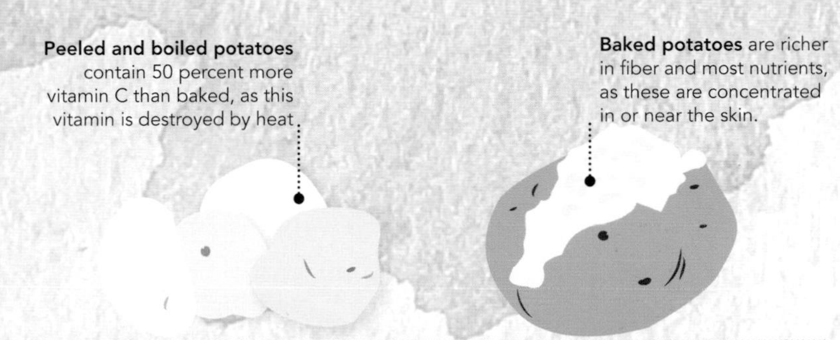

BOILED POTATOES HAVE MORE		BAKED POTATOES HAVE MORE
	FIBER	38%
	POTASSIUM	39%
	MAGNESIUM	33%
	PHOSPHORUS	31%
	IRON	46%
	ZINC	50%
5%	THIAMIN	
	VITAMIN B6	45%
50%	VITAMIN C	

THE BRAIN | VISION | HEARING & BALANCE | ORAL HEALTH
IMMUNITY | BONES & MUSCLES | SKIN & SENSATION | THE LUNGS
HEART & BLOOD | GUT HEALTH | URINARY HEALTH | MEN/WOMEN

BEET, PEPPER, AND CHUNKY HUMMUS WRAP

This gloriously technicolored lunch boasts superior levels of dietary nitrates, potassium, antioxidants, and fiber—what's more, it tastes delicious.

SERVES **2**

Ingredients

1 red bell pepper
1 yellow bell pepper
2 beets
1 tbsp olive oil
3 whole-wheat wraps
2¾oz (80g) watercress
½–1 tsp ground cumin
14oz (400g) can chickpeas in water, rinsed and drained
good handful of cilantro
freshly ground black pepper

For the hummus

2 tbsp tahini
3 tbsp lemon juice
4 tbsp olive oil
1 garlic clove, crushed

1 Preheat the oven to 400°F (200°C). Halve and seed the bell peppers, then chop them into large chunks. Peel the beets and cut them into quarters or chunks ¾in (2cm) across.

2 Once chopped, put all of the vegetables onto a baking sheet and drizzle them with the olive oil. Roast on the top rack of the oven for 20 minutes until the beets are cooked, but still have some bite. Once the vegetables have roasted, remove them from the oven and set them aside to cool a little.

3 Meanwhile, place the tahini and lemon juice into a food processor and blend for 1 minute to cream the tahini. Use a spatula to scrape down the sides, then add the olive oil, garlic, and ground cumin. Blend again, then pour in three-quarters of the chickpeas and mix until smooth. Add the cilantro, plenty of black pepper, and the remaining chickpeas. Pulse to roughly mix, but keep the hummus chunky. Season with more cumin, lemon, and black pepper, to taste. Warm the wraps.

4 Spread the hummus on the wraps, using 2–3 tablespoons per wrap. Add a handful of watercress in a line down the center of the wrap and top with the warm roasted vegetables. Season with more black pepper and a little lemon if desired, then roll up the wrap and serve. Any leftover hummus can be stored in a covered container in the refrigerator for another meal (see also page 115).

NUTRITION PER SERVING Calories **514** Total fat **23.3g** Saturated fat **5g** Cholesterol **0mg** Carbohydrates **59.4g** Dietary fiber **15.5g** Sugars **14.7g** Protein **15.8g** Sodium **426mg**

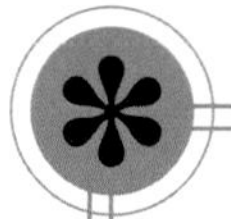

Smart swaps

- Swap the roasted beets for **carrot** batons (cut them into batons about ½in/1cm) thick) to boost the wrap's levels of beta-carotene, which the body uses to make immune-boosting vitamin A.
- Replace the watercress with **arugula leaves** to double the brain-friendly folate levels.

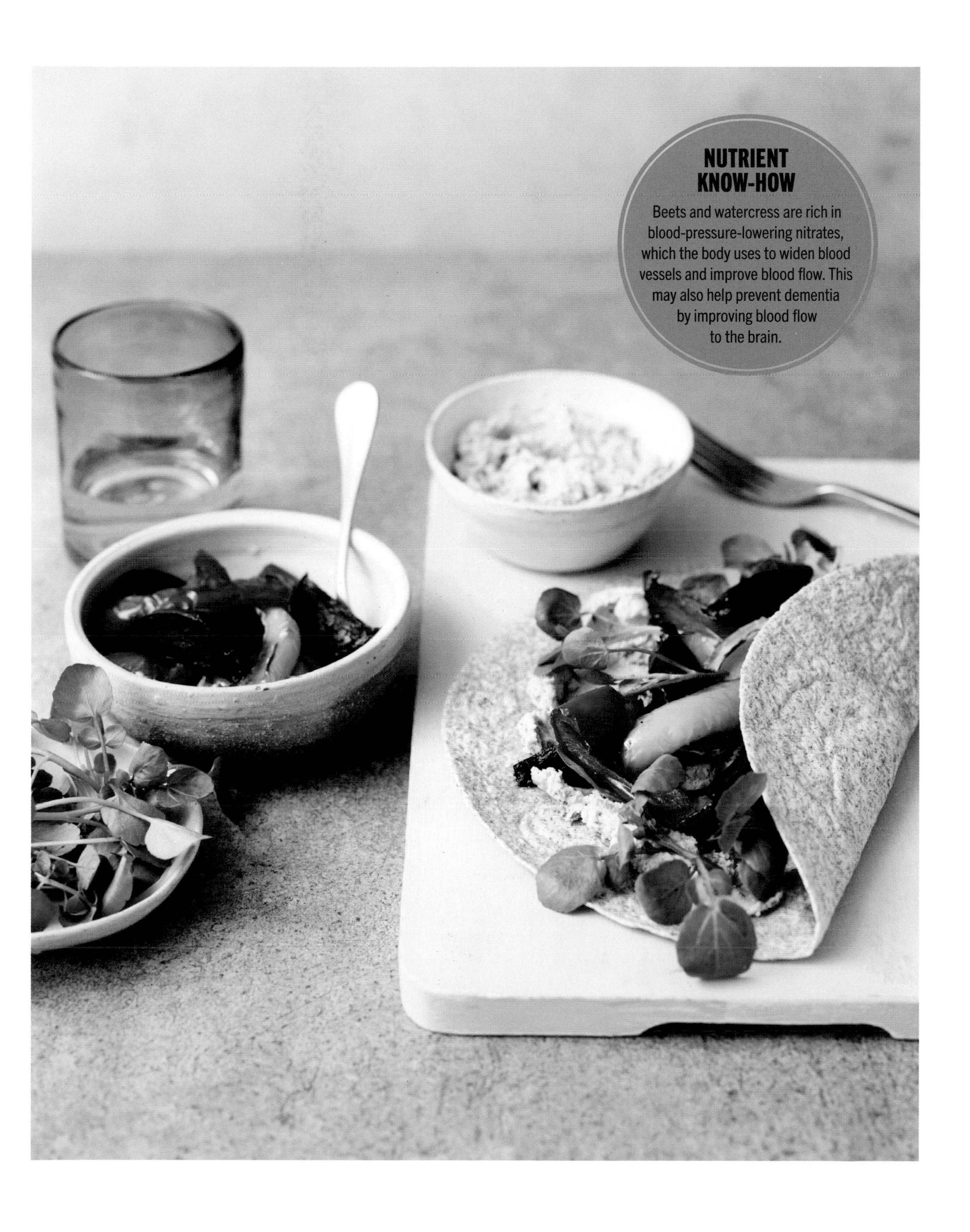

NUTRIENT KNOW-HOW

Beets and watercress are rich in blood-pressure-lowering nitrates, which the body uses to widen blood vessels and improve blood flow. This may also help prevent dementia by improving blood flow to the brain.

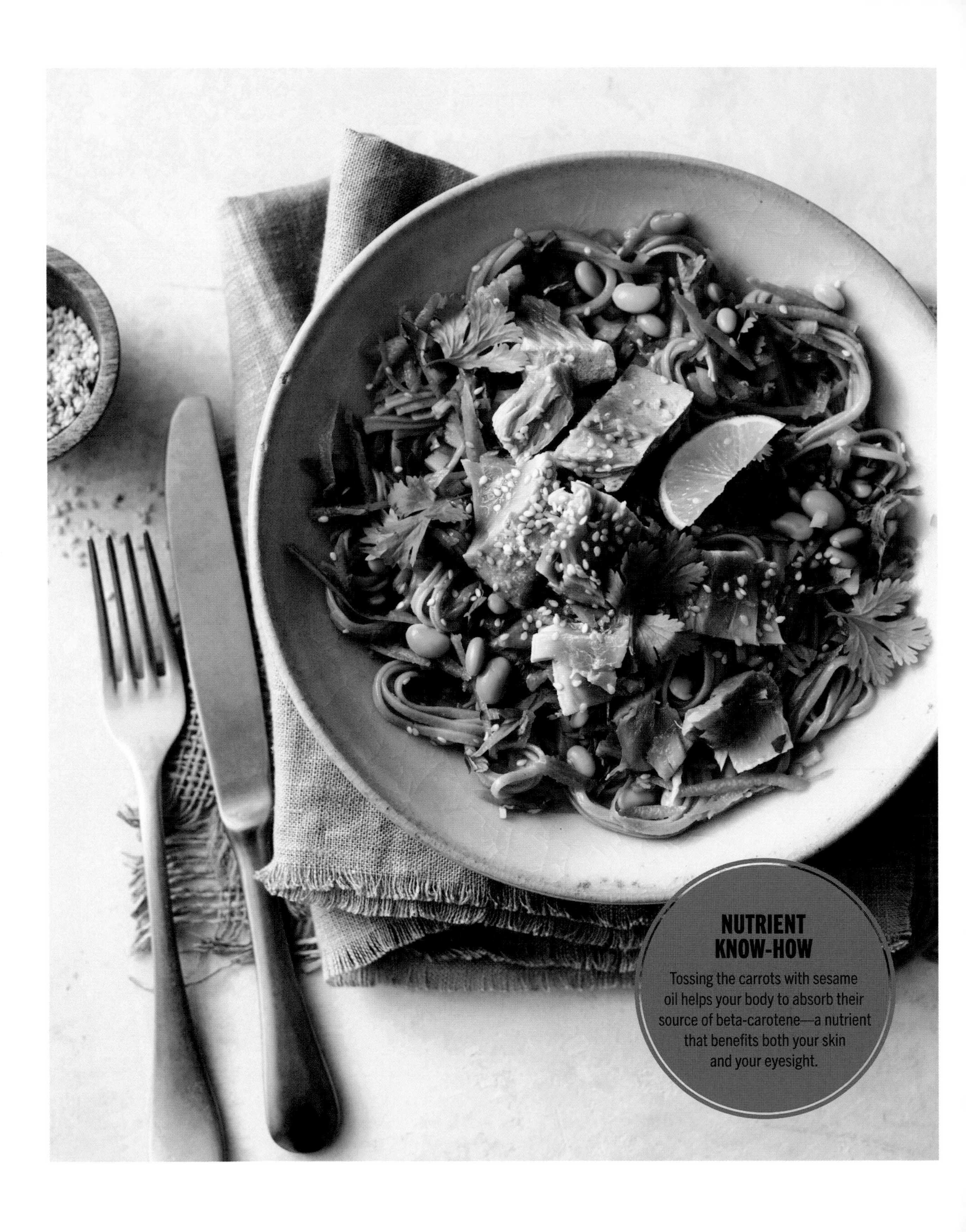

NUTRIENT KNOW-HOW

Tossing the carrots with sesame oil helps your body to absorb their source of beta-carotene—a nutrient that benefits both your skin and your eyesight.

ASIAN–STYLE TUNA SALAD

When you want a nourishing and uplifting lunchtime meal with added crunch, this salad delivers. It works particularly well as a nutrient-dense packed lunch.

THE BRAIN	VISION	HEARING & BALANCE	ORAL HEALTH
IMMUNITY	BONES & MUSCLES	SKIN & SENSATION	THE LUNGS
HEART & BLOOD	GUT HEALTH	URINARY HEALTH	MEN/ WOMEN

SERVES **2**

Ingredients

- 2 tsp sesame seeds
- 3½oz (100g) buckwheat soba noodles
- 2 medium carrots
- 4½oz (125g) edamame, defrosted if frozen
- 1in (2.5cm) fresh ginger, peeled
- 2 tbsp sesame oil
- 4¼oz (120g) fresh tuna steak
- 1 small red onion, finely diced
- ½ green bell pepper, finely chopped
- 2 tbsp cilantro leaves, roughly chopped
- lime wedges, to serve

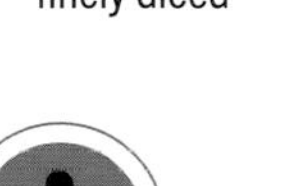

Smart swaps

- Swap the carrots for **zucchini** to get an extra boost of zeaxanthin and lutein. Both of these micronutrients protect against age-related macular degeneration.
- Using a **red bell pepper** in place of the green will boost the amounts of brain-friendly folate and heart-friendly potassium.
- Use **canned salmon** (instead of the tuna) to bump up levels of omega-3 fats.

1 Heat a small frying pan over medium heat and add the sesame seeds. Toast for 1–2 minutes until they start to turn pale golden brown. Remove from the heat and leave them to cool.

2 Put a small pan of water over high heat and, when the water is boiling, add the soba noodles. Cook the noodles for 5 minutes, stirring occasionally, then drain them and rinse with cold water. Set the noodles aside to continue to drain.

3 While the noodles are boiling, peel and grate the carrots and place them in a medium bowl with the edamame. Then grate the ginger and add the sesame oil. Mix well to coat all of the grated carrot and edamame in the oil.

4 Cook the tuna on a griddle or in the oven so it's cooked to your liking. Once cooked, let it rest and flake it into large pieces.

5 Stir the now well-drained noodles into the carrot along with the red onion, green bell pepper, and cilantro leaves. Divide the salad between two bowls or plates, and top with the tuna. Add a squeeze of lime juice and a sprinkle of the toasted sesame seeds.

NUTRITION PER SERVING Calories **504** Total fat **20.3g** Saturated fat **4g** Cholesterol **21mg** Carbohydrates **48.3g** Dietary fiber **12g** Sugars **11.7g** Protein **31.8g** Sodium **72mg**

-WONDERFOOD-

SOY

Soy is a popular food in Japan, the country with the highest life expectancy according to the World Health Organization. Studies show soy can lower cholesterol and ease hot flashes, and may protect against breast cancer and osteoporosis.

WHICH SOY?

Soy comes in many forms, so it's easy to include in your diet every day.

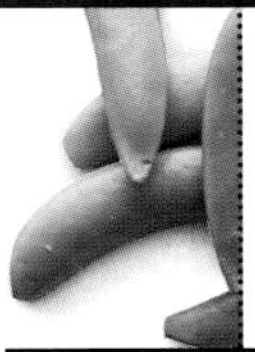

Edamame

- Are much higher in protein than other legumes and are rich in fiber, so you feel fuller for longer

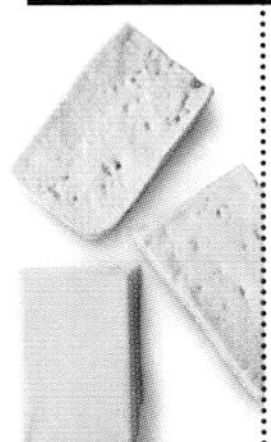

Tofu (firm)

- Is a nutritional powerhouse—it's packed with protein, as well as containing good amounts of copper, selenium, calcium, and phosphorus

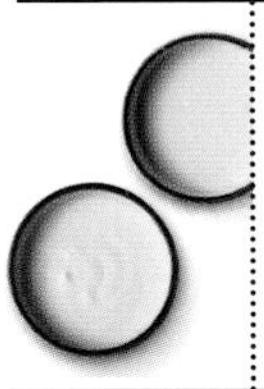

Soy milk and yogurt

- Are heart-friendly, as they contain mostly unsaturated fats and are rich in cholesterol-lowering soy protein

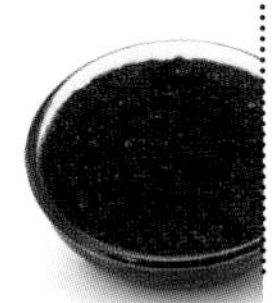

Miso

- Is made from fermented soybeans and is packed with probiotics, so it benefits digestion

HOW MUCH?

Enjoy 25g of soy protein daily.

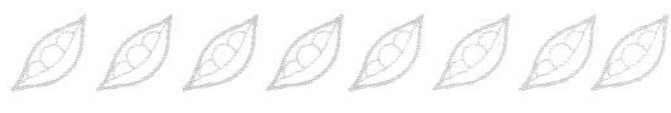

Soy protein per serving:

- 9.5g in 2¾oz (80g) edamame
- 1.9g in 1 tbsp of miso
- 4.8g in 7fl oz (200ml) soy milk
- 6g in 5½oz (150g) soy yogurt
- 9g in 3½oz (100g) firm tofu

BEST BOUGHT

Buy plain, unsweetened soy products.

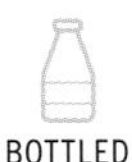

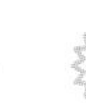

HOW TO STORE

Store fresh products in the refrigerator and dried or canned products in a pantry.

RAW OR COOKED?

Eat raw or cooked, depending on type.

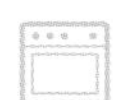
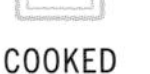

Breast cancer protection

In the past there were concerns that isoflavones in soy might promote tumor growth, but newer research suggests soy products may protect against breast cancer. Studies based in Asian countries have confirmed that higher intakes of soy products seem to reduce the risk of the disease by about a third in pre- and postmenopausal women.

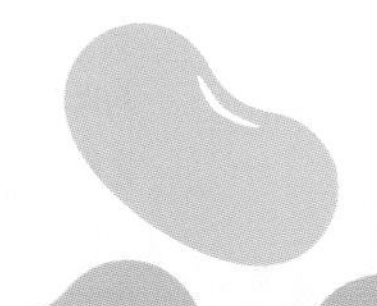

Researchers found that women who ate at least 13g of soy protein a day (compared with 5g) were 11 percent less likely to develop breast cancer.

Eases menopausal hot flashes

Evidence shows eating foods rich in isoflavones—such as soy products—can help reduce menopausal hot flashes. A review of 17 studies found drinking the equivalent of two glasses of soy milk daily decreased the frequency of hot flashes by 20 percent and their severity by 26 percent.

Better bone health

Soy foods—and their isoflavones—seem to promote stronger bones in postmenopausal women. This is important, as estrogen levels decline during menopause, causing bones to lose strength and putting women at an increased risk of osteoporosis and fractures. Two large Asian studies found good intakes of soy reduced the risk of all fractures by about a third in women.

Decreases the risk of prostate cancer

Compared with Western countries, the incidence of prostate cancer (much like breast cancer, see left) is much lower in Asian countries where soy is regularly eaten. Isoflavones are phyto-estrogens, and these seem to slow down the growth of cancer cells.

⇩50%

reduction in the risk of prostate cancer in those with higher intakes of soy.

Heart friendly

Soy protein is known to reduce LDL (bad) cholesterol and triglycerides (a type of fat in blood). Other studies suggest isoflavones in soy improve artery health (see below for soy's heart benefits); plus replacing saturated fats with unsaturated fats is beneficial for the heart. A large study found those women who ate soy foods at least five times a week were a third less likely to die of cardiovascular disease than those who ate it twice a week or less. In another study of 65,000 postmenopausal Chinese women, those with the highest intakes of soy protein had an 86 percent lower risk of having a nonfatal heart attack than those with the lowest intakes.

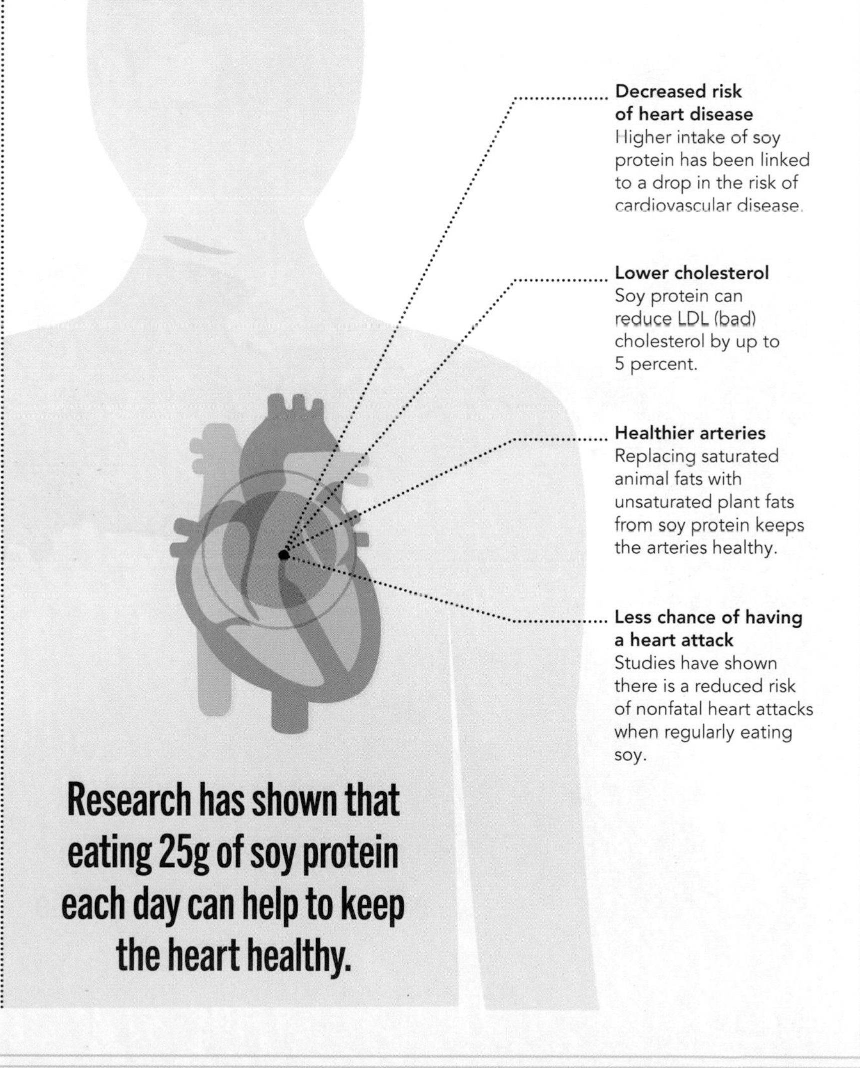

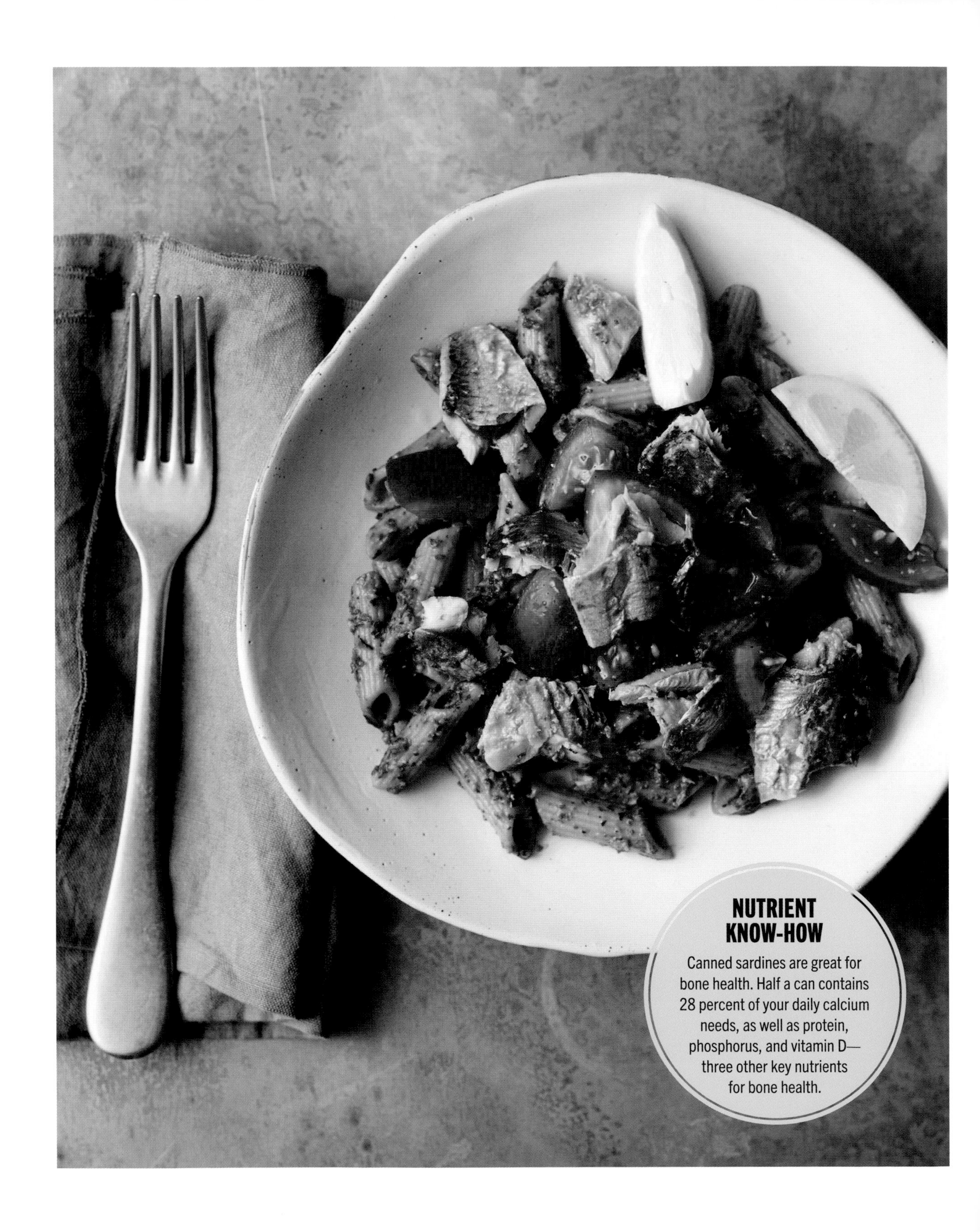
NUTRIENT KNOW-HOW
Canned sardines are great for bone health. Half a can contains 28 percent of your daily calcium needs, as well as protein, phosphorus, and vitamin D—three other key nutrients for bone health.

WHOLE-WHEAT PASTA SALAD WITH SARDINES

Bursting with flavor and color, this dish checks a lot of longevity boxes. The canned fish offers dual benefits via healthy omega-3 fats and extra calcium.

THE BRAIN | VISION | HEARING & BALANCE | ORAL HEALTH
IMMUNITY | BONES & MUSCLES | SKIN & SENSATION | THE LUNGS
HEART & BLOOD | GUT HEALTH | URINARY HEALTH | MEN/ WOMEN

SERVES **2**

Ingredients

5½oz (150g) whole-wheat penne pasta

4 vine-ripened tomatoes

freshly ground black pepper

4¼oz (120g) canned sardines in olive oil, drained

2 lemon wedges, to serve

For the pesto

good handful of basil

good handful of mint leaves

½ green chili, roughly chopped

1 tbsp olive oil

1 ripe small avocado, halved and pitted

lemon juice, to taste

1 Put a large pan of water on to boil. When boiling, add the pasta and cook for 10–12 minutes until it is al dente. Drain the pasta well and allow to cool a little.

2 While the pasta is cooking, make the pesto. Place the basil stalks and leaves, mint leaves, green chili, and oil into a blender. Blend the mixture to a pulp, then add in the avocado flesh and blend again until you have a smooth paste. Season with black pepper and lemon juice, to taste.

3 Roughly chop the tomatoes into ¾in (2cm) chunks, transfer to a plate, and season with black pepper. Flake or chunk the sardines and add to the tomatoes.

4 Add the pesto to the pasta, stirring to mix thoroughly. Spoon the pasta into serving bowls, then arrange the tomatoes and sardines on top. Serve with lemon wedges. This dish works well both as a hot lunch or a cold one the next day.

NUTRITION PER SERVING Calories **519** Total fat **23.7g** Saturated fat **4.7g** Cholesterol **30mg** Carbohydrates **57.8g** Dietary fiber **12.7g** Sugars **8.3g** Protein **22.2g** Sodium **190mg**

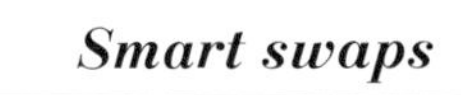

Smart swaps

- Swap the mint in the pesto for a handful of **pine nuts** for a nuttier flavor and a micronutrient boost—you'll get more potassium, phosphorus, iron, zinc, manganese, and vitamin E.
- For a different texture, replace half of the pasta with a 14oz (400g) can of **green lentils** (rinsed and drained). They contain more than double the protein and a third more fiber than the pasta, making this a perfect hunger-busting swap.

-WONDERFOOD-

AVOCADOS

Creamy and delicious, avocados are loaded with good fats that lower cholesterol and protect against wrinkles. They are also packed with a variety of vitamins and minerals that help with everything from keeping eyes healthy to regulating blood pressure.

WHICH AVOCADOS?

There's little nutritional difference between different varieties such as hass or fuerte avocados. However, many of the phytonutrients are concentrated in the dark green flesh closest to the skin, so don't leave any of this behind when you peel them.

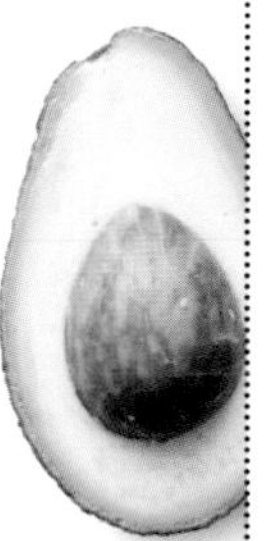

Avocados

- Are high in monounsaturated fat, which benefits the skin and heart
- Are great for the eyes, as they are rich in lutein and zeaxanthin
- Contain potassium, essential for blood pressure regulation

HOW MUCH?

Eat half an avocado three to four times a week. Although avocados have many health benefits, remember that they are high in calories.

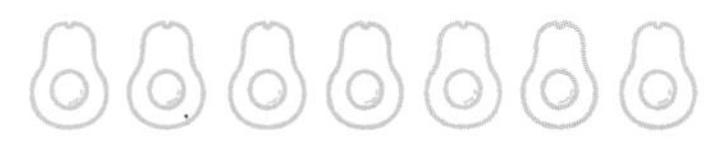

BEST BOUGHT

Look for avocados with unblemished skin. Those with a slight "neck" rather than a rounded top may have ripened longer on the tree and will be more flavorful.

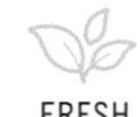

HOW TO STORE

If your avocado is not ripe, leave it at room temperature to ripen or put it in a paper bag or the fruit bowl with a banana to speed up the ripening process. Don't refrigerate avocados until they are ripe.

RAW OR COOKED?

Best eaten raw. To check if they're ready to eat, gently squeeze—if the flesh yields slightly, it's ripe.

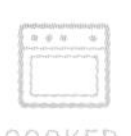

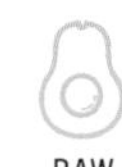

Wrinkle reducer

One study of people over 70 found a good intake of monounsaturated fats was linked to fewer wrinkles; almost two thirds of the fat in an avocado is monounsaturated. Avocados also contain vitamin E, an antioxidant that helps protect against cell damage to the skin—for example, from the sun's ultraviolet (UV) rays.

Maintains vision

Avocados are rich in the carotenoids lutein and zeaxanthin, which support eye health and have been linked to a lower risk of cataracts and macular degeneration. Plus, the monounsaturated fats in avocados benefit the eyes by helping improve the absorption of eye-friendly carotenoids.

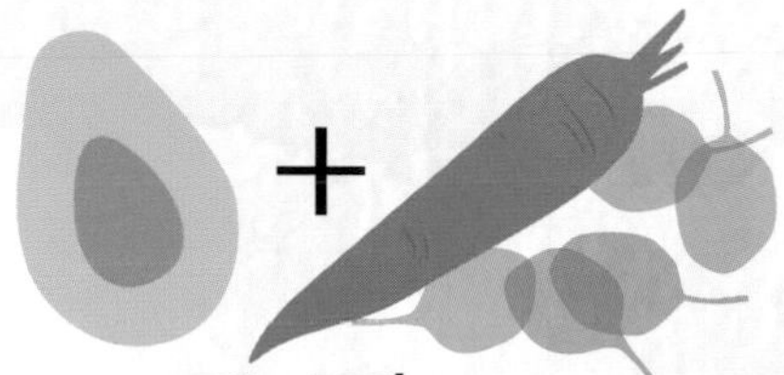

15x

Avocados help the body absorb significantly more carotenoids from foods such as carrots and spinach when eaten together.

Prostate health

Enjoy a salad of lycopene-rich tomatoes and lutein-containing avocados to protect against prostate cancer. In lab-based tests, lutein reduced the growth of prostate cancer cells by 25 percent, while lycopene reduced cell growth by 20 percent. Combining the two resulted in an even larger reduction in cell growth.

32%

reduction in prostate cancer cell growth with a combination of lutein and lycopene.

Reduces cholesterol

Adding avocado to diets has been shown to reduce total cholesterol, LDL (bad) cholesterol, and triglycerides, while also boosting HDL (good) cholesterol. These heart-healthy benefits are most likely thanks to avocados being high in monounsaturated fat. Avocados also contain heart-friendly phytosterols, such as beta-sitosterol, which help to lower blood cholesterol levels.

Provides and boosts nutrients

Not only do avocados contain good amounts of fiber; potassium; copper; and vitamins B6, E, and K (see below for how these nutrients benefit the body), but studies also show that people who eat them tend to have better diets overall. In one study, avocado eaters had lower body weights and waist circumferences and were less likely to suffer from metabolic syndrome. Better still, avocados enable us to get more out of the other foods we eat them with, maximizing the absorption of carotenoids.

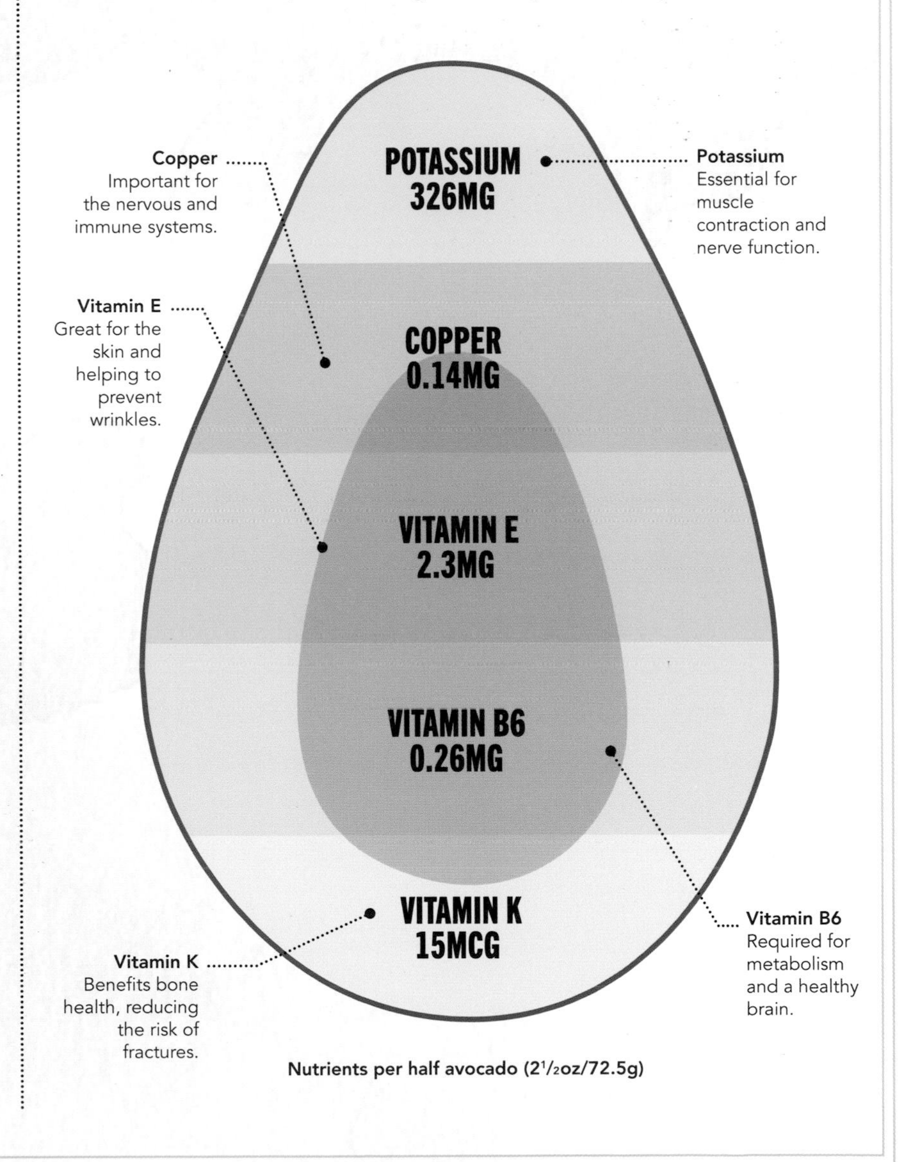

Nutrients per half avocado (2½oz/72.5g)

DINNERS

One of the biggest adjustments to the plan can be eating a smaller dinner. But both the plan and these meals won't leave you longing for more—you'll feel fully satisfied. What's more, you will wake up hungry in the morning, ready for a hearty breakfast.

11%

Eating fewer calories at the end of the day helps weight loss. In a 2013 study of overweight women, weight, BMI, and waistlines were all reduced—weight by 11 percent.

TURKEY STIR-FRY

Short on time? This stir-fry checks off plenty of longevity benefit boxes and is super-quick.

SERVES **2**

Ingredients

3½oz (100g) brown rice
1 tbsp sunflower oil
1 garlic clove, crushed
2in (5cm) fresh ginger, peeled and finely chopped
1 red chili, seeds removed and finely chopped
10oz (300g) turkey breast strips
1 small package (10–12oz/ 300–350g) stir-fry vegetables mix
2 handfuls of bean sprouts
1oz (30g) cashew nuts
2 tsp reduced-sodium soy sauce
1 tbsp sesame seeds, to serve

1 Cook the rice according to the package instructions in unsalted water. When cooked, drain and keep warm.

2 Meanwhile, heat the oil in a nonstick frying pan or wok over medium heat. Add the garlic, ginger, and chili and fry for 1 minute, taking care that they don't burn.

3 Add the turkey and fry until cooked through. Next, add the vegetables and bean sprouts and fry for 3 minutes.

4 Add the nuts, soy sauce, and rice, and toss together for 1 minute until hot. Serve sprinkled with sesame seeds.

NUTRITION PER SERVING Calories **589** Total fat **20.7g** Saturated fat **3.9g** Cholesterol **86mg** Carbohydrates **55g** Dietary fiber **9.5g** Sugars **10.2g** Protein **49.2g** Sodium **317mg**

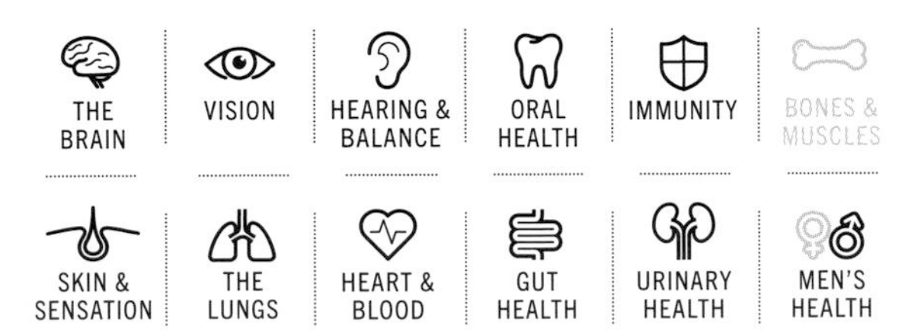

TASTY TOFU WRAPS

Devour these wraps and fill up on cholesterol-lowering and antioxidant phytochemicals.

SERVES **2**

Ingredients

10oz (300g) firm tofu, cut into strips
1 tbsp fajita seasoning
2 tbsp canola oil
1 garlic clove, crushed
1 red onion, cut into wedges
1 red bell pepper and 1 yellow bell pepper, cut into strips
squeeze of lime juice
freshly ground black pepper
4 small whole-wheat wraps, warmed
4 tbsp plain soy yogurt
2½oz (70g) arugula leaves

1 Toss the tofu with the fajita seasoning and half the oil. Set aside for 20 minutes; meanwhile, get the prep done.

2 Fry the tofu in a nonstick frying pan for 3–5 minutes, then set aside. Heat the remaining oil, then cook the garlic, onion, and bell peppers for 5–7 minutes, returning the tofu to heat through. Add the lime juice and black pepper.

3 Fill each of the warmed wraps with the tofu and vegetable mixture, a spoonful of soy yogurt, and a quarter of the arugula.

NUTRITION PER SERVING Calories **608** Total fat **26.4g** Saturated fat **4.7g** Cholesterol **0mg** Carbohydrates **61.8g** Dietary fiber **14.6g** Sugars **16.8g** Protein **28.3g** Sodium **505mg**

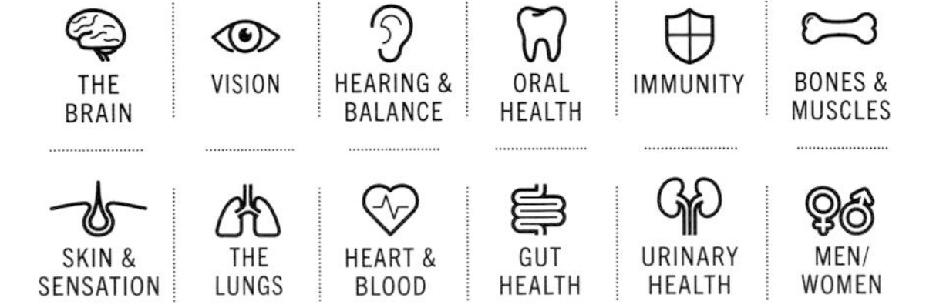

-SUPERGROUP-

LEAFY GREEN VEGETABLES

People who live long lives need no encouragement to "eat their greens." Vegetables such as broccoli, kale, and spinach are packed with nutrients and help protect against heart disease and cancer.

WHICH LEAFY GREENS?

These commonly eaten leafy greens provide a spectrum of nutrients.

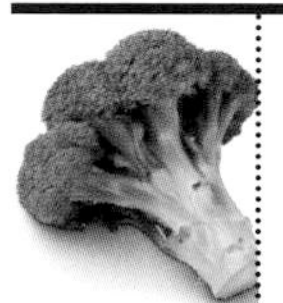

Broccoli

- Is well-rounded, providing vitamins C and E, as well as lutein and zeaxanthin

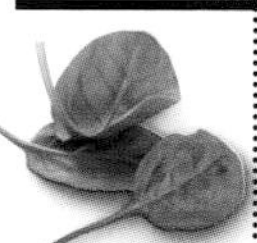

Spinach

- Is very rich in blood pressure–lowering potassium

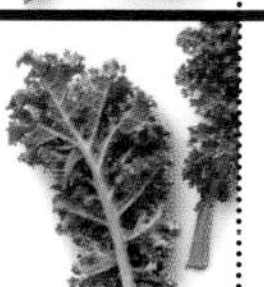

Kale

- Helps to strengthen bones and teeth, as it is high in calcium and vitamin K

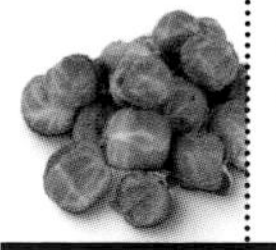

Brussels sprouts

- Are particularly high in cancer-fighting glucosinolates

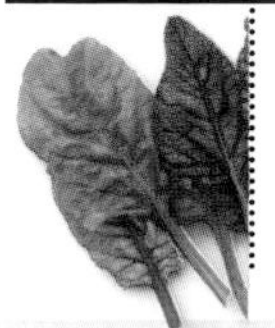

Swiss chard

- Is one of the best sources of lutein and zeaxanthin, both vital for good eye health

HOW MUCH?

Eat three to four servings a week.

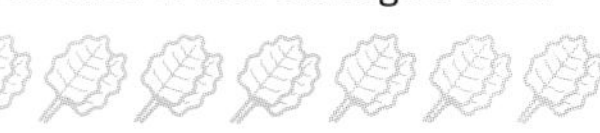

BEST BOUGHT

Buy either fresh or frozen. Don't buy fresh preprepared vegetables, as they start losing vitamin C once cut.

FRESH

FROZEN

HOW TO STORE

Keep fresh or frozen veggies in suitable containers in the refrigerator or freezer.

RAW OR COOKED?

Eat raw or steam or stir-fry quickly to preserve nutrients. Eat the dark outer leaves, as they are rich in nutrients.

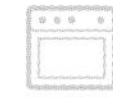

COOKED

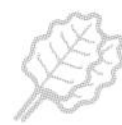

RAW

Good eye health

Many of the antioxidants typically found in leafy greens—vitamins C and E, beta-carotene, lutein, and zeaxanthin—help to slow the progression of eye conditions such as age-related macular degeneration, cataracts, and glaucoma. In one study, women who ate more than one serving of kale (or collard greens) a week were 57 percent less likely to have glaucoma than those who ate them no more than once a month.

29%

reduced risk of age-related macular degeneration from eating at least one serving of cooked spinach a week.

Memory booster

One study of adults with an average age of 81 years found those who ate one to two daily servings of green leafy vegetables had the cognitive function of a person 11 years younger compared with those who avoided them, probably due to the folate, beta-carotene, and vitamin K.

Ultimate health promoters

Cruciferous vegetables or *Brassicas*, such as broccoli, Brussels sprouts, and kale, and leaves such as spinach, Swiss chard, and lettuce are powerhouses of health-protecting nutrients (see below for the diverse array of body-wide benefits). Unsurprisingly, a large Chinese study found adults who ate the most cruciferous vegetables had a 22 percent reduced risk of dying from any medical cause.

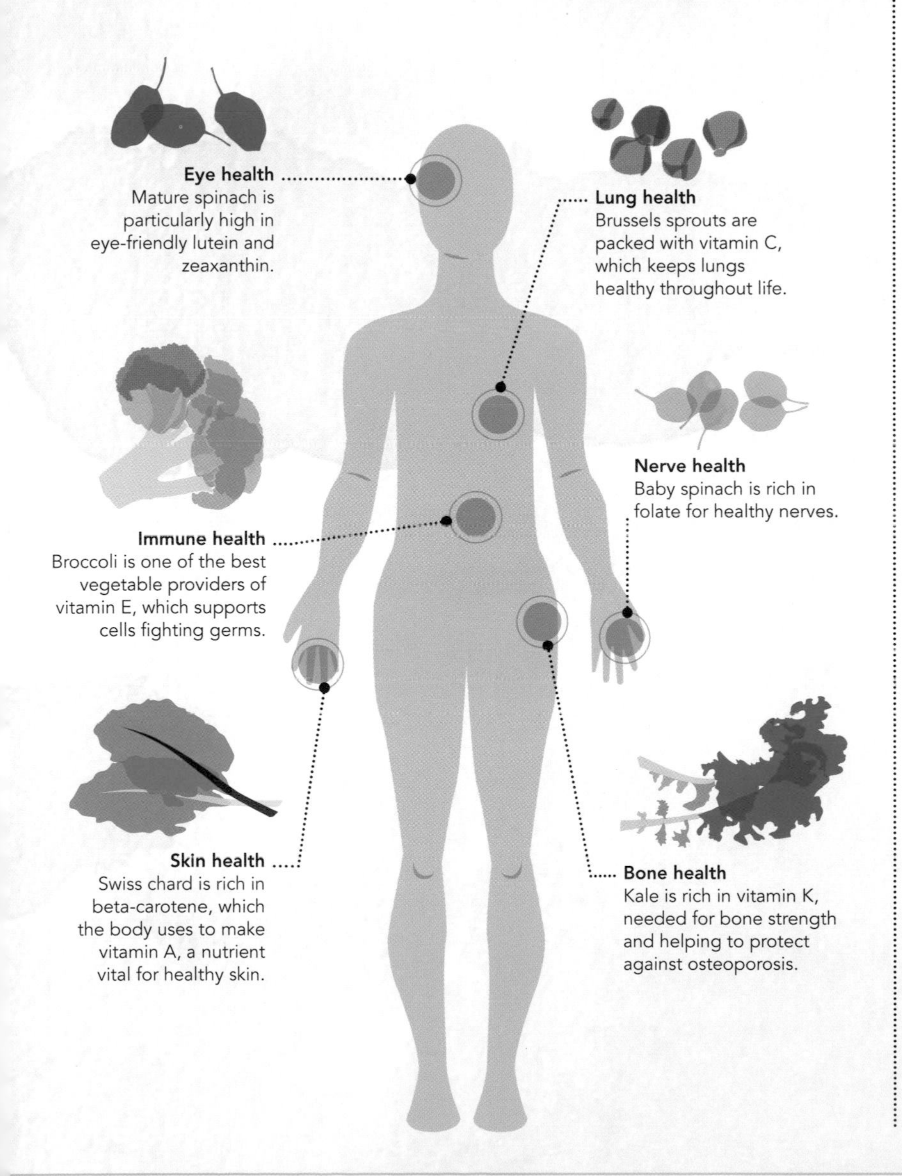

Heart health

Leafy greens contribute to a healthy heart in a number of ways. They contain potassium, which lowers high blood pressure; fiber, which keeps cholesterol in check; and folate, which protects against heart disease and stroke. Their extensive range of antioxidants can also protect against free radical damage, a key contributor for atherosclerosis.

Cancer prevention

Studies confirm that higher intakes of cruciferous vegetables are linked to a lower risk of many cancers, including those in the bladder, breast, colon, stomach, lungs, ovaries, pancreas, prostate, and kidneys. These green vegetables are rich in unique compounds called glucosinolates, which break down to form cancer-busting compounds, and are packed with cancer-fighting flavonoids and carotenoids.

18%

reduction in the risk of colon cancer for people eating the most cruciferous vegetables.

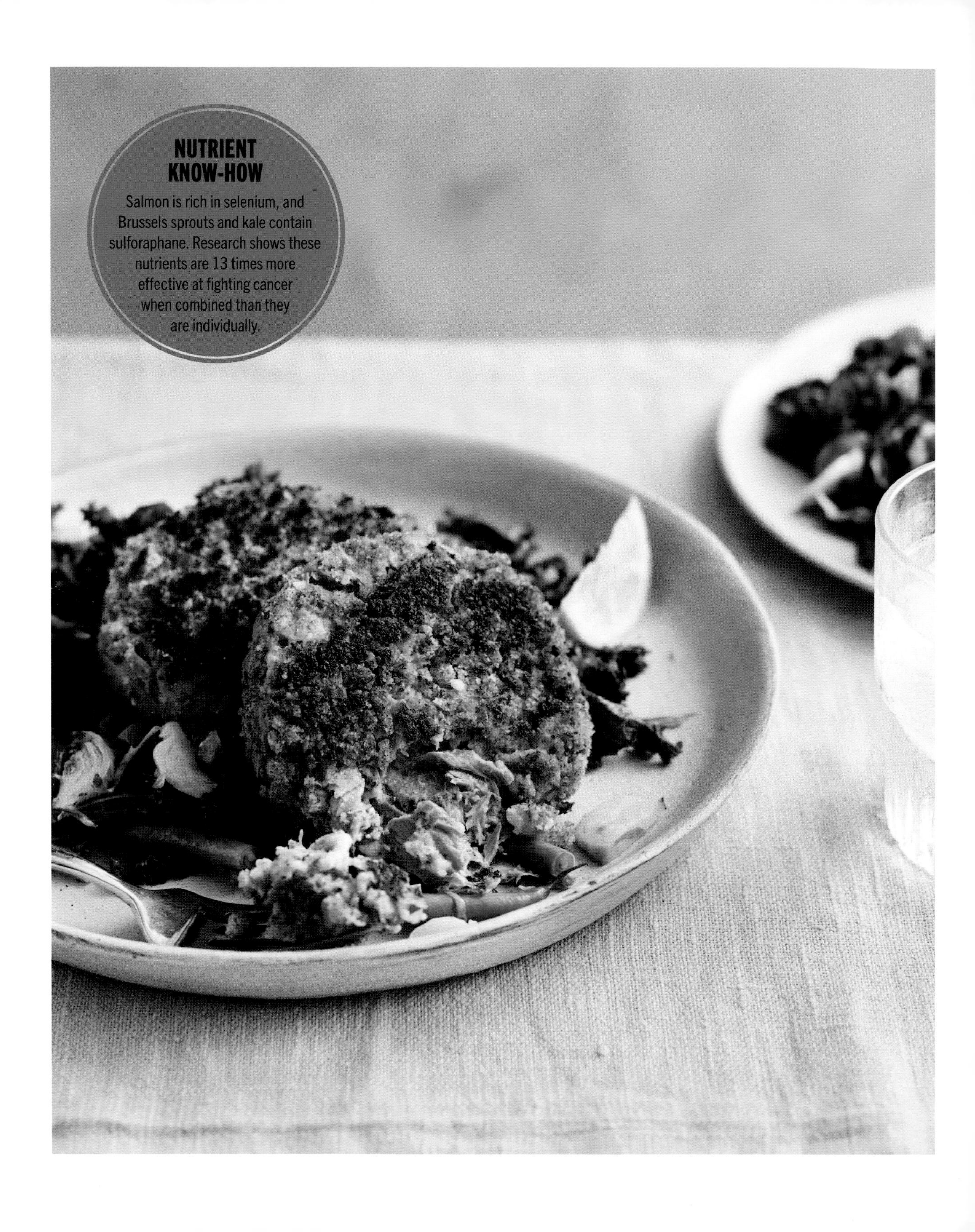
NUTRIENT KNOW-HOW
Salmon is rich in selenium, and Brussels sprouts and kale contain sulforaphane. Research shows these nutrients are 13 times more effective at fighting cancer when combined than they are individually.

SUMAC FISHCAKES WITH GREENS

It's good to know that Brussels sprouts rank highest among the cruciferous vegetables in glucosinolates—chemicals that protect against cancer.

THE BRAIN	VISION	HEARING & BALANCE	ORAL HEALTH
IMMUNITY	BONES & MUSCLES	SKIN & SENSATION	THE LUNGS
HEART & BLOOD	GUT HEALTH	URINARY HEALTH	MEN/ WOMEN

SERVES **2**

Ingredients

1 potato (5¾oz/170g), any type, scrubbed

2 wild Alaskan salmon fillets (4¾oz/130g each)

2 tsp sumac

1 slice whole-wheat bread

1 ripe small avocado

zest of 1 lemon

2 tbsp chopped parsley

freshly ground black pepper, to taste

1 garlic clove, grated

1 tbsp olive oil

For the greens

1 tbsp olive oil

3½oz (100g) fine green beans, cut into thirds

3½oz (100g) Brussels sprouts, shredded

3½oz (100g) kale, shredded

2 garlic cloves, chopped

1 Preheat the oven to 350°F (180°C). Chop the potato into chunks, and place in a pan of water over high heat. Bring to a boil and cook the potato for 15 minutes. Meanwhile, put the salmon fillets skin side down on a baking sheet, sprinkle with sumac, and rub the spice into the fish. Bake the fish in the oven for 12–15 minutes until cooked through and the flesh is opaque. Set aside to cool a little.

2 Toast the bread in the warm oven for 3–4 minutes and set aside. Meanwhile, put the avocado flesh, lemon zest (keep the lemon to serve), chopped parsley, and some black pepper into a mixing bowl. Mash everything together. When the potatoes are soft enough, drain and mash them, then add them to the avocado mix.

3 Remove the skin from the salmon and flake the flesh into the mixture. With damp hands, divide the mixture into four, shaping it into even-sized patties. Then, set aside.

4 Blend the toast into fine breadcrumbs in a food processor. Mix them with the grated garlic, then coat the fishcakes with the mixture, pressing it into the patties on all sides. Heat the olive oil in a frying pan and fry the fish cakes for 3 minutes on each side (cover with a lid for last minutes), so they are golden brown.

5 For the greens, heat the oil in a wok and, when hot, add the green beans and sprouts. Stir-fry for 2 minutes, so they start to color, then add the kale. Stir-fry for another 2 minutes, then add the garlic and season with pepper. Serve with the fishcakes and lemon wedges.

NUTRITION PER SERVING Calories **603** Total fat **36.7g** Saturated fat **6.9g** Cholesterol **66mg** Carbohydrates **31.4g** Dietary fiber **13.6g** Sugars **5g** Protein **38.1g** Sodium **210mg**

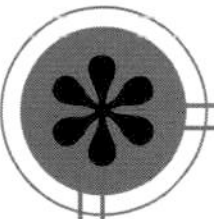

Smart swaps

- Swap the salmon for **haddock** or any other white fish fillets. They may have fewer omega-3 fats, but they have 16 times more iodine, vital for cognitive function.
- Use **spinach leaves** (big leaves are best rather than baby leaf spinach) if you can't get ahold of sprouts. Both are rich in eye-friendly lutein and zeaxanthin; in fact, spinach has seven times more.

-SUPERGROUP-

FISH AND SHELLFISH

All fish and shellfish contain health-promoting omega-3 fats. Good intakes of fish protect against dementia and arthritis, while shellfish are a particularly rich source of antioxidants.

WHICH FISH/SHELLFISH?

Here are some of the most popular and beneficial types of fish and shellfish.

LEVELS OF OMEGA-3 FATS INCREASES

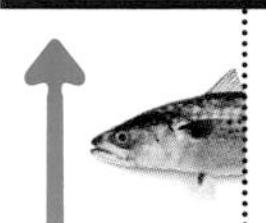

Mackerel
- Is the richest source of omega-3 fats, vital for a healthy heart

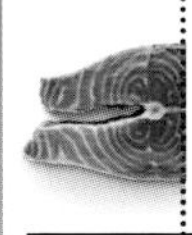

Salmon
- Is a good source of omega-3 fats, which aid cognitive function

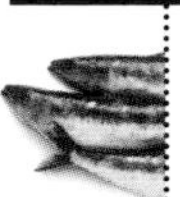

Sardines
- Are rich in calcium, so help bone density

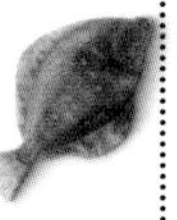

Flounder
- Is particularly good for skin- and eye-friendly biotin

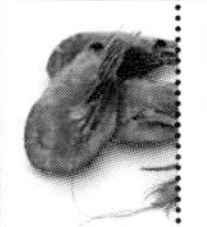

Shrimp
- Are rich in zinc, which benefits the immune system

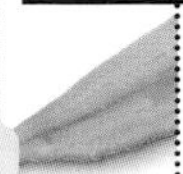

Haddock
- Is rich in iodine, for thyroid function

HOW MUCH?

Eat two portions of fish or shellfish a week, one of which should be oily.

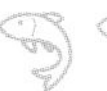
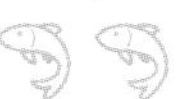

BEST BOUGHT

Buy sustainable fresh, frozen, or canned fish or shellfish (check sodium content of canned). Frozen is as nutritious as fresh.

CANNED

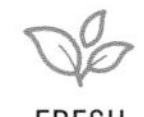
FRESH

FROZEN

HOW TO STORE

Store in the refrigerator, freezer, or pantry, depending on the type bought.

RAW OR COOKED?

Cook fish or, if preferred, eat raw if sushi grade. Cook shellfish before eating.

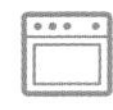
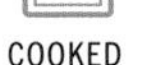
COOKED

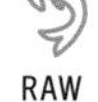
RAW

Immune efficiency

Shellfish provide good amounts of iron, copper, zinc, and selenium—all essential for a strong immune system. The immune system becomes less efficient as we age, making us more prone to infections, allergies, and even cancer. Except for iron, these nutrients also act as antioxidants, mopping up harmful free radicals.

Protecting against dementia

All fish is brain food. A French study found in those people who weren't genetically predisposed to Alzheimer's disease, eating fish once a week reduced their risk of this condition by 35 percent. While omega-3 fats are often hailed for slowing cognitive decline, fish are also rich in iodine and vitamins B3, B6, and B12, all of which are important for a healthy brain and reducing the risk of dementia.

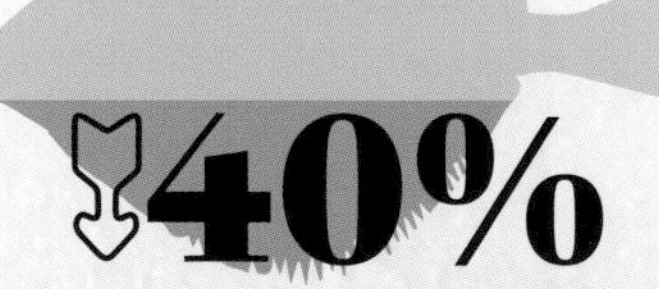

40%

reduction in the risk of any form of dementia from eating fish once a week.

Strong bones, teeth, and muscles

Oily fish is naturally rich in vitamin D, a nutrient many of us are deficient in, especially in our more senior years (see also page 36). It helps the body absorb calcium, so it is vital for strong bones and teeth, plus it's crucial for healthy muscles. Vitamin D supplements can help, but eating oily fish is best.

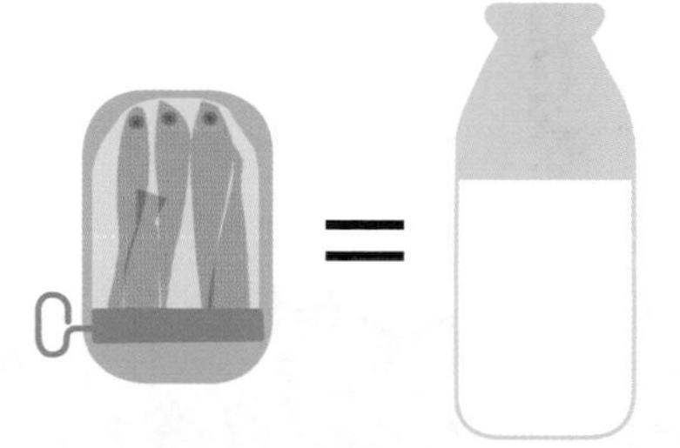

3½oz (100g) of drained canned sardines in oil provides the same amount of calcium as 14fl oz (400ml) of skim milk.

Cholesterol-friendly

The cholesterol in shellfish doesn't affect blood cholesterol levels (unless you have familial hypercholesterolemia, see page 70). Instead, it is high intakes of saturated and trans fats that affect blood cholesterol. Shellfish are low in these—and better still, they also contain omega-3 fats.

Boost heart health

All fish and shellfish, but particularly oily fish, contain omega-3 fats. According to the American Heart Association, these reduce the risk of an abnormal heartbeat, lower triglycerides (a type of fat found in the blood), slow down atherosclerosis (artery hardening), and reduce blood pressure. Vitamins B6 and B12 in fish also help control homocysteine levels.

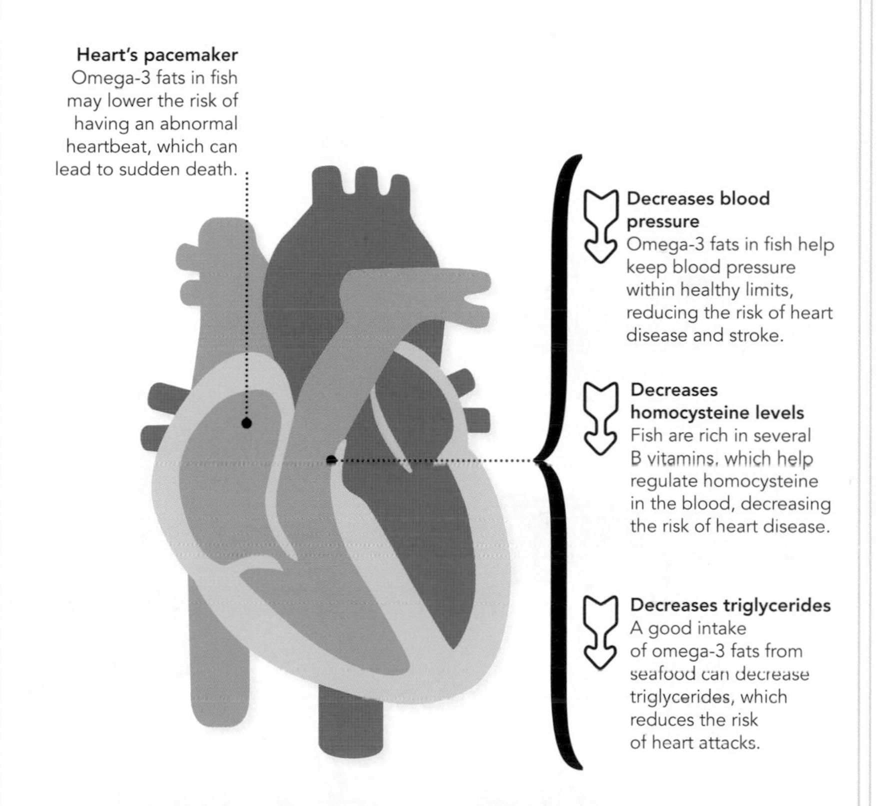

Good eyesight

One of the omega-3 fats—docosahexaenoic acid (DHA)—is important for healthy eyes. Studies have shown that having a good intake of fish and seafood, especially oily fish, helps protect the eyes from age-related macular degeneration.

Relief from arthritis

Both fish and shellfish are rich sources of omega-3 fats, which seem to have an anti-inflammatory effect and may help reduce the swelling and pain associated with arthritis, particularly for people suffering from rheumatoid arthritis.

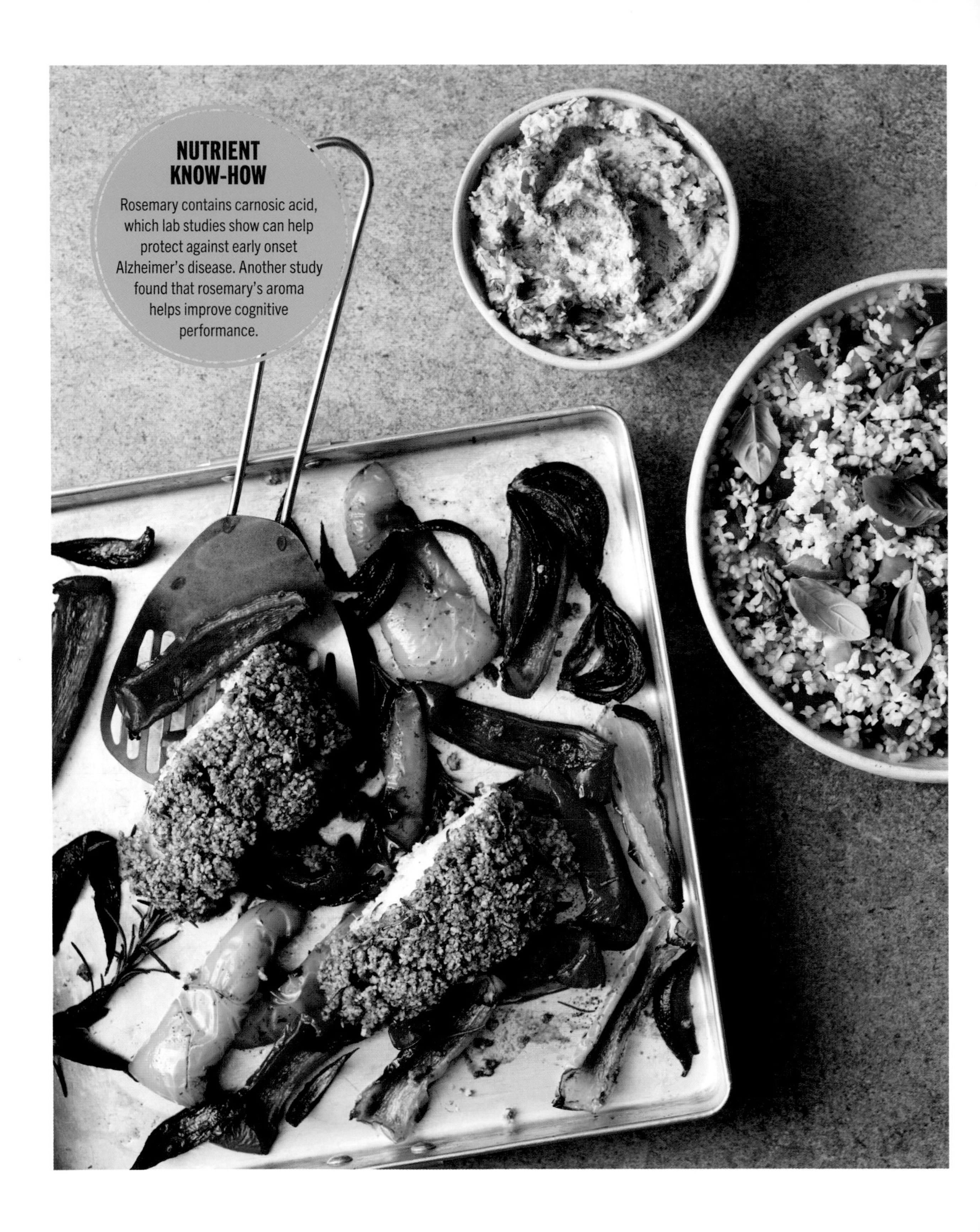

NUTRIENT KNOW-HOW

Rosemary contains carnosic acid, which lab studies show can help protect against early onset Alzheimer's disease. Another study found that rosemary's aroma helps improve cognitive performance.

THE BRAIN	VISION	HEARING & BALANCE	ORAL HEALTH
IMMUNITY	BONES & MUSCLES	SKIN & SENSATION	THE LUNGS
HEART & BLOOD	GUT HEALTH	URINARY HEALTH	MEN/ WOMEN

ROASTED HADDOCK WITH A HERBY CRUMB

This brain-friendly fish dinner boasts great levels of vitamin C, from the bell peppers and orange, as well as other antioxidants, such as lycopene in the tomatoes.

SERVES **2**

Ingredients

3½oz (100g) bulgur wheat

1 small red onion, sliced into wedges

1 red bell pepper, sliced

1 yellow bell pepper, sliced

2 tbsp olive oil

1 tsp paprika

4 sprigs rosemary

⅓ cup (30g) pecan nuts

1 garlic clove

2 unsmoked haddock loins (about 6¼oz/180g in total)

chunky hummus (see page 96), to serve

For the dressing

4 ripe medium tomatoes, chopped

handful of basil leaves, shredded, plus extra to garnish

handful of mint leaves, shredded

juice and zest of 1 orange

freshly ground black pepper

1 Preheat the oven to 400°F (200°C). Put the bulgur wheat into a pan over high heat with 1 cup (250ml) water. Bring to a boil, reduce to a simmer, and cook for 20 minutes until soft.

2 Put the onion and bell peppers on a roasting pan. Drizzle them with the oil, season with paprika, and toss well. Tuck 2 rosemary sprigs in among the onion and peppers, and transfer the pan to the oven for 20 minutes until the vegetables are soft.

3 Meanwhile, put the nuts, garlic, and the leaves from the other sprigs of rosemary into a small food processor. Blend for 1 minute, so that the mixture is a rough crumb. Place the haddock loins on a board and use spoonfuls of the nut mix to top the fish, pressing the crumb down well.

4 Take the pan out of the oven and carefully place the haddock fillets on top of the vegetables. Return to the oven for another 8–10 minutes until the fish is cooked and its flesh is opaque.

5 For the dressing, combine the chopped tomatoes (including the juice and seeds) with the basil, mint, orange juice, orange zest, and plenty of black pepper.

6 When the bulgur wheat is cooked, drain any excess water and return it to the pan. Pour over the dressing and stir it in well. Serve the fish, paprika vegetables (removing the rosemary sprigs), and bulgur wheat with a spoonful of homemade chunky hummus.

NUTRITION PER SERVING Calories **577** Total fat **27.4g** Saturated fat **3.3g** Cholesterol **44mg** Carbohydrates **59.7g** Dietary fiber **11.9g** Sugars **17.5g** Protein **27.2g** Sodium **74mg**

Smart swaps

- Swap the pecans for **Brazil nuts** to get a different micronutrient mix—extra potassium, calcium, magnesium, phosphorus, iron, copper, vitamin E, and selenium.
- Replace the haddock with fresh **mackerel** fillets for a huge boost in omega-3 fats, iron, and vitamin D.

STEAK AND WEDGES

This "steak and fries" delivers big on benefits.

SERVES **2**

Ingredients

2 large potatoes, any type, 1lb 2oz (500g), skin-on, cut into wedges
2 tbsp olive oil
2 lean fillet steaks (5oz/140g each)
2 large ripe tomatoes, halved
2 portobello mushrooms
2 corn-on-the-cob
freshly ground black pepper

1 Preheat the oven to 425°F (220°C) and the grill and a nonstick baking sheet to high. Rinse the cut potatoes well and pat dry. Toss them in a baking dish in 1 tablespoon of the oil. Bake for 30 minutes, shaking the pan midway.

2 In a large bowl, coat the steaks, tomatoes, mushrooms, and corn with the remaining oil and some black pepper. Place the corn on the preheated sheet on the grill for 8 minutes. Remove the sheet, turn the corn and add the steak, tomatoes, and mushrooms; return to the grill.

3 Once the steaks are done (5 minutes each side for medium doneness), remove to rest, and put the sheet of vegetables back on the grill for a few more minutes. Serve the steak, grilled vegetables, and potato wedges together.

NUTRITION PER SERVING Calories **588** Total fat **22.1g** Saturated fat **5.9g** Cholesterol **85mg** Carbohydrates **61.4g** Dietary fiber **9.6g** Sugars **7.8g** Protein **39.5g** Sodium **72mg**

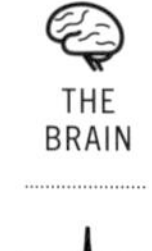
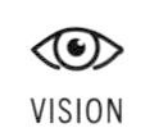
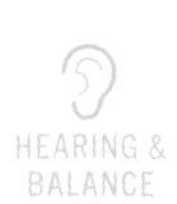
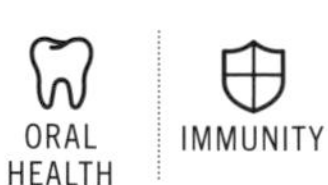
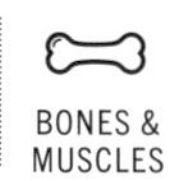

THE BRAIN | VISION | HEARING & BALANCE | ORAL HEALTH | IMMUNITY | BONES & MUSCLES

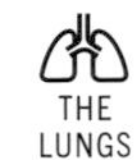
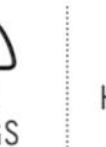
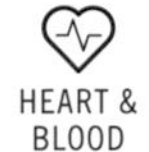
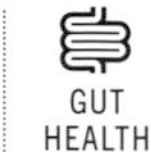
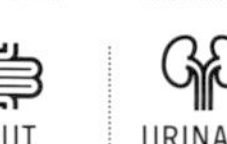
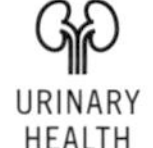
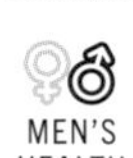
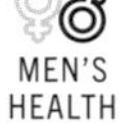

SKIN & SENSATION | THE LUNGS | HEART & BLOOD | GUT HEALTH | URINARY HEALTH | MEN'S HEALTH

LEMON CHICKEN PASTA

A fresh and crunchy dinner that provides plenty of protein and fiber to ward off night-time hunger.

SERVES **2**

Ingredients

2 small skinless chicken breasts (about 4½oz/125g each)
freshly ground black pepper
2 tbsp olive oil infused with garlic (homemade, if possible)
7oz (200g) whole-wheat pasta
5¾oz (160g) tenderstem broccoli, broken into florets, stalks chopped
5¾oz (160g) green beans, cut into thirds
zest of 1 lemon and juice of ½ lemon

1 Pound the chicken between two pieces of plastic wrap until equal in thickness; season with black pepper.

2 Heat 1 tablespoon of oil in a large nonstick frying pan over medium heat. Cook the chicken for 3 minutes each side, then turn the heat to low and cover the pan for 3 minutes; next, remove from the heat and let rest.

3 Cook the pasta according to the instructions. In the last 3 minutes, steam the broccoli and green beans over the pasta water. Drain all and mix together; set aside.

4 Using two forks, shred the chicken into its cooking juices, then mix in the pasta, green vegetables, lemon zest and juice, the remaining oil, and black pepper. Serve.

NUTRITION PER SERVING Calories **608** Total fat **15.3g** Saturated fat **2.5g** Cholesterol **88mg** Carbohydrates **73g** Dietary fiber **17.4g** Sugars **7.3g** Protein **47.3g** Sodium **84mg**

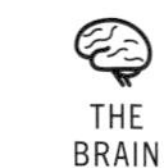
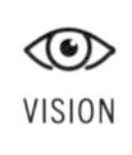
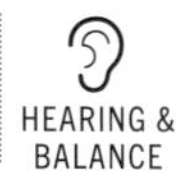
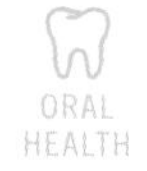
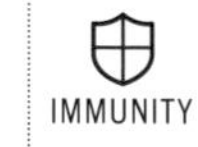
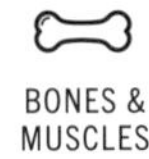

THE BRAIN | VISION | HEARING & BALANCE | ORAL HEALTH | IMMUNITY | BONES & MUSCLES

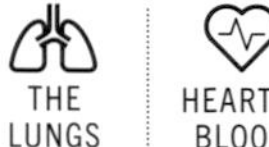
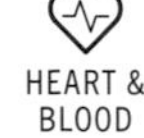
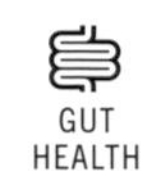
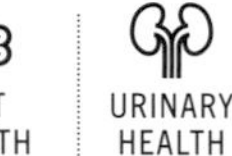
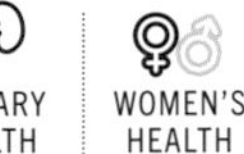

SKIN & SENSATION | THE LUNGS | HEART & BLOOD | GUT HEALTH | URINARY HEALTH | WOMEN'S HEALTH

ROAST PORK AND VEGGIES

A healthy take on a traditional roast dinner that maximizes nutrition, as well as flavor.

SERVES **2**

Ingredients

4 small potatoes (11oz/320g in total), any type, skin-on, pricked
½ small cauliflower, broken into florets
1 tbsp canola oil, plus extra for pork
2 lean pork loin steaks (6oz/170g each), rubbed with oil and freshly ground black pepper
2 soft eating apples, peeled and roughly chopped
2 carrots, diced
5¾oz (160g) shredded kale
1 tbsp reduced-sodium gravy granules (from packet)

1 Preheat the oven to 350°F (180°C). Coat the potatoes and cauliflower with oil; roast the potatoes for 50 minutes and the cauliflower for 35 minutes.

2 Pan fry the pork for 2 minutes each side. Transfer to the oven and roast for 15 minutes; rest for 5 minutes.

3 Microwave the chopped apples, partly covered, for 3–4 minutes. Mash with a fork and set aside.

4 Steam the carrots for 10 minutes and the kale for just 3 minutes. Dissolve the gravy granules in ⅓ cup (100ml) boiling water. Serve the pork with the roasted and steamed vegetables and the applesauce on the side.

NUTRITION PER SERVING Calories **592** Total fat **18.8g** Saturated fat **4g** Cholesterol **107mg** Carbohydrates **61.6g** Dietary fiber **14.9g** Sugars **26.5g** Protein **47.8g** Sodium **390mg**

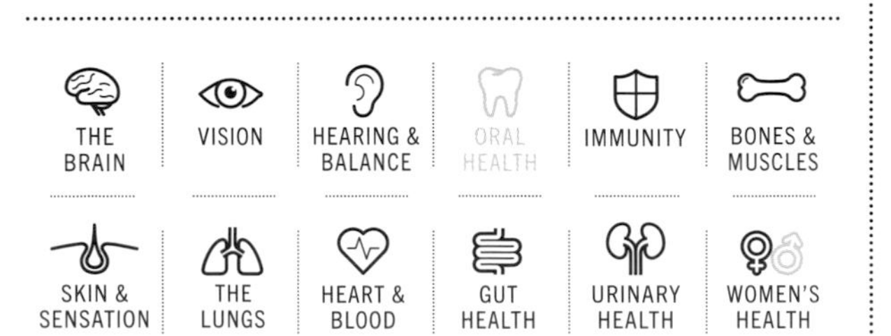

MUSHROOM STEW

Even hardened carnivores will love this fiber-filled and immune-boosting stew.

SERVES **2**

Ingredients

5oz (140g) brown rice
2 tbsp olive oil
10oz (300g) mixed mushrooms
1 onion, thickly sliced
1 leek, thickly sliced
1–2 garlic cloves, finely chopped
1 tbsp each of tomato paste and plain flour
¾ cup (160ml) homemade vegetable stock (see page 120)
14oz (400g) can chopped tomatoes with herbs
freshly ground black pepper
chopped tarragon and 2 tbsp fat-free Greek yogurt, to serve

1 Cook the rice according to the package instructions. Heat half the oil in a nonstick pan over medium heat. Fry the mushrooms for 8 minutes until browned; set aside.

2 Add the remaining oil to the pan. Cook the onions, leeks, and garlic gently over low heat for 10 minutes. Coat the vegetables in the tomato paste and flour. Add the stock and simmer for 5 minutes.

3 Add the mushrooms along with the black pepper; simmer for 15 minutes. Then, stir through the tarragon and serve with the yogurt.

NUTRITION PER SERVING Calories **498** Total fat **13.3g** Saturated fat **2g** Cholesterol **2mg** Carbohydrates **82.4g** Dietary fiber **9.6g** Sugars **18g** Protein **17.4g** Sodium **79mg**

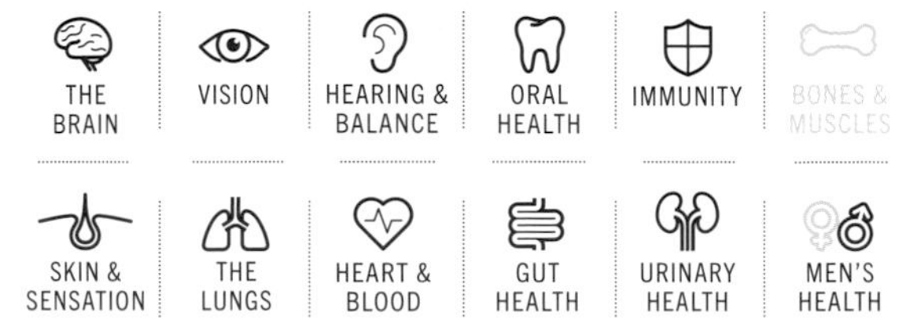

-SUPERGROUP-

MUSHROOMS

Throughout history, mushrooms have been used as medicine to treat many ailments. Now modern science backs up their many health-promoting roles, which include boosting immunity, regulating blood pressure, and reducing inflammation.

WHICH MUSHROOMS?

Discover how these commonly eaten mushrooms benefit health and longevity via their phytochemicals.

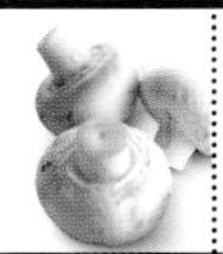

Button
- Are an excellent low-fat source of antioxidants

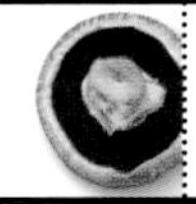

Portobello
- Are rich in selenium, a key antioxidant

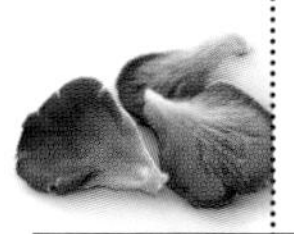

Oyster
- Provide B vitamins, which are important for metabolism

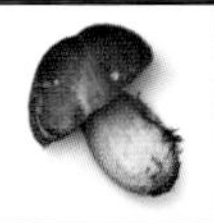

Porcini
- Contain ergosterol, an anti-inflammatory

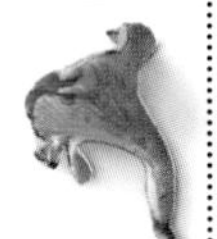

Chanterelle
- Are rich in potassium, which helps regulate blood pressure

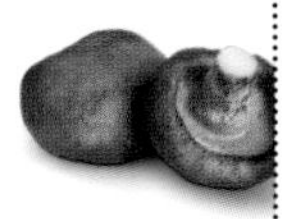

Shiitake
- Are good for boosting vitamin B6, low levels of which have been linked to depression

HOW MUCH?

Enjoy two to three times a week. One serving is about 10 button mushrooms or 4 medium mushrooms.

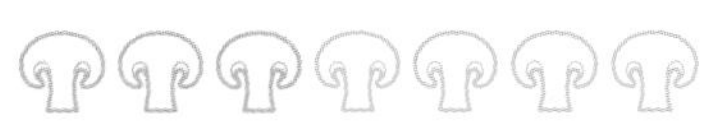

BEST BOUGHT

Choose firm fresh or dried mushrooms, or canned in water without added salt. Wild types contain more vitamin D2.

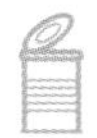
CANNED

FRESH

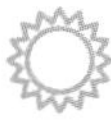
DRIED

HOW TO STORE

Keep fresh mushrooms in a paper (not plastic) bag in the refrigerator; store canned or dried mushrooms in a pantry.

RAW OR COOKED?

Eat raw or cooked: it's best to grill or microwave if cooking. Soak dried first.

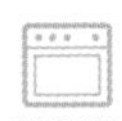
COOKED

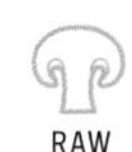
RAW

Cancer competitors

Many lab-based studies have suggested some phytochemicals in mushrooms help to prevent, stop the growth of, or even treat cancer. Much of the focus has been on lentinan, found in shiitake mushrooms. A study of Chinese women found those who ate ¼oz (10g) of fresh mushrooms or more each day were 64 percent less likely to have breast cancer than those who didn't eat any.

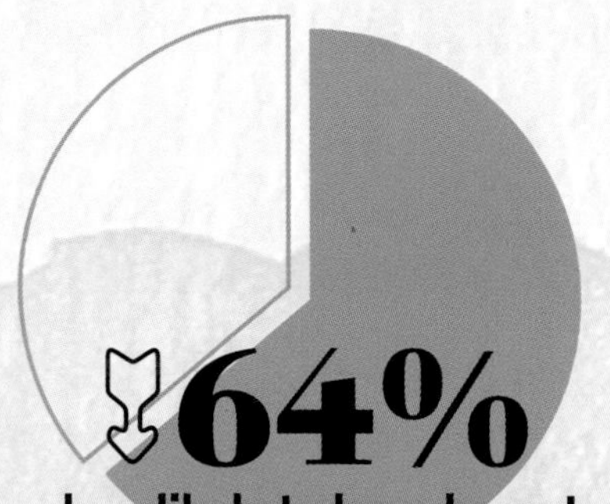

64%

less likely to have breast cancer if you eat mushrooms daily (rather than not at all), according to one study.

Antioxidant powers

Lab-based studies show that all varieties of mushrooms provide phytochemicals that can boost immunity. One study found that when adults ate ⅛oz (5g) of dried shiitake mushrooms every day for 4 weeks (equivalent to 3oz/84g of fresh mushrooms), immune function was enhanced.

Calorie reducer

Studies found replacing meat with button mushrooms meant adults consumed 420 fewer calories in those meals and only had an extra 50 calories later in the day. That's a calorie deficit of 370 calories per day—enough to lose 5lb (2.25kg) if that change was made once a week for a year. It's the fact that mushrooms are low in calories but still satiating that gives them their waistline magic.

Ultimate health protectors

Mushrooms contain phytochemicals that fight bacteria and viruses, and help to lower inflammation—good news, as chronic inflammation is at the root of many diseases, including heart disease and type 2 diabetes. Plus, mushrooms contain good levels of copper, an antioxidant that helps to protect our cells from damage caused by free radicals.

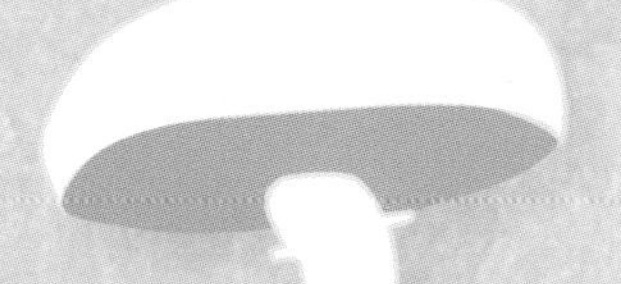

Chanterelle, portobello, and white mushrooms all provide significant amounts of copper.

Bone density booster

UV light converts ergosterol in mushrooms into vitamin D2, which can boost often-lacking vitamin D intakes (see pages 36–37). Sunshine can offer a certain increase, but pure UVB creates the most (see below).

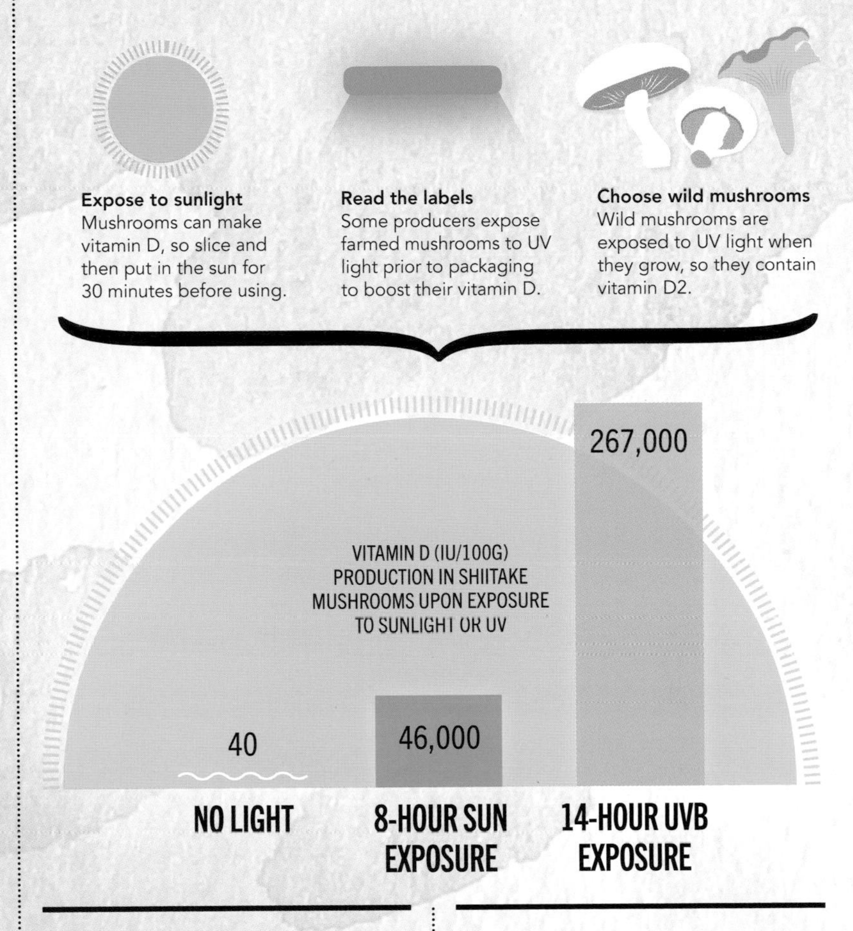

Great for the heart

Mushrooms keep the heart healthy in several ways. They contain substances that act as anti-inflammatories, and they are rich in antioxidants that protect blood vessels. Studies also show that mushrooms can lower total and LDL (bad) cholesterol.

Blood pressure regulators

Shiitake mushrooms are rich in a chemical called eritadenine, which seems to block the activity of an enzyme that constricts blood vessels. As blood vessels remain widened, blood pressure is more likely to remain at normal levels.

BARLEY RISOTTO WITH ROASTED SQUASH

This new twist on a classic dish swaps in whole-grain barley. Rich in soluble fiber, it's great for protecting against insulin resistance and type 2 diabetes.

THE BRAIN | VISION | HEARING & BALANCE | ORAL HEALTH | IMMUNITY | BONES & MUSCLES | SKIN & SENSATION | THE LUNGS | HEART & BLOOD | GUT HEALTH | URINARY HEALTH | WOMEN'S HEALTH

SERVES **2**

Ingredients

For the low-sodium stock (about 1½ pints/ 900ml)

- 2 carrots, halved
- 2 leeks, cut into thirds
- 3 shallots, halved
- 4 celery sticks, cut into thirds
- 2 tbsp olive oil
- bouquet garni: 2–3 thyme sprigs; 3 bay leaves; a small bunch of flat-leaf parsley
- freshly ground black pepper

For the risotto

- 3 tbsp olive oil
- 1 red onion, chopped
- 1 celery stick, sliced
- 2 garlic cloves, crushed
- 4½oz (125g) hulled pearl barley
- ½ squash (about 12oz/350g), scrubbed and seeded
- 3½oz (100g) baby spinach leaves
- 1 tbsp sage leaves, shredded, plus extra to garnish (optional)
- 1 tbsp thyme leaves
- balsamic vinegar, to serve

1 Preheat the oven to 375°F (190°C). Toss the stock vegetables in the oil and place on a baking sheet. Roast for 25 minutes until the carrots are soft. Transfer the vegetables to a large pan, cover them with 1½ pints (900ml) boiling water, and add a bouquet garni of thyme, bay leaves, and parsley, along with plenty of black pepper. Bring to a boil, cover, and simmer for 15 minutes. Strain the stock (keep the vegetables for another meal), and set aside.

2 Next, make the risotto. Heat 2 tablespoons of oil in a large pan and fry the onion for 3–4 minutes until soft. Put the celery and a crushed garlic clove into the pan, and cook for another 2 minutes. Next, add the barley and stir well to coat the grains, before pouring in 1 pint (600ml) of stock. Bring to a boil, stirring intermittently, then reduce the heat, cover, and simmer for 45–50 minutes until the grains are tender. You may need to add more liquid occasionally.

3 Meanwhile, roast the squash. Turn the oven up to 400°F (200°C). Place the squash half on a baking sheet. Rub the remaining crushed garlic over the cut surface of the squash. Drizzle with 1 tablespoon of oil, season with black pepper, and roast for 25–30 minutes until very soft. Remove the squash from the oven and allow to cool a little.

4 When the barley is cooked, add the spinach leaves, and stir in the sage and thyme. Use a spoon to scoop out bite-sized pieces of squash flesh and stir them into the barley. Divide the risotto between two bowls and drizzle with balsamic vinegar to serve.

NUTRITION PER SERVING Calories **503** Total fat **20.2g** Saturated fat **2.9g** Cholesterol **0mg** Carbohydrates **75.8g** Dietary fiber **6.4g** Sugars **14.6g** Protein **9.4g** Sodium **36mg**

Smart swaps

- Swap the baby spinach for **kale** for extra vitamins A, C, and E.
- Use **red bell peppers** instead of squash for a boost of folate, which helps brain function.

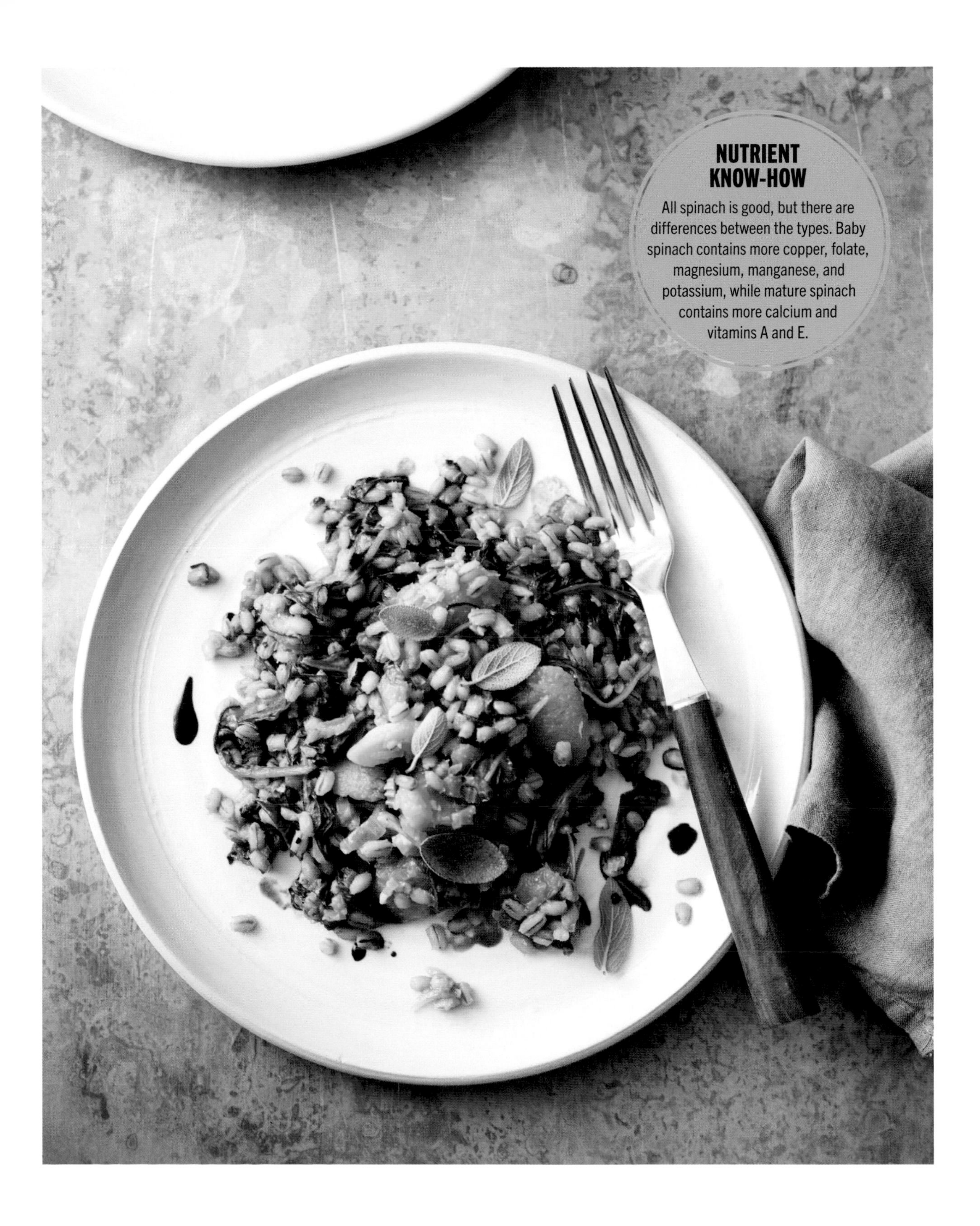

NUTRIENT KNOW-HOW

All spinach is good, but there are differences between the types. Baby spinach contains more copper, folate, magnesium, manganese, and potassium, while mature spinach contains more calcium and vitamins A and E.

-SUPERGROUP-

ONIONS, GARLIC, AND LEEKS

All members of the allium family are great for flavor, plus they are packed with naturally occurring plant chemicals that help keep the heart healthy, regulate blood sugar levels, and protect against cancer.

WHICH ALLIUMS?

These popular and easy-to-source alliums have powerful health properties.

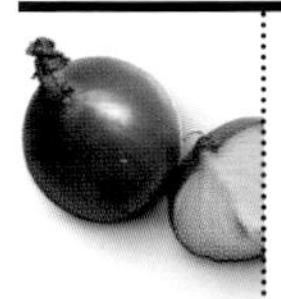

Onions

- Contain sulfur compounds, which give them many of their health benefits

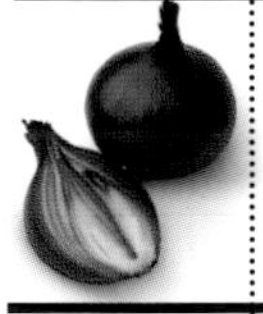

Red onions

- Are a great source of heart-healthy and cancer-fighting quercetin

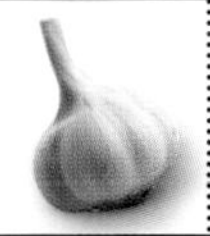

Garlic

- Lowers blood pressure and cholesterol levels, so is heart-friendly

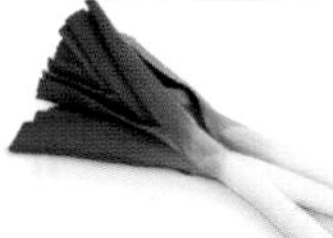

Leeks

- Contain good levels of the flavonoid kaemperfol, which acts as an antioxidant

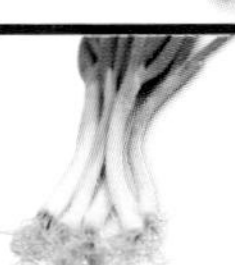

Scallions

- Contain 62 times more skin-friendly vitamin A than regular onions

HOW MUCH?

Eat at least one serving of alliums a day.

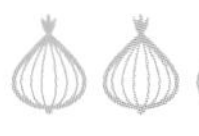
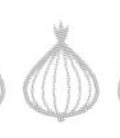
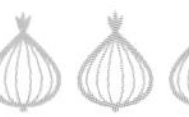
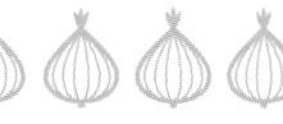

BEST BOUGHT

Choose fresh, firm, dry produce.

HOW TO STORE

Only leeks and scallions need to be refrigerated. Keep onions in a cool, dry, dark place with a good air flow.

RAW OR COOKED?

Most alliums can be eaten raw or cooked. For optimum benefits, finely chop or crush garlic to release the sulfur compounds.

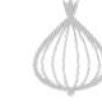

Anti-inflammatories

Inflammation is thought to be at the root of many long-term health problems, including heart disease, type 2 diabetes, Alzheimer's disease, rheumatoid arthritis, and inflammatory bowel diseases. The flavonoid quercetin, which is found particularly in onions, has been shown in many lab-based studies to help reduce inflammation—in particular, it may inhibit the enzymes that generate substances such as prostaglandins, which cause inflammation and pain.

Allergy minimizers

Onions are a very good source of quercetin, which has many health benefits. One advantage is that it helps to prevent histamine being released from cells, so it may have a role to play in protecting against allergies such as hayfever. This is very important, as allergies are increasingly being seen in older people, probably due to lower immunity and cell aging.

Quercetin acts as a natural antihistamine, and may help to minimize the effects of allergies such as hayfever.

Heart friendly

Research shows that regularly eating alliums is linked to a lower risk of cardiovascular disease. One study found higher intakes of these vegetables were linked to a 64 percent reduced risk of the disease over 6 years. In another study, those who ate at least one serving of onions a week were 22 percent less likely to suffer a heart attack than those who had no onions. Alliums are packed with sulfur compounds, as well as flavonoids such as kaempferol and quercetin (the most abundant flavonoid in alliums), which acts as an antioxidant. See how they compare below.

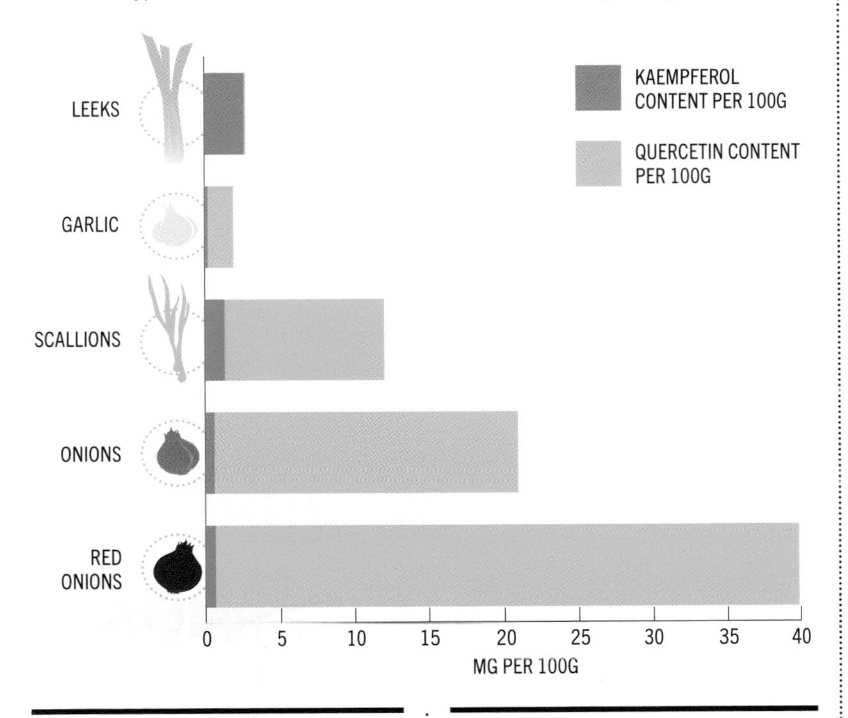

Cancer protective

Alliums are rich in sulfur-containing compounds which, when crushed, are transformed into new compounds, such as allicin (in garlic). These give them their familiar flavor, odor, and potential health benefits. These benefits may include protection against cancer—in particular, of the digestive tract (such as the stomach and colon)—although further research is needed.

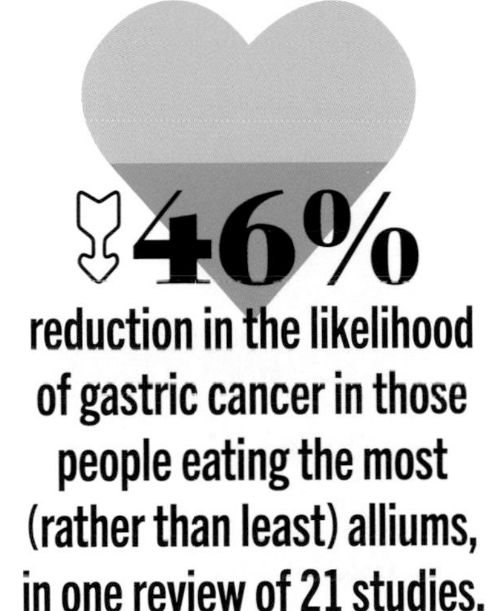

reduction in the likelihood of gastric cancer in those people eating the most (rather than least) alliums, in one review of 21 studies.

Good gut health

Onions, garlic, and leeks are prebiotics. This means they're rich in indigestible fiber, which provides food for "friendly" probiotic bacteria in the large intestine, enabling them to grow, flourish, and crowd out bad bacteria. This helps to keep the digestive system working well.

Memory aids

Alliums may help with memory; for example, scallions contain good levels of memory-boosting nutrients such as folate and lutein. Plus, leeks contain five times more folate than onions, which is great news, as good intakes of folate may help to protect us from Alzheimer's disease.

Blood sugar control

Garlic and onions may help to lower blood sugar levels, making them beneficial for people with insulin resistance (the precursor for type 2 diabetes) or diabetes. In one study of patients with diabetes, a 3½oz (100g) serving of red onion significantly reduced blood sugar levels.

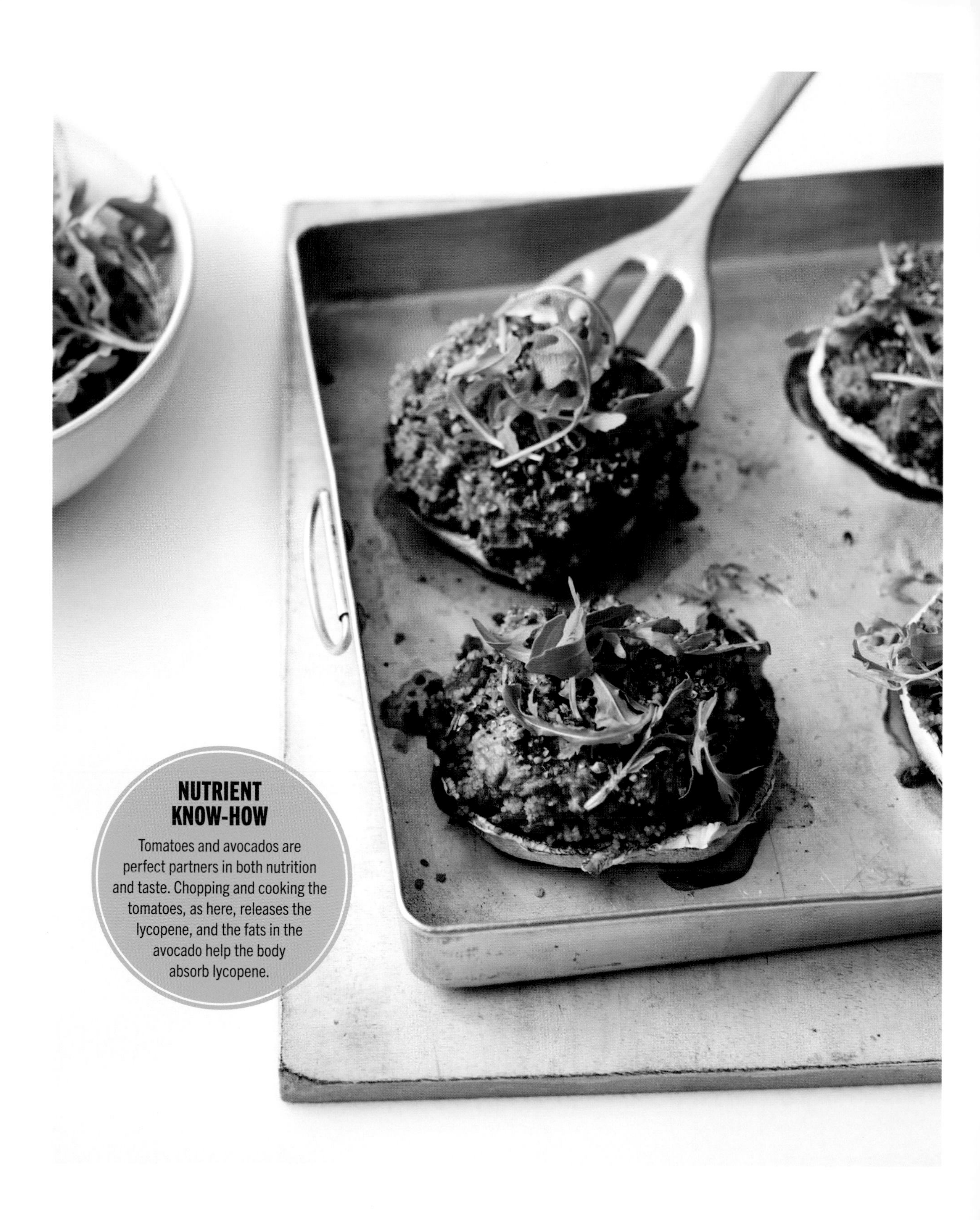

NUTRIENT KNOW-HOW

Tomatoes and avocados are perfect partners in both nutrition and taste. Chopping and cooking the tomatoes, as here, releases the lycopene, and the fats in the avocado help the body absorb lycopene.

MUSHROOMS STUFFED WITH TOMATO COUSCOUS

You may never cook couscous in water again. Here, it's "cooked" in tomatoes for a heart-friendly dinner that's high in soluble fiber and cancer-protective lycopene.

THE BRAIN | VISION | HEARING & BALANCE | ORAL HEALTH | IMMUNITY | BONES & MUSCLES | SKIN & SENSATION | THE LUNGS | HEART & BLOOD | GUT HEALTH | URINARY HEALTH | MEN'S HEALTH

SERVES **2**

Ingredients

- 2½oz (75g) whole-wheat couscous
- 8oz (227g) can chopped tomatoes, a good-quality brand
- 3 tbsp extra-virgin olive oil
- handful of chives, finely cut
- freshly ground black pepper
- 1 ripe avocado
- zest and juice of 1 lemon
- 4 large field mushrooms
- 2 tbsp (30g) dukkah seed mix
- 1oz (30g) arugula leaves, to serve

1 Put the couscous in a medium bowl with the chopped tomatoes and olive oil, and give them a good stir to coat all of the grains. Add the chives and a good seasoning of freshly ground black pepper. Stir and set aside for 10–15 minutes.

2 Preheat the oven to 350°F (180°C). Meanwhile, halve the avocado and remove the pit. Use a spoon to scoop out the flesh and put it in a bowl with the lemon zest and juice, mashing it all together to make a smooth paste.

3 Discard the mushroom stalks and place the mushrooms, stalk side upward, on a lightly greased baking sheet.

4 When the couscous has softened, divide it between the four mushrooms, filling each well, and leveling the top with the back of the spoon. Next, spread the mashed avocado over the top of the couscous, repeating for all the mushrooms. Sprinkle the mushrooms with dukkah seeds so that the tops are well covered.

5 Put the sheet in the oven for 15–20 minutes until the mushrooms have cooked through but not softened completely. Serve with the arugula leaves.

NUTRITION PER SERVING Calories **511** Total fat **34.4g** Saturated fat **5.8g** Cholesterol **0mg** Carbohydrates **36.3g** Dietary fiber **12g** Sugars **7.4g** Protein **12.8g** Sodium **139mg**

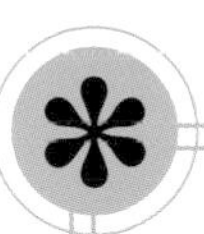

Smart swaps

- Swap the mushrooms for halved **orange bell peppers** or **beef tomatoes**, scooping out the insides and filling with the couscous mix as before. You'll get a hit of antioxidant vitamin C, which is good news for boosting collagen to keep skin looking smooth and line free.
- For a protein boost, swap the couscous for **quinoa**. Cook it according to package instructions, then mix with the chopped tomatoes, olive oil, chives, and pepper.

-WONDERFOOD-

TOMATOES

An integral part of the Mediterranean diet, tomatoes are a great source of health-promoting vitamins A and C. They also contain a powerful antioxidant called lycopene, which may improve heart health and protect against a number of cancers. Better still, cooking seems to boost the lycopene-related benefits of tomatoes, as does serving them with a little fat—for example, olive oil.

WHICH TOMATOES?

All tomatoes are packed with health-promoting vitamins, but these tomatoes and tomato products are particularly high in the beneficial antioxidant lycopene.

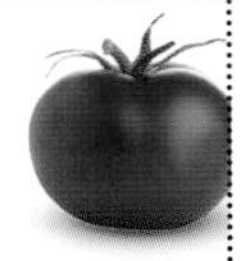

Regular tomatoes

- Contain high levels of vitamin C, which is important for the immune system

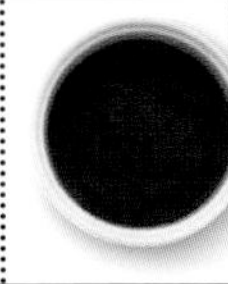

Tomato purée

- Is a great provider of beta-carotene, which the body uses to make vitamin A

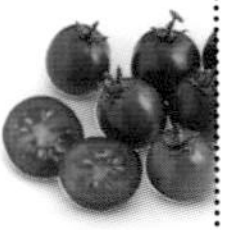

Cherry tomatoes

- Are rich in beta-carotene, which benefit the eyes and immunity

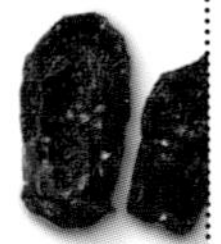

Sun-dried tomatoes

- Are higher in most nutrients, as drying concentrates the vitamins and minerals

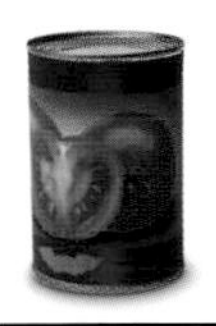

Chopped or whole canned tomatoes

- Are a great source of lycopene due to the heat treatment used during processing

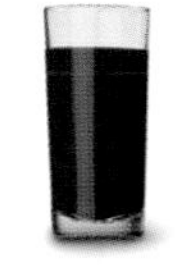

Tomato juice

- Is extremely high in lycopene, which has many anticancer and heart-boosting effects

HOW TO STORE

Leave tomatoes on your work surface to ripen. Once ripe, keep them in a cool place, away from sunlight, but don't refrigerate: cold temperatures damage their cells, affecting the tomatoes' flavor permanently.

HOW TO EAT

Eat both raw and cooked tomatoes, but note cooking and processing tomatoes actually boosts their lycopene content.

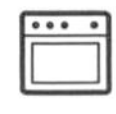
COOKED

RAW

HOW MUCH?

A daily serving of tomatoes or tomato products is ideal. However, consuming tomatoes only a few times a week still offers many health benefits.

1 serving equals

- 1 whole regular tomato
- 6 cherry tomatoes
- 7oz (200g) chopped canned tomatoes
- 2 canned plum tomatoes
- 4 sun-dried tomatoes
- 1 small glass of tomato juice
- 2 level tablespoons of tomato purée

BEST BOUGHT

When buying fresh, choose ripe, dark red tomatoes, as they contain the most lycopene. Canned, sun-dried, and puréed tomato products are good choices, as they have high levels of lycopene, but look out for hidden sodium in any processed products.

CANNED

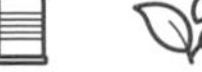
FRESH

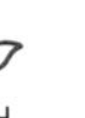
DRIED

JUICED

Perfect partners

Tomatoes' benefits are enhanced by other foods. Fat helps the body absorb carotenoids such as lycopene, and one study found adding avocado to a tomato salsa boosted lycopene absorption by four times. Another great partnership, which studies have found may prevent cancer, is eating tomatoes with broccoli.

+

⇩52%

reduction in size of prostate cancer tumor in lab-based tests when broccoli and tomatoes were eaten together.

Fights cancer

Lycopene may protect against many cancers, including those of the lung, pancreas, stomach, mouth, colon, and breast. The most compelling evidence is its effect on prostate cancer, the second most common cancer in men—a review of 26 studies found higher lycopene intakes are generally linked to a lower incidence of this disease.

Heart health

Many studies suggest tomatoes—and, in particular, the lycopene they contain—help keep the heart healthy. Research shows higher intakes of tomatoes and tomato products reduce LDL (bad) cholesterol, increase HDL (good) cholesterol, and may lower blood pressure. One review of studies also found lycopene decreased the risk of stroke by 19 percent. Discover how different tomatoes and tomato products compare in terms of their lycopene content below to see how to get your daily supply.

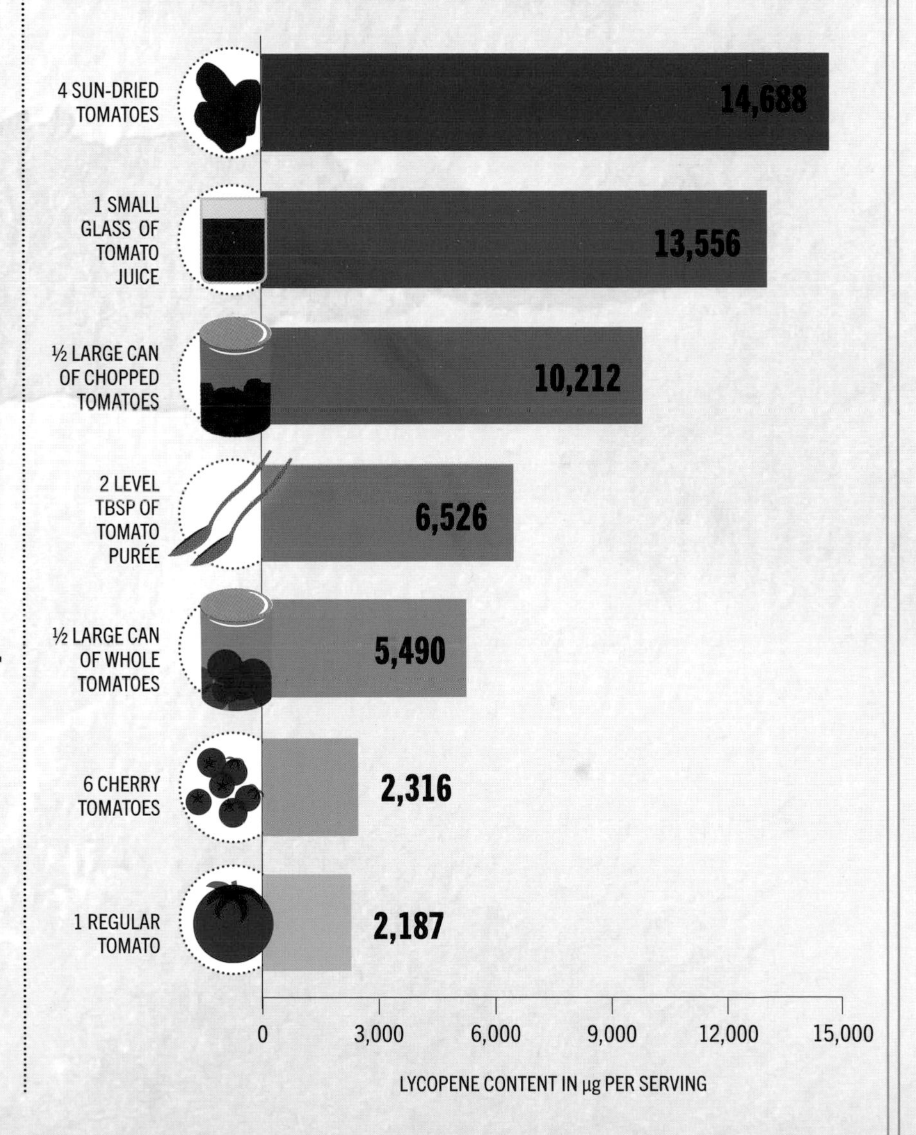

COD WITH SWEET POTATO WEDGES

Olive oil promotes the uptake of beta-carotene from the sweet potatoes and kale.

SERVES **2**

Ingredients

2 large sweet potatoes (9oz/250g each), skin-on, cut into wedges
2 tbsp olive oil
1 tsp paprika
5¾oz (160g) cauliflower, broken into smaller florets
5¾oz (160g) green beans, cut into thirds
5¾oz (160g) shredded kale
2 cod loins (about 6oz/170g each)
freshly ground black pepper

1 Preheat the oven to 425°F (220°C). Coat the sweet potato wedges with 1½ tablespoons of oil and the paprika and roast in a nonstick dish for 30 minutes.

2 Preheat the grill to high and bring a large pan of water to a boil. Steam the vegetables above this water, adding in 2-minute intervals: first, the cauliflower, then the green beans, and finally the kale for the final 2 minutes.

3 While the vegetables are steaming, pat the cod dry, coat in the remaining oil, season with black pepper, and grill for 5–6 minutes. Serve the cod and wedges on warmed plates with the steamed vegetables.

NUTRITION PER SERVING Calories **513** Total fat **14.9g** Saturated fat **2.4g** Cholesterol **88mg** Carbohydrates **60.4g** Dietary fiber **16g** Sugars **19.5g** Protein **39.4g** Sodium **296mg**

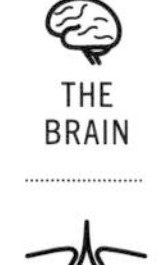
THE BRAIN

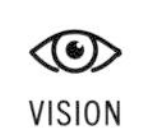
VISION

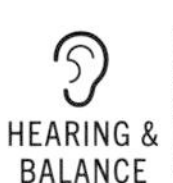
HEARING & BALANCE

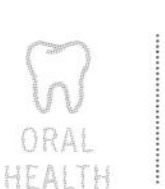
ORAL HEALTH

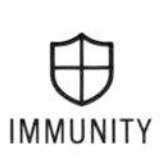
IMMUNITY

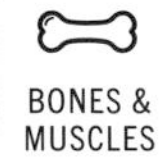
BONES & MUSCLES

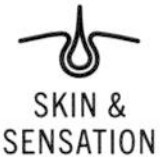
SKIN & SENSATION

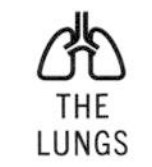
THE LUNGS

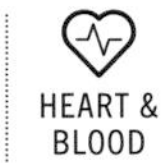
HEART & BLOOD

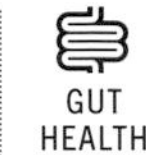
GUT HEALTH

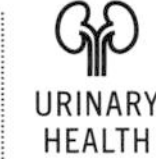
URINARY HEALTH

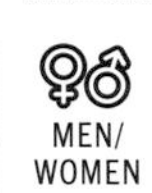
MEN/ WOMEN

RATATOUILLE

A vegetable feast brimming with anti-aging antioxidants that's a breeze to make.

SERVES **2**

Ingredients

2 tbsp olive oil
1 small onion, thickly sliced
2 garlic cloves, finely chopped
1 red bell pepper and 1 yellow bell pepper, diced
1 small eggplant, diced
1 zucchini, sliced
7oz (200g) cherry tomatoes
14oz (400g) can chopped tomatoes
1 tbsp each of tomato paste and balsamic vinegar
1 tsp dried mixed herbs
freshly ground black pepper
5½oz (150g) brown rice
handful of basil, roughly torn, to garnish

1 Heat the oil in a large nonstick pan over medium-low heat. Fry the onion and garlic gently until softened. Add the bell peppers, eggplant, and zucchini and cook for 5 minutes. Next, add all the tomatoes, the paste, balsamic, and dried herbs. Season with black pepper, bring to a boil, cover, and simmer for 30 minutes.

2 Meanwhile, cook the rice according to the package instructions. Serve hot, garnished with basil.

NUTRITION PER SERVING Calories **511** Total fat **14.3g** Saturated fat **2.2g** Cholesterol **0mg** Carbohydrates **86.9g** Dietary fiber **14.3g** Sugars **27.6g** Protein **14.4g** Sodium **25mg**

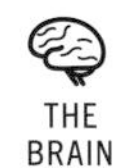
THE BRAIN

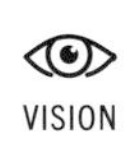
VISION

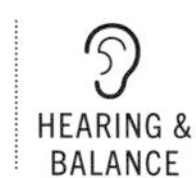
HEARING & BALANCE

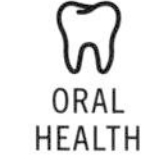
ORAL HEALTH

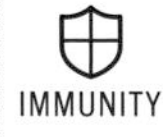
IMMUNITY

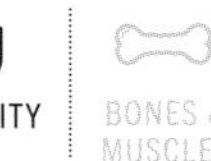
BONES & MUSCLES

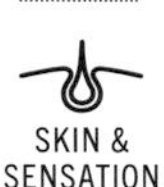
SKIN & SENSATION

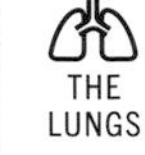
THE LUNGS

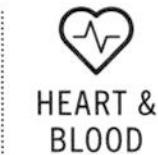
HEART & BLOOD

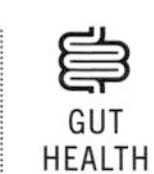
GUT HEALTH

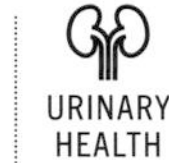
URINARY HEALTH

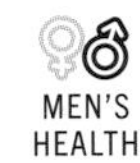
MEN'S HEALTH

PASTA WITH TUNA AND ROASTED VEGGIES

An antioxidant-rich vegetable medley partnered with healthy omega-3 fats.

SERVES **2**

Ingredients

9oz (250g) butternut squash flesh, cut into chunks

6¼oz (180g) cherry tomatoes

1 zucchini, thickly sliced

1 red onion, cut into wedges

1 yellow bell pepper, cut into chunks

1 tbsp olive oil

4½oz (125g) whole-wheat pasta

2 fresh tuna steaks (about 4oz/120g each), seasoned with freshly ground black pepper

handful of chives, finely chopped

½ lemon, cut into wedges to serve

1 Preheat the oven to 400°F (200°C). Toss all of the vegetables in 1 tablespoon of oil in a large nonstick roasting pan and roast for 30–40 minutes. Next, cook the pasta according to the package directions and drain; set aside.

2 Heat a nonstick frying pan and sear the tuna on both sides until done to your liking.

3 Mix the pasta and roasted vegetables together with the chives. Serve topped with the tuna and a lemon wedge.

NUTRITION PER SERVING Calories **512** Total fat **9.1g** Saturated fat **1.5g** Cholesterol **42mg** Carbohydrates **67.9g** Dietary fiber **15.9g** Sugars **21.3g** Protein **43.8g** Sodium **94mg**

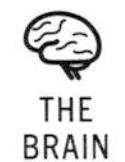

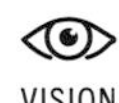
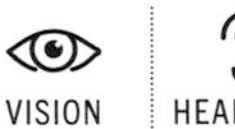

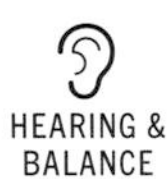

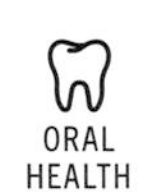

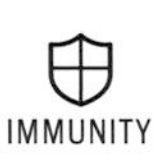

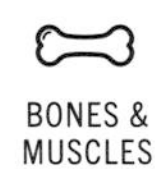

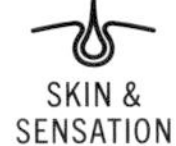

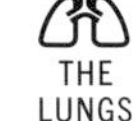
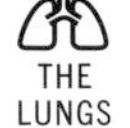

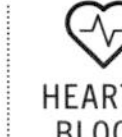
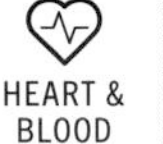

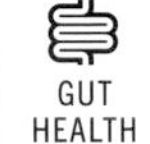

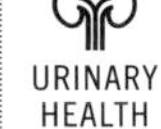

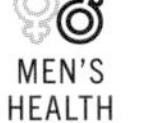

ROSEMARY LAMB

This dish helps to fight off free-radical damage in the brain, thanks to rosemary's carnosic acid.

SERVES **2**

Ingredients

2 lean lamb steaks (about 4oz/120g each)

1½ tbsp olive oil

freshly ground black pepper

2 sweet potatoes (about 8oz/225g each) skin-on, cut into chunks

1 sprig rosemary

5¾oz (160g) broccoli

5¾oz (160g) baby sweetcorn

1 Preheat the oven to 425°F (220°C). Pat the lamb dry, rub with ½ tablespoon of oil, and season with freshly ground black pepper.

2 Coat the potatoes with the remaining oil and torn rosemary, and roast in the oven for 25 minutes.

3 Heat a large nonstick frying pan until searingly hot and cook the lamb for 2 minutes on each side, then remove to rest on a warm plate.

4 Steam the broccoli and baby sweetcorn for 5 minutes, then serve with the potatoes and lamb, along with any juices from resting the meat.

NUTRITION PER SERVING Calories **500** Total fat **19.3g** Saturated fat **5.7g** Cholesterol **89mg** Carbohydrates **52.6g** Dietary fiber **13.2g** Sugars **15.9g** Protein **32.4g** Sodium **181mg**

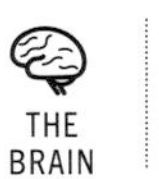

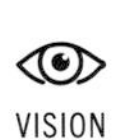

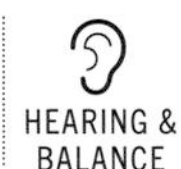

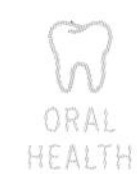

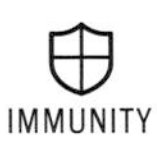

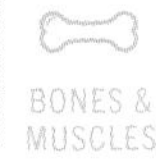

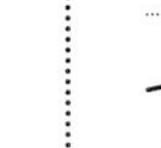
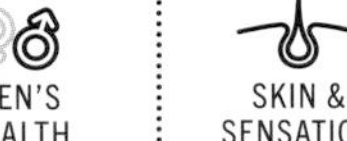

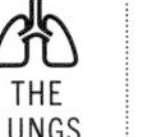

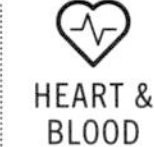

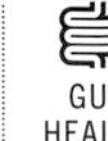
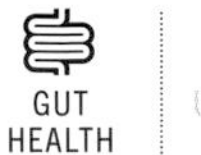

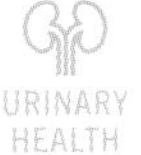

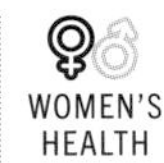

-WONDERFOOD-

OLIVE OIL

Olive oil is a well-known ingredient of the Mediterranean diet and has many bonuses relating to cholesterol, blood pressure, age-related diseases, and cognitive function. The benefits don't stop there though—it may also help to prevent certain types of cancer.

WHICH OLIVE OILS?

All olive oils are rich in heart-healthy monounsaturated fats and contain the same good amount of vitamin E. Extra-virgin is the purest and best enjoyed raw, while virgin and pure olive oils are less expensive and have a lower smoke point, so are good for cooking with.

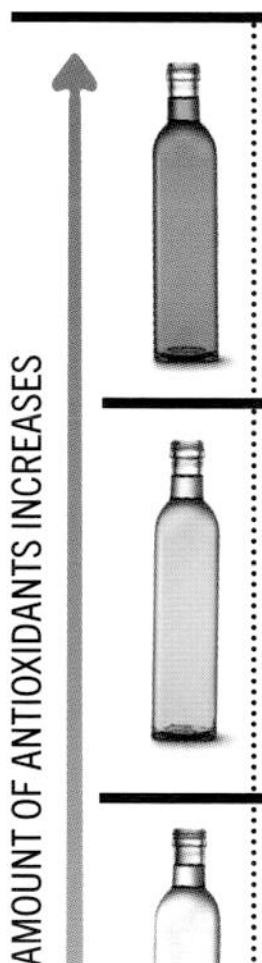

Extra-virgin olive oil

- Comes from the first pressing of the olives
- Is very rich in polyphenols and antioxidants

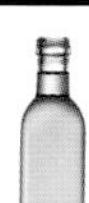

Virgin olive oil

- Is also from the first pressing, but using riper olives
- Is only moderately high in antioxidants

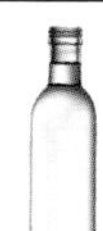

Olive oil/Pure olive oil

- Is usually a mix of extra-virgin and refined olive oils
- Is more processed and so contains fewer polyphenols

HOW MUCH?

One tablespoonful a day. It's high in calories—a tablespoonful has 100 calories—so be aware of this.

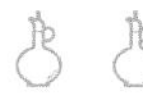
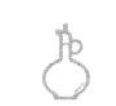
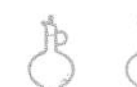

BEST BOUGHT

Extra-virgin is the best choice for maximum health benefits.

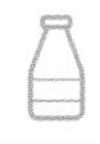

HOW TO STORE

Olive oil can become rancid if exposed to light and heat, so buy in tinted bottles and keep out of sunlight in a cool area.

RAW OR COOKED?

Extra-virgin is ideally consumed raw, while virgin and olive oil are best to cook with.

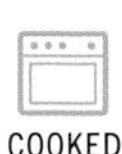

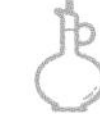

Cancer protector

Olive oil may help protect against cancer. A review of studies found people with the highest intakes of olive oil compared with the lowest intakes were 34 percent less likely to have any type of cancer, particularly breast cancer. It's not clear exactly how olive oil makes this happen, although lab-based studies show that polyphenols in olive oil may help to prevent the initiation and progression of cancer through their antioxidant action.

37%

People with the highest (rather than lowest) intakes of olive oil were 37 percent less likely to have breast cancer.

Cognitive enhancer

One large study found that elderly people who regularly used olive oil in cooking and as a dressing were less likely to suffer from cognitive decline, particularly when it came to visual memory—the ability to remember the characteristics of things they'd seen.

Antioxidant powers

All olive oil is rich in vitamin E, a vitamin with potent antioxidant ability. Extra-virgin olive oil is also packed with polyphenols, many of which act as antioxidants and anti-inflammatories. This is a powerful combination—the antioxidants mop up cell-damaging free radicals, while anti-inflammatories combat unwanted inflammation in the body.

Stroke prevention

There's good evidence that olive oil, and particularly one of the main monounsaturated fats in it—oleic acid—helps to reduce high blood pressure, which in turn can help to protect against stroke. Indeed, many studies show a lower incidence of stroke in people who have good intakes of olive oil.

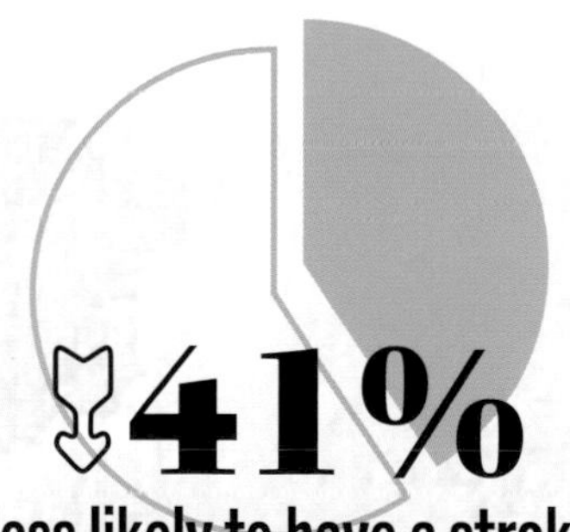

41%

less likely to have a stroke if you use olive oil in cooking and as a dressing (rather than never using it), according to one study.

Cholesterol controller

Diets high in saturated fat are known to raise LDL (low-density lipoprotein) or "bad" cholesterol, while diets rich in unsaturated fat tend to lower LDL levels. Studies show that swapping saturated for monounsaturated fat (a switch from butter to olive oil) helps cut LDL and total cholesterol by 6–10 percent.

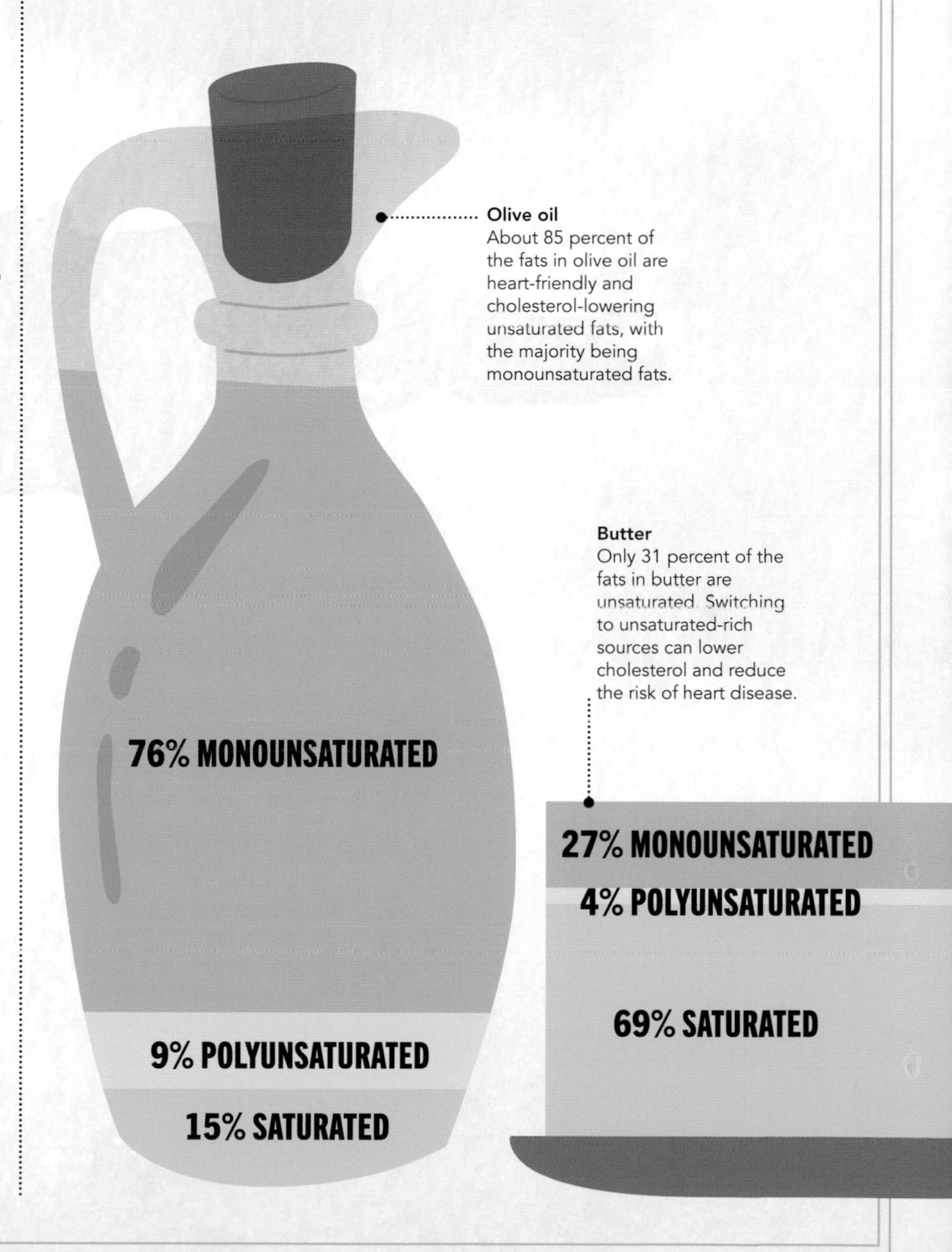

THE BRAIN | VISION | HEARING & BALANCE | ORAL HEALTH
IMMUNITY | BONES & MUSCLES | SKIN & SENSATION | THE LUNGS
HEART & BLOOD | GUT HEALTH | URINARY HEALTH | MEN/WOMEN

ROASTED FLOUNDER WITH SWEET POTATO NOODLES

Look after your sight with a plate packed with eye-friendly nutrients—lutein and zeaxanthin in the bok choy and zucchini, and beta-carotene-rich sweet potatoes.

SERVES **2**

Ingredients

2 sweet potatoes (about 5½oz/150g each), scrubbed but not peeled

4 tbsp olive oil

2 flounder fillets

freshly ground black pepper

juice of 1 lemon, plus lemon wedges to serve

1 tbsp capers in brine, drained and roughly chopped

1 medium zucchini

1 head bok choy

2 garlic cloves, crushed

flat-leaf parsley, chopped, to garnish

1 Use a julienne peeler, mandoline, spiralizer, or sharp chef's knife to cut the sweet potato into thin strips (like noodles), and place them in a bowl with 2 tablespoons of olive oil. Toss well, so that the "noodles" are well coated.

2 Preheat the oven to 350°F (180°C). Using a sharp knife, trim the flounder fillets so that they are evenly sized. Put the fillets skin side down on a lightly oiled nonstick baking sheet, pat dry, and season with black pepper and a squirt of lemon juice. Roast them in the oven for 10–15 minutes until the flesh is opaque.

3 Meanwhile, heat 1 tablespoon of oil in a nonstick pan. When hot, add the sweet potato "noodles" and cook for 4–5 minutes, stirring continuously. Once cooked, transfer to a bowl and dress them with the capers and the juice of half a lemon. Mix well, and keep warm until ready to serve.

4 Make long ribbons of zucchini by cutting off the ends and running a vegetable peeler down its length repeatedly. Separate the bok choy leaves and cut them in half lengthwise, ensuring that they remain long and chunky. Return the pan to the heat with the last tablespoon of oil. When hot, toss in the zucchini ribbons, garlic, and bok choy. Fry for 2 minutes, then remove from the heat.

5 Divide the "noodles" between two plates or bowls. Add a mound of garlicky greens and top each with a flounder fillet. Use the chopped parsley to garnish.

NUTRITION PER SERVING Calories **488** Total fat **25g** Saturated fat **3.8g** Cholesterol **112mg** Carbohydrates **35.5g** Dietary fiber **7.5g** Sugars **11.4g** Protein **32.7g** Sodium **526mg**

Smart swaps

- Swap the flounder for **tilapia** fillets. Tilapia is rich in vitamin B12, omega-3s, and protein, the last being important in cellular repair and metabolic activity.
- **Brown rice** makes a satisfying swap for the sweet potato noodles and comes with added selenium to boost immunity.

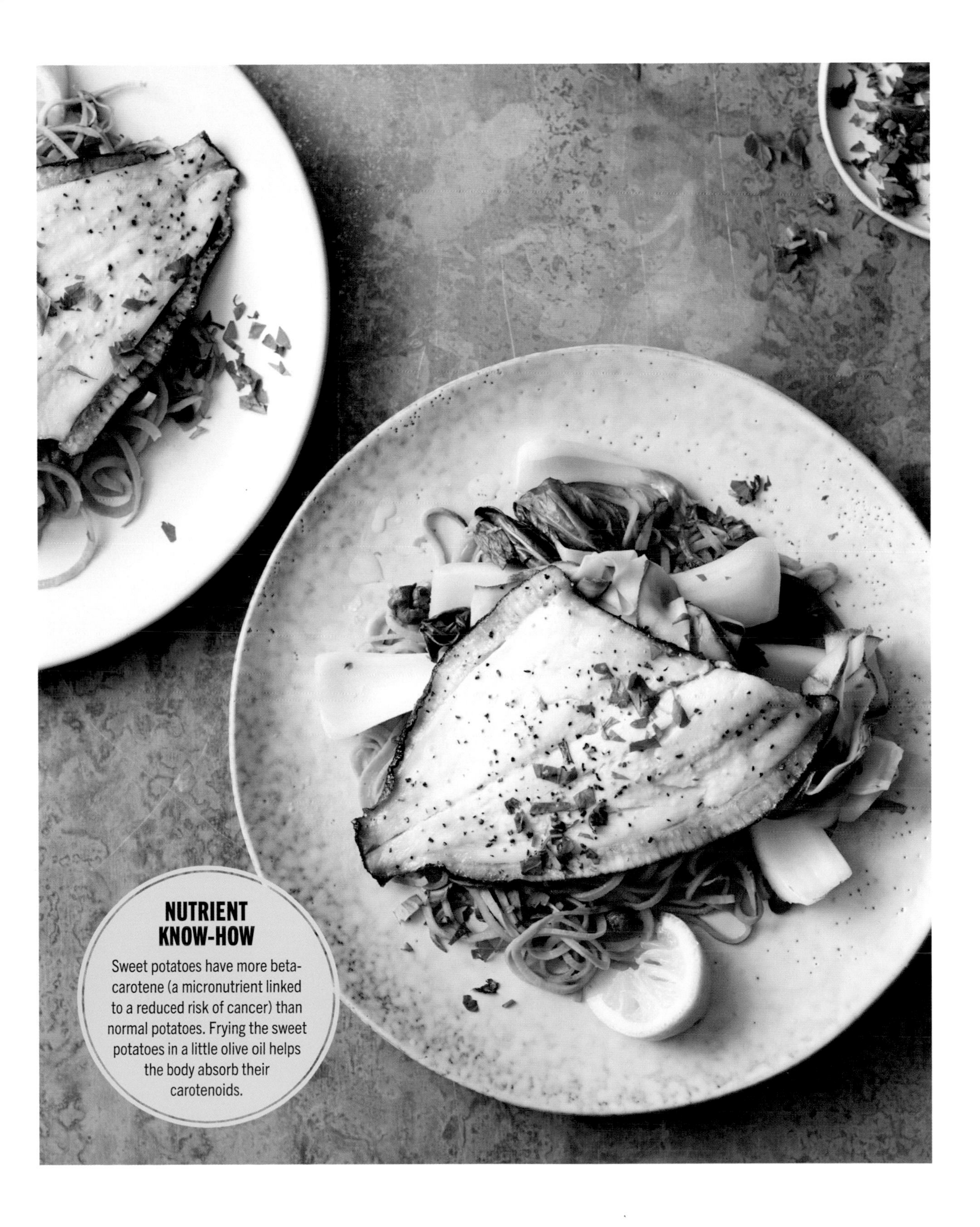

NUTRIENT KNOW-HOW

Sweet potatoes have more beta-carotene (a micronutrient linked to a reduced risk of cancer) than normal potatoes. Frying the sweet potatoes in a little olive oil helps the body absorb their carotenoids.

-SUPERGROUP-

CITRUS FRUITS

Best known for containing vitamin C, which supports the immune system, citrus fruits do far more than just fight infections. They are linked with everything from protection against heart disease and cancer to slowing down cataract development.

WHICH CITRUS FRUITS?

These popular citrus fruits are eaten worldwide and are great providers of vitamin C, a powerful antioxidant.

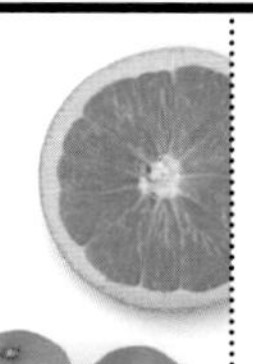

Oranges, mandarins, and tangerines

- Contain over 170 phytochemicals with anti-inflammatory, antitumor, and antioxidant functions
- Are rich in hesperidin, which may lower cholesterol levels
- Are a good source of beta-cryptoxanthin, for lung health

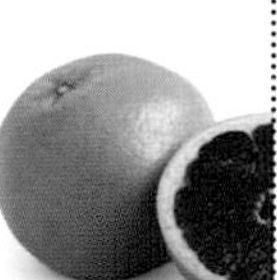

Grapefruit

- Help to lower cholesterol levels
- Come in pink, red, and blond varieties. Pink and red are rich in lycopene, a powerful antioxidant

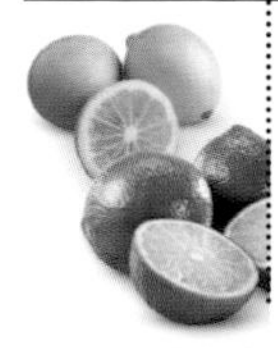

Lemons and limes

- Benefit the heart, as they enhance flavors of food without having to add salt

HOW MUCH?

Aim to have one portion of citrus fruits every day.

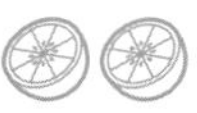
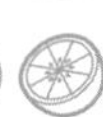
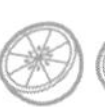
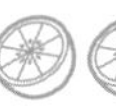
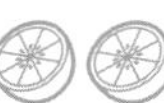

BEST BOUGHT

Choose unwaxed citrus fruits for zesting.

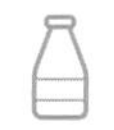
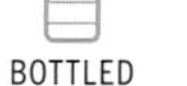

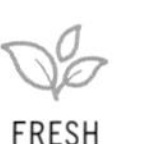

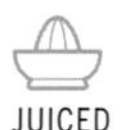

HOW TO STORE

Citrus fruits release more juice when warm, so keep at room temperature.

RAW OR COOKED?

Best eaten raw. Enjoy the whole fruits (rather than just having a glass of juice) so you get the fiber. The peel contains considerably more antioxidants than the juice, so use the grated zest to add flavor to your dishes.

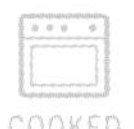

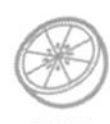

Cataract protection

Studies show eating vitamin C–rich foods, such as citrus fruits, can reduce the risk of cataracts. Because vitamin C is an antioxidant, having more vitamin C in the eye fluid helps to prevent oxidation that clouds the lens. In one 2016 study, scientists found diets rich in vitamin C reduced the risk of developing cataracts by a fifth, and, over a decade, stopped them progressing by a third.

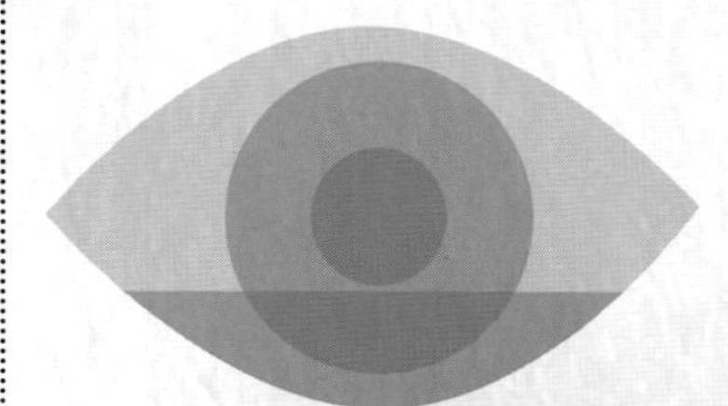

33%

reduced risk of cataract progression for those with a diet rich in vitamin C.

Collagen strengthener

Vitamin C is used to make collagen, which is vital for ligaments, tendons, blood vessels, and bones, and has an important role in healing wounds and repairing tissues. It also helps skin look smooth and plump: one study of American women found high intakes of vitamin C reduced wrinkles by 11 percent.

Heart helper

Various studies link higher intakes of vitamin C and the phytochemicals found in fruits with a reduced risk of heart disease. One large study of almost 115,000 adults found people who had the highest amounts of citrus fruits in their diet (compared with the lowest) had a 28 percent reduced risk of stroke, while for those with the highest levels of citrus juices, the risk decreased by 35 percent.

Lowers cholesterol

Studies show that components of citrus fruits may help lower cholesterol. Consuming citrus juices regularly has also been linked to lower cholesterol levels in humans. It is best, however, to eat the whole orange rather than just have orange juice, as much of the hesperidin (which is thought to lower cholesterol) is found in the white pith and peel.

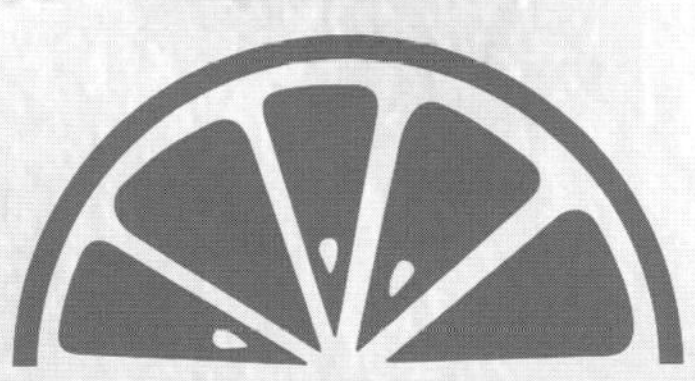

In a study, red grapefruit reduced total and LDL (or bad) cholesterol twice as much as the yellow variety.

All-around health hero

Numerous studies show diets high in citrus fruits protect against many diseases, including cancer, arthritis, heart disease, cataracts, and diabetes. The evidence suggests citrus fruits may help reduce the risk of cancer of the esophagus, mouth, larynx, pharynx, and stomach by 40–50 percent. The protective nutrients of citrus fruits—fiber, vitamin C, potassium, folate, and flavonoids—are located in different parts.

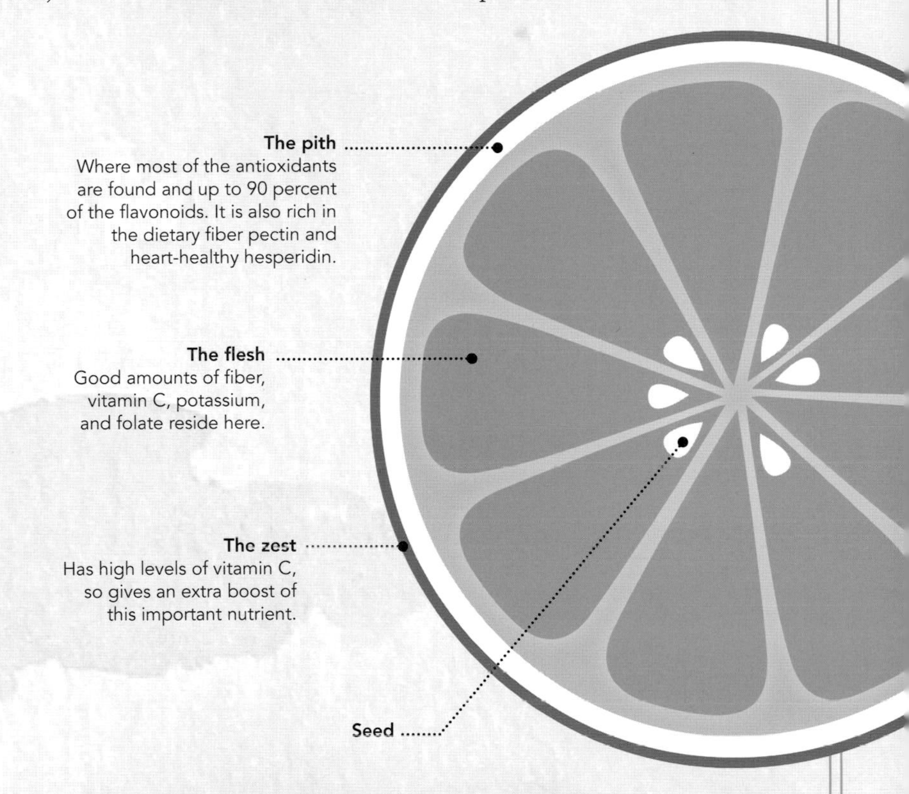

Dementia protector

A 2017 study found that over 6 years, the risk of dementia was reduced by 23 percent in those who ate citrus fruits most days. More research is needed, but citrus fruits contain vitamin C and phytochemicals that may help brain cells to stay healthy.

Infection fighter

Citrus fruits are especially rich in vitamin C, which is vital for strong immunity. This vitamin has been found to stimulate the functions of white blood cells called leucocytes, while as an antioxidant it protects immune cells from the damaging effects of free radicals.

PASTA WITH CHILI AND GARLIC SHRIMP

You'll smell the aromatic phytochemicals in the garlic—it's these that reduce cholesterol levels.

SERVES **2**

Ingredients

5¾oz (160g) whole-wheat spaghetti
5¾oz (160g) peas
2 tbsp olive oil
1–2 garlic cloves, finely chopped
1 red chili, finely chopped
5½oz (150g) peeled, raw jumbo shrimp, patted dry
7oz (200g) cherry tomatoes, halved
handful of parsley, chopped
juice and zest of 1 lemon
freshly ground black pepper

1 Cook the pasta according to the package instructions; add the peas for the last minute. Drain and set aside. Meanwhile, put the oil, garlic, and chili in a large nonstick frying pan and heat gently for 2 minutes.

2 Add the shrimp and cook for 3–4 minutes until they are pink and cooked through. Add the tomatoes and cook for a few minutes until softened. Then, add in the peas and cooked pasta to the pan, together with the parsley and the lemon zest and lemon juice. Mix and season with black pepper.

NUTRITION PER SERVING Calories **501** Total fat **14.7g** Saturated fat **2.2g** Cholesterol **113mg** Carbohydrates **67.4g** Dietary fiber **15.3g** Sugars **11.7g** Protein **29g** Sodium **173mg**

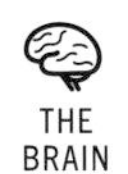
THE BRAIN
VISION
HEARING & BALANCE
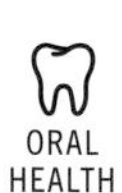
ORAL HEALTH
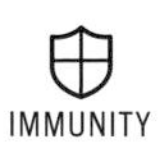
IMMUNITY
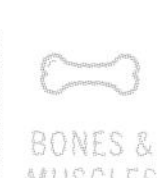
BONES & MUSCLES
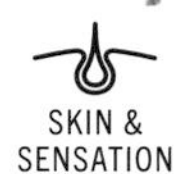
SKIN & SENSATION
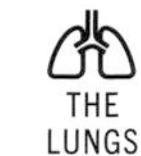
THE LUNGS
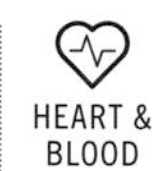
HEART & BLOOD
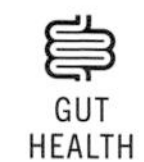
GUT HEALTH
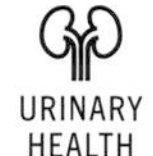
URINARY HEALTH
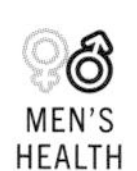
MEN'S HEALTH

TOFU SKEWERS

Marinating tofu imparts great flavors in a dish that offers anti-aging benefits for everyone.

SERVES **2**

Ingredients

9oz (250g) firm tofu, cut into cubes
1 tbsp olive oil
1 fat garlic clove, finely grated
1 red chili, finely chopped
5½oz (150g) brown rice
1 green bell pepper and 1 red bell pepper, cut into chunks
7oz (200g) cherry tomatoes
freshly ground black pepper
4½oz (125g) plain soy yogurt
3½oz (100g) cucumber, grated (squeeze out the excess moisture)
juice of ½ lemon
2 tbsp chopped mint leaves

1 Toss the tofu with the oil, garlic, and chili in a nonmetallic dish. Leave to marinate for 30 minutes.

2 Cook the rice according to the package instructions. Preheat the grill to medium. Thread the tofu onto 6 metal skewers with the bell peppers and cherry tomatoes. Season with black pepper and grill for 15 minutes.

3 Combine the yogurt, cucumber, lemon juice, and mint, and serve alongside the tofu kebabs and rice.

NUTRITION PER SERVING Calories **485** Total fat **13.7g** Saturated fat **2.5g** Cholesterol **0mg** Carbohydrates **72.3g** Dietary fiber **8.8g** Sugars **12.6g** Protein **22.1g** Sodium **36mg**

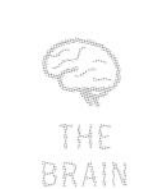
THE BRAIN
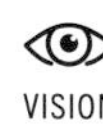
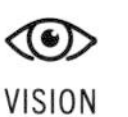
VISION

HEARING & BALANCE
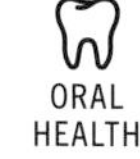
ORAL HEALTH
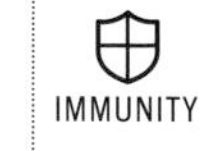
IMMUNITY
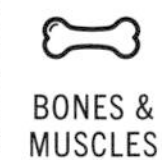
BONES & MUSCLES
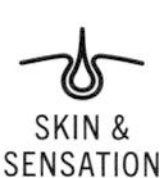
SKIN & SENSATION
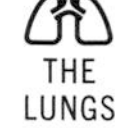
THE LUNGS
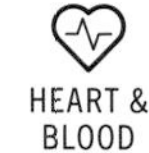
HEART & BLOOD
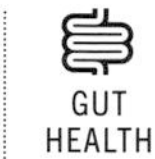
GUT HEALTH
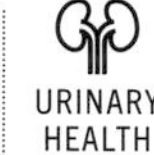
URINARY HEALTH
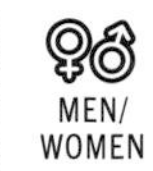
MEN/ WOMEN

VEGETABLE CHILI

A vibrant and vitamin-rich veggie-only version.

SERVES **2**

Ingredients

1 tbsp canola oil
1 onion, any type, diced
pinch each of chili powder, cumin seeds, and smoked paprika
1–2 garlic cloves, finely chopped
1 red bell pepper and 1 green bell pepper, cut into chunks
1 zucchini, cut into cubes
3½oz (100g) button mushrooms
14oz (400g) can chopped tomatoes
1 tbsp tomato paste
freshly ground black pepper
14oz (400g) can kidney beans in water, rinsed and drained
2 whole-wheat wraps, cut into small triangles
4 tbsp plain soy yogurt

1 Heat the oil in a nonstick pan over low heat. Fry the onion, spices, and garlic for 3–4 minutes. Next, add the bell peppers and zucchini and fry for another 5 minutes. Add the mushrooms and fry for 2–3 minutes. Next, add the tomatoes and the paste. Season with black pepper, bring to a boil, and simmer for 15 minutes until the sauce is thick. Add the kidney beans and heat through.

2 Meanwhile, lightly toast the wrap triangles until crisp. Serve with the chili, topped with the yogurt.

NUTRITION PER SERVING Calories **487** Total fat **13.4g** Saturated fat **2.8g** Cholesterol **0mg** Carbohydrates **69.4g** Dietary fiber **24.3g** Sugars **24.3g** Protein **24.2g** Sodium **312mg**

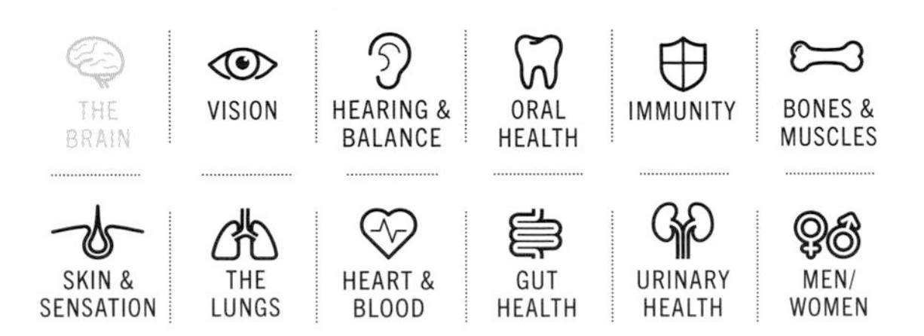

FISH AND CHIPS WITH PEAS

The anti-aging twist on this dish serves up baked sweet potato "chips," packed with beta-carotene and high in fiber for full-on health.

SERVES **2**

Ingredients

1lb (450g) sweet potatoes, skin-on, cut into medium chips
2 tbsp canola oil
1½ tbsp plain flour
freshly ground black pepper
2 cod loins or fillets (about 6oz/170g each), cut in half
5¾oz (160g) frozen peas
½ lemon cut into wedges, to serve

1 Preheat the oven to 425°F (220°C). Coat the sweet potato chips in half the oil and then put in the oven to bake for 25–30 minutes. Meanwhile, in a large shallow bowl, mix together the flour and black pepper.

2 Pat the cod dry and dust the pieces in flour, shaking off the excess then discarding the remaining flour. Fry the fish in the remaining oil in a large nonstick frying pan for 3 minutes each side. Switch off the heat and rest the cod in the pan with a lid on for 1 minute.

3 Boil the peas for 2 minutes, then drain and serve with the cod, sweet potato chips, and a wedge of lemon.

NUTRITION PER SERVING Calories **508** Total fat **13.4g** Saturated fat **1.4g** Cholesterol **88mg** Carbohydrates **63.8g** Dietary fiber **12.5g** Sugars **17.4g** Protein **37.5g** Sodium **248mg**

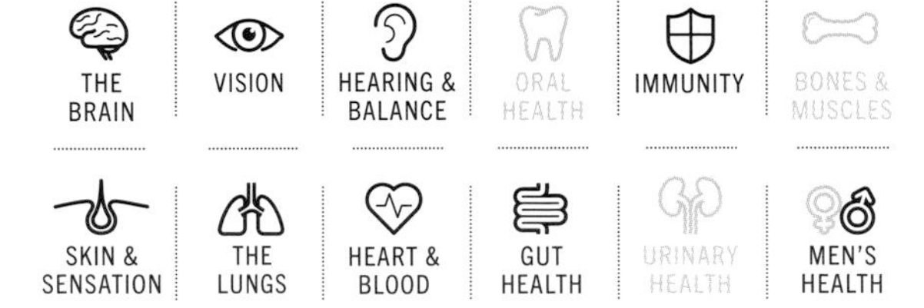

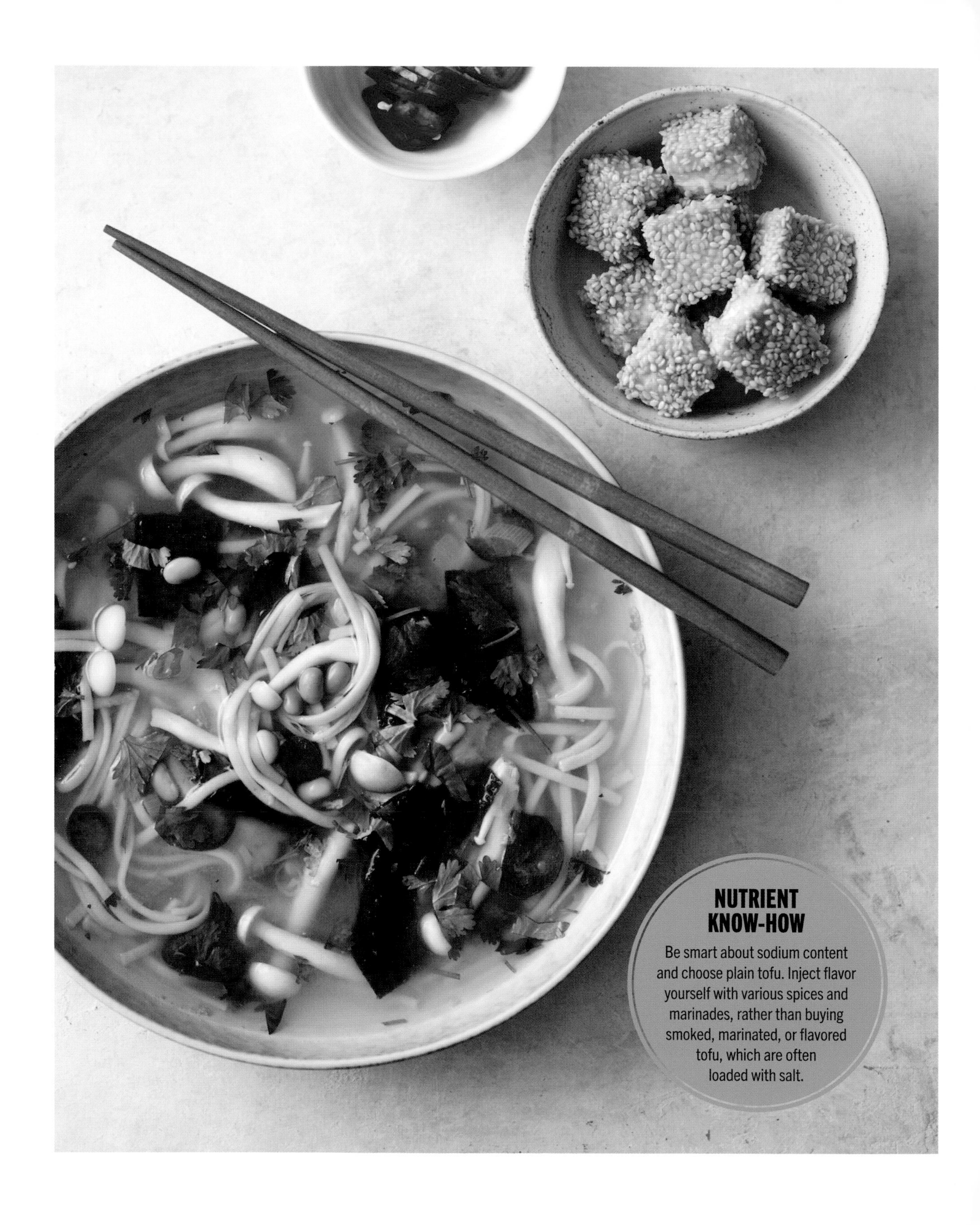

NUTRIENT KNOW-HOW

Be smart about sodium content and choose plain tofu. Inject flavor yourself with various spices and marinades, rather than buying smoked, marinated, or flavored tofu, which are often loaded with salt.

THE BRAIN | VISION | HEARING & BALANCE | ORAL HEALTH
IMMUNITY | BONES & MUSCLES | SKIN & SENSATION | THE LUNGS
HEART & BLOOD | GUT HEALTH | URINARY HEALTH | MEN/WOMEN

JAPANESE-STYLE NOODLE SOUP

This dish's star is soy—in the miso, the tofu, and the edamame. Enjoy this satisfying soup and fill up on its benefits—stronger bones and lower blood cholesterol.

SERVES **2**

Ingredients

- 2 tsp miso paste, any type
- 2 garlic cloves, grated
- 4 scallions, shredded
- ½ red chili, sliced in rings
- 2 tsp grated fresh root ginger
- 1¾oz (50g) brown soba noodles
- 2oz (60g) edamame
- 3½oz (100g) enoki mushrooms (or other Asian variety), broken into individual pieces
- 5½oz (150g) firm tofu, drained
- 1 egg, beaten
- 3 tbsp (30g) sesame seeds
- 1 tbsp vegetable oil
- 2 sheets of nori seaweed
- handful of cilantro leaves
- juice of ½ lime
- 2 tsp sesame oil

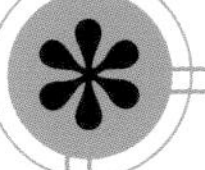

Smart swaps

- Replace the edamame with **fava beans** if you are watching your weight; fava beans have fewer calories and more fiber, which keeps you feeling full for longer.
- If you don't mind a nonvegetarian option, use fresh **jumbo shrimp** instead of tofu, coating them with sesame seeds in the same way. You'll get twice as much protein, potassium, and vitamin E.

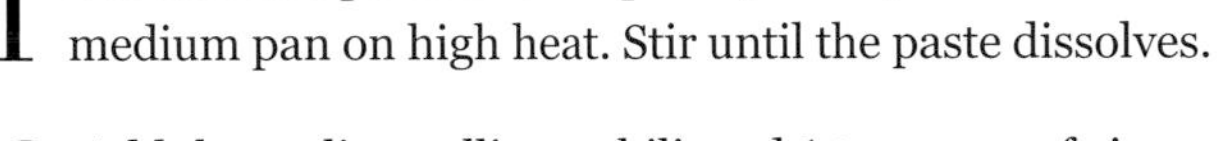

1 Put the miso paste and 1½ pints (900ml) of water into a medium pan on high heat. Stir until the paste dissolves.

2 Add the garlic, scallions, chili, and 1 teaspoon of ginger. Bring to a gentle boil and throw in the noodles, edamame, and mushrooms. Reduce the heat and simmer for 5 minutes, stirring occasionally, until the noodles are cooked. Remove from the heat.

3 Meanwhile, cut the tofu into ¾in (2cm) cubes and pat them dry with paper towel. Put the beaten egg and sesame seeds into separate shallow bowls. Dip the tofu cubes into the egg, then into the sesame seeds, coating each cube well.

4 Heat the oil in a small frying pan and, when hot, toss in the tofu cubes. Fry them for 1–2 minutes until the seeds turn golden brown, then flip the tofu and repeat. The sides should brown without needing to turn the cubes repeatedly. Once golden and crisp, remove the cubes to a plate lined with paper towel.

5 Shred or cut the seaweed sheets into strips and scatter them over the soup to soften. Stir in the remaining grated ginger, the cilantro, and the lime juice.

6 Divide the soup between two bowls and season each with 1 teaspoon of sesame oil. Put the tofu cubes into two small side dishes and serve them alongside the soup.

NUTRITION PER SERVING Calories **396** Total fat **24.8g** Saturated fat **3.9g** Cholesterol **46mg** Carbohydrates **21.7g** Dietary fiber **7.6g** Sugars **2g** Protein **21.1g** Sodium **283mg**

-SUPERGROUP-

NUTS

Nuts are little wonders, loaded with minerals, phytochemicals, and essential fats that keep the heart healthy, as well as helping to prevent colon cancer, gallstones, and type 2 diabetes. In addition, eating them regularly may help with weight management, and "cleaning up your diet." Plus, new research shows they may also slow down the aging process.

WHICH NUTS?

Nuts vary in the vitamins, minerals, and phytochemicals they contain, so enjoy eating a selection to gain the maximum health-promoting nutrients. Here are some of the most commonly available nuts that are best for longevity.

Almonds

- Have considerably more bone-strengthening calcium than other nuts, which may help prevent osteoporosis
- Are one of the best for eye-friendly vitamin E

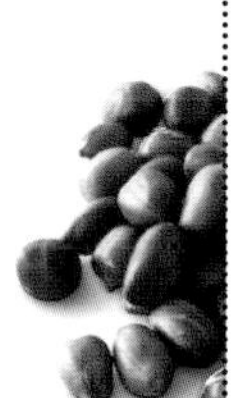

Peanuts

- Contain fewer calories, less fat, and more B vitamins than other nuts
- Are a very good source of folate, containing around double the amount of almonds and pistachios and four times more than Brazil nuts

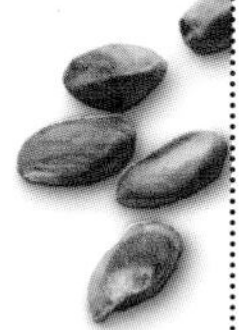

Pistachios

- Are the only nut to contain significant amounts of the antioxidants lutein and zeaxanthin, which are important for good eye health

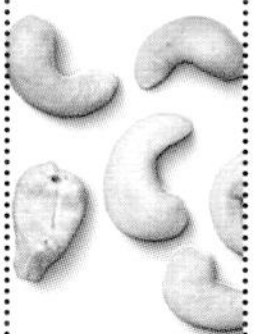

Cashew nuts

- Contain more immune system–boosting copper than most other nuts—around twice as much as almonds, peanuts, and pistachios

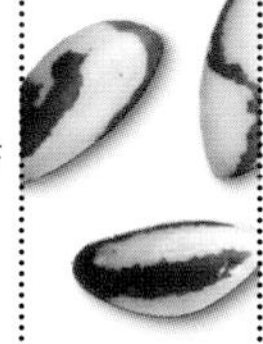

Brazil nuts

- Are exceptionally high in the antioxidant selenium, which is essential for a healthy immune system and protects against disease-causing free radical damage

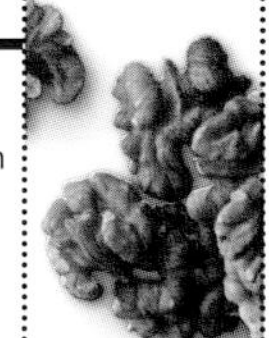

Walnuts

- Are rich in a poly-unsaturated fat called alpha-linolenic acid, which the body uses to make the omega-3 fats (EPA and DHA) that occur naturally in oil-rich fish

HOW MUCH?

Eat one 1oz (28g) serving of nuts a day.

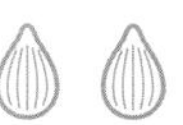

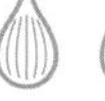
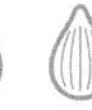

HOW TO STORE

Keep in a sealed package or an airtight container in a cool, dark place.

BEST BOUGHT

Always choose unflavored, plain nuts, as flavored nuts contain seasonings, salt, honey, and/or sugar.

RAW OR COOKED?

Nuts are nutritious both raw and cooked; roast or bake at a low temperature.

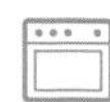

Aging slowdown

It sounds too good to be true, but early research suggests eating nuts helps to slow down the shortening of telomeres (see page 11). After studying the DNA of more than 5,000 adults, scientists found those who consumed 5 percent of their calories from nuts and seeds had more than 18 months of reduced cell aging.

Prevention of colon cancer

Eating peanuts may help protect against colorectal cancer—a study of 24,000 adults found the risk of colon cancer was cut by 58 percent in women and 27 percent in men when peanuts were eaten twice a week. It's believed phytic acid, phytosterols, and resveratrol may protect against cancer.

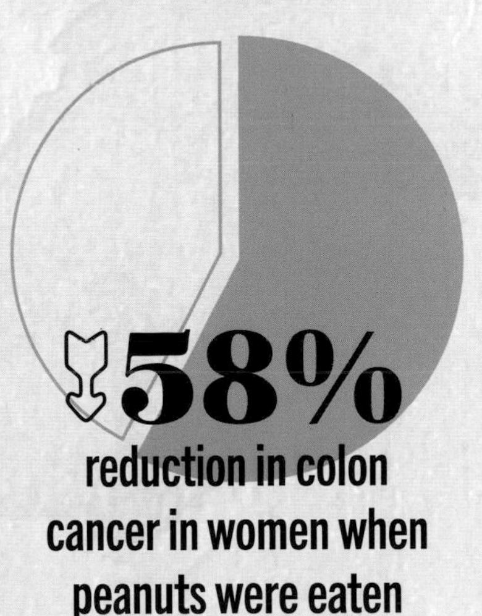

58% reduction in colon cancer in women when peanuts were eaten twice a week.

Disease protector

Nuts can protect against a wide range of diseases, from cancer to gallstones. A study of 120,000 Americans over a 26–30-year time period found daily nut eaters were a fifth less likely to have died than those who avoided them. Plus, a review of 29 studies found eating 1oz (28g) of nuts each day cut the risk of cancer by 15 percent and cardiovascular disease by 21 percent. The same review concluded eating 1oz (28g) of nuts each day reduced the risk of dying from various diseases:

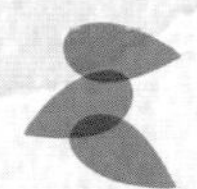

BENEFITS OF EATING 1OZ (28G) OF NUTS A DAY:

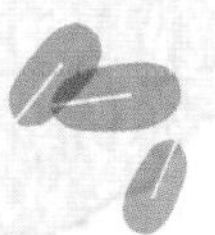

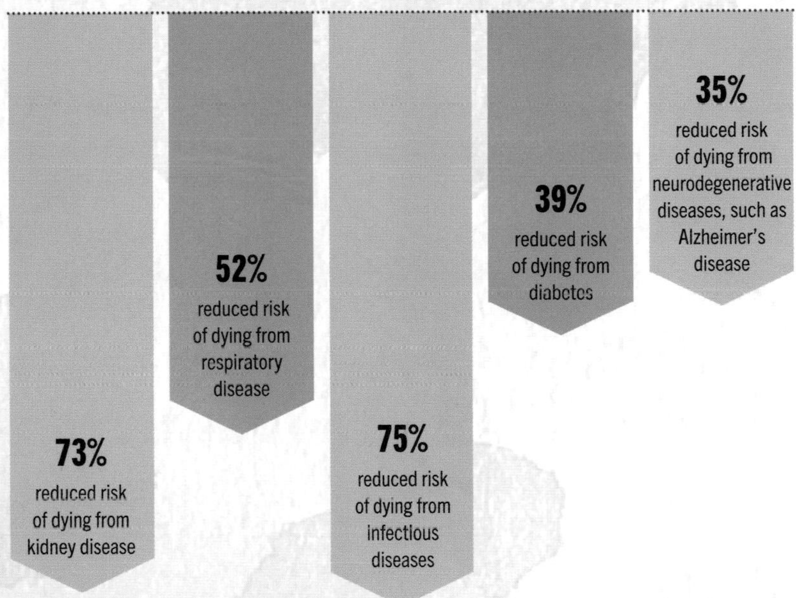

Helping tackle obesity

Research confirms that eating nuts regularly doesn't cause weight gain and may aid weight loss. In one study of 51,000 women, those who ate nuts at least twice a week gained less weight over 8 years than those who avoided them.

Prevent gallstones

One large study found that women who ate at least 1oz (28g) of nuts five times a week had a 25 percent lower risk of getting gallstones. Another study found that for nut-eating men, the risk of getting gallstones was 30 percent lower.

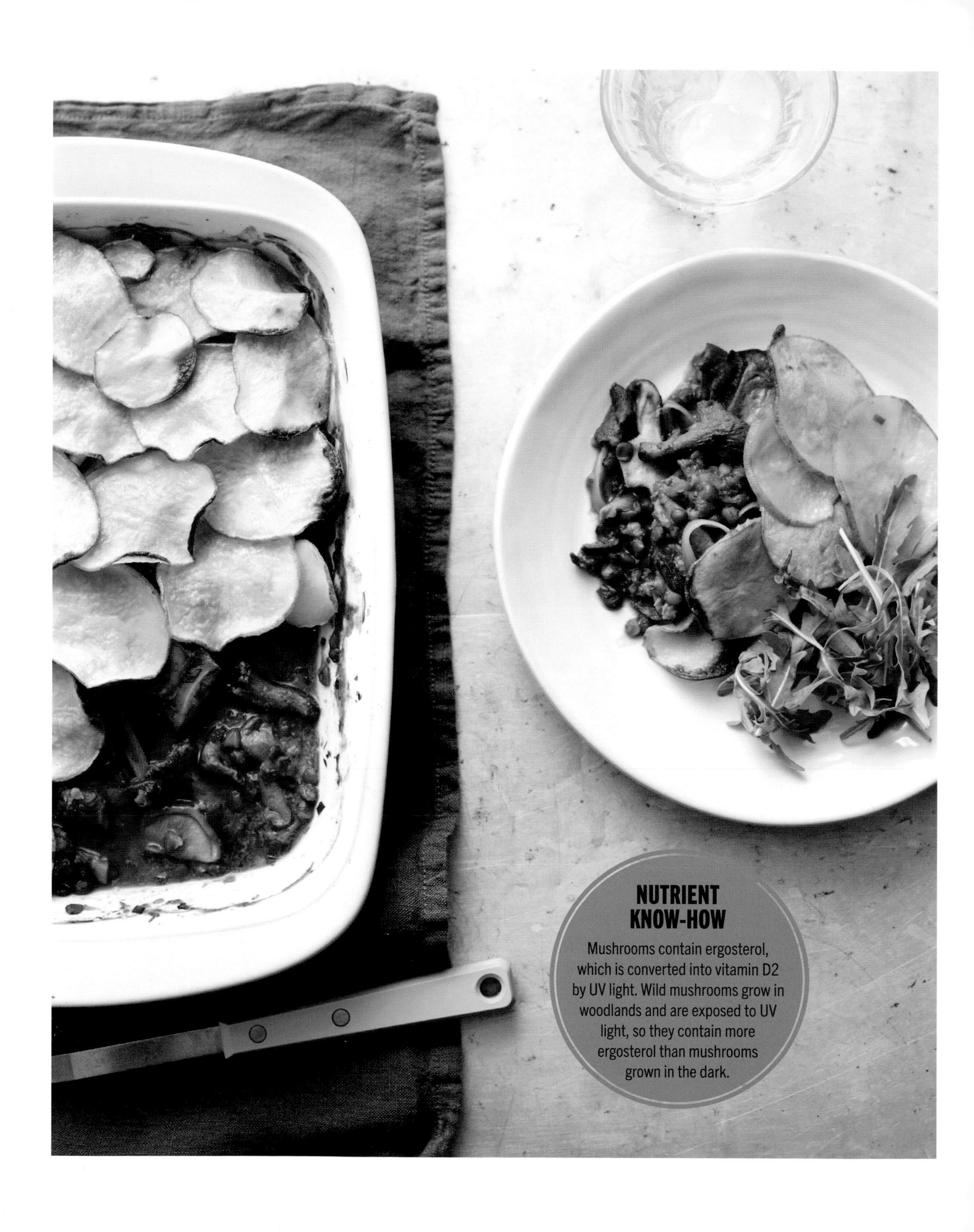

NUTRIENT KNOW-HOW

Mushrooms contain ergosterol, which is converted into vitamin D2 by UV light. Wild mushrooms grow in woodlands and are exposed to UV light, so they contain more ergosterol than mushrooms grown in the dark.

THE BRAIN | VISION | HEARING & BALANCE | ORAL HEALTH | IMMUNITY | BONES & MUSCLES | SKIN & SENSATION | THE LUNGS | HEART & BLOOD | GUT HEALTH | URINARY HEALTH | WOMEN'S HEALTH

WILD MUSHROOM PIE

A heart-warming and health-giving pie that, thanks to the mushrooms, supports immunity and counters the inflammation that promotes aging.

SERVES **2**

Ingredients

- ¾oz (20g) dried porcini mushrooms
- 2 tbsp olive oil, plus 1 tbsp extra
- 2 echalion or banana shallots, cut into wedges
- 2 garlic cloves, sliced
- 10oz (300g) mixed mushrooms (such as shiitake, oyster, or forestière)
- 14oz (400g) can green lentils, rinsed and drained
- 2 tbsp chopped tarragon leaves
- 1 tsp Szechuan peppercorns, ground
- 3½oz (100g) low-fat Greek yogurt
- 1 medium potato (6¾oz/190g), any type, scrubbed
- 2oz (50g) arugula leaves, to serve

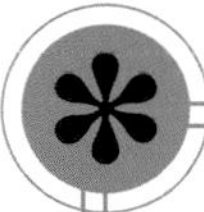

Smart swaps

- Swap the lentils for **kidney beans** to get extra fiber and calcium. Canned kidney beans contain 39 percent more heart-friendly fiber and three times more bone-building calcium than canned lentils.
- Replace the tarragon with diced **red chili** if you want to lose weight and like it spicy. Capsaicin, the compound in chili that gives it its heat, has been found to help us burn more calories.

1 Soak the porcini mushrooms in ⅔ cup (150ml) of hot water for 15–20 minutes until softened. Preheat the oven to 400°F (200°C).

2 Meanwhile, heat 2 tablespoons of oil in a frying pan over medium heat. Cook the shallots for 4–5 minutes until soft, then add the garlic and cook for 1 minute.

3 When the porcini mushrooms have rehydrated, remove them from their liquid, setting aside the soaking water. Thickly slice the porcini and the other mushrooms and add them to the pan. Lower the heat and cook gently for 5 minutes, stirring occasionally.

4 Strain the porcini's soaking water, and pour it into the pan along with the lentils, tarragon, and Szechuan peppercorns. Stir and cook for 2–3 minutes, then remove the pan from the heat and stir in the Greek yogurt. Transfer the mushroom mixture to an ovenproof dish (8in/20cm).

5 Slice the potato very thinly (about ⅛in/3mm) and arrange the slices over the mushrooms, overlapping the edges of potato and filling the gaps, so that the pie doesn't dry out in the oven.

6 Use a pastry brush to coat the potato topping with the remaining oil. Then put the dish in the oven for 20–25 minutes until the potato is cooked and starting to crisp. Serve with arugula.

NUTRITION PER SERVING Calories **438** Total fat **18.6g** Saturated fat **2.9g** Cholesterol **1mg** Carbohydrates **51.2g** Dietary fiber **10.3g** Sugars **6.7g** Protein **19.5g** Sodium **111mg**

OVEN-ROASTED CHICKEN AND VEGGIES

A low-fat, high-protein meal with a triumvirate of vegetables, which ups heart and digestive benefits.

SERVES **2**

Ingredients

2 skinless chicken breasts (about 5½oz/150g each)
freshly ground black pepper
1½ tbsp canola oil
14oz (400g) sweet potato, skin-on, cut into chunks
5¾oz (160g) cauliflower, broken into florets
5¾oz (160g) green cabbage, shredded
5¾oz (160g) snow peas
1 tbsp reduced-sodium gravy granules (from packet; optional)

1 Preheat the oven to 400°F (200°C). Place the chicken into a snug ovenproof dish and season with black pepper. Lightly oil a piece of parchment paper and lay it oil side down on top and tuck in around the chicken.

2 Coat the potato chunks in the remaining oil in another oven dish. Roast the chicken and the potatoes for 25–30 minutes, or until the chicken is cooked through.

3 Steam the cauliflower and cabbage for 5 minutes and the snow peas for the final 2–3 minutes. If using the gravy, make up with ⅓ cup (100ml) of cooking juices and boiling water. Serve the chicken with vegetables and gravy.

NUTRITION PER SERVING Calories **499** Total fat **11.9g** Saturated fat **1.9g** Cholesterol **105mg** Carbohydrates **56g** Dietary fiber **14.2g** Sugars **20.6g** Protein **45.3g** Sodium **389mg**

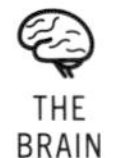
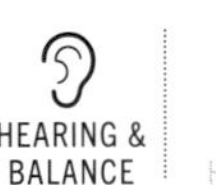
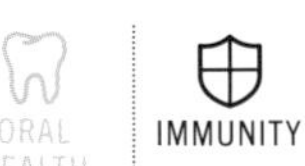
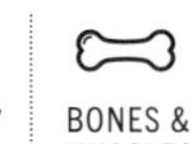
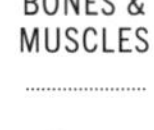
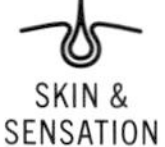
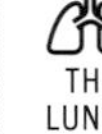
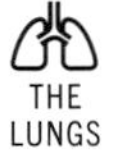
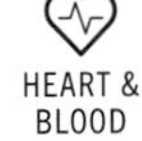
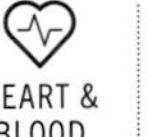
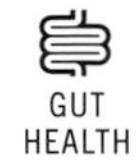
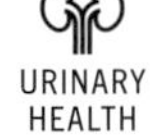
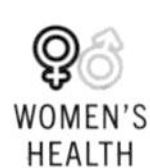

THE BRAIN | VISION | HEARING & BALANCE | ORAL HEALTH | IMMUNITY | BONES & MUSCLES
SKIN & SENSATION | THE LUNGS | HEART & BLOOD | GUT HEALTH | URINARY HEALTH | WOMEN'S HEALTH

ROASTED GREEK VEGGIES WITH FETA

This rainbow of vegetables offers a powerful mix of health-promoting antioxidants.

SERVES **2**

Ingredients

1 small red onion, cut into wedges
1 red bell pepper and 1 green bell pepper, cut into chunks
1 small eggplant, thickly sliced
1 zucchini, thickly sliced
1 tbsp olive oil
1 tbsp balsamic vinegar
oregano, to taste
freshly ground black pepper
½ x 14oz (400g) can green beans in water, rinsed and drained
1¼oz (40g) reduced-fat feta cheese
2 whole-wheat pita breads, toasted
4 tbsp fat-free Greek yogurt

1 Preheat the oven to 400°F (200°C). Toss the vegetables with the oil, balsamic, and oregano. Season with black pepper. Roast for 30–40 minutes until the vegetables are browned, adding the beans for the last 5 minutes.

2 Divide the vegetables between two plates and crumble over the feta. Serve with the pita breads and yogurt.

NUTRITION PER SERVING Calories **414** Total fat **10.3g** Saturated fat **3.4g** Cholesterol **23mg** Carbohydrates **56g** Dietary fiber **16.7g** Sugars **18.9g** Protein **25.9g** Sodium **617mg**

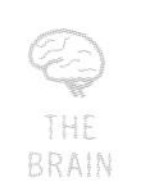
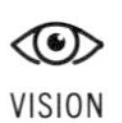
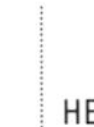
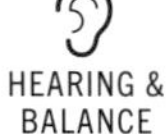
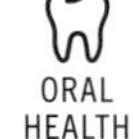
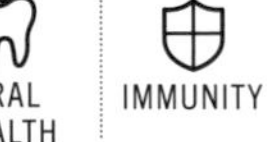
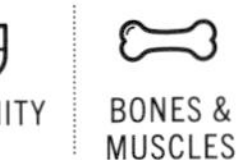
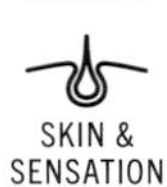
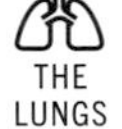
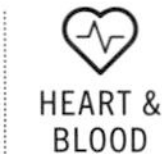
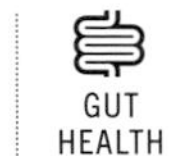
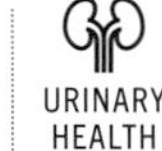
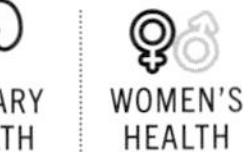

THE BRAIN | VISION | HEARING & BALANCE | ORAL HEALTH | IMMUNITY | BONES & MUSCLES
SKIN & SENSATION | THE LUNGS | HEART & BLOOD | GUT HEALTH | URINARY HEALTH | WOMEN'S HEALTH

HOT AND CRISPY SALMON

Tangy on the tastebuds and packed with omega-3 fats, this satisfying dish supports brain health.

SERVES **2**

Ingredients

9oz (250g) new potatoes
2 skinless wild salmon fillets (about 4oz/120g each), patted dry
6 tbsp breadcrumbs from 1 slice whole-wheat bread
1 tbsp horseradish sauce
zest of ½ lemon (reserve the lemon to cut into wedges as a garnish)
freshly ground black pepper
5¾oz (160g) carrots, cut into batons
5¾oz (160g) green cabbage, finely shredded

1 Preheat the oven to 400°F (200°C). Put the potatoes into a large pan (one which can hold a steaming basket), cover with water, bring to a boil, then simmer the potatoes for 20 minutes.

2 Mix the breadcrumbs with the horseradish and lemon zest. Lay the salmon fillets in a nonstick baking sheet and press the breadcrumb mix equally on top with a few grinds of black pepper; bake for 10–12 minutes.

3 Steam the carrots (above the potatoes) for 10 minutes, adding the cabbage for the last 2 minutes. Serve the salmon with the potatoes, vegetables, and lemon wedges.

NUTRITION PER SERVING Calories **403** Total fat **13.9g** Saturated fat **2.9g** Cholesterol **62mg** Carbohydrates **37.8g** Dietary fiber **10.2g** Sugars **12.1g** Protein **33.2g** Sodium **237mg**

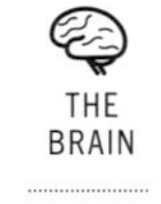
THE BRAIN
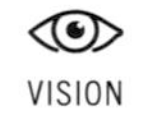
VISION
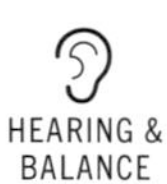
HEARING & BALANCE
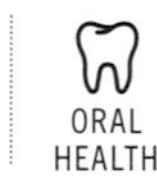
ORAL HEALTH
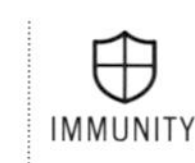
IMMUNITY
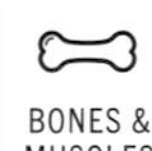
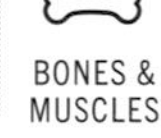
BONES & MUSCLES
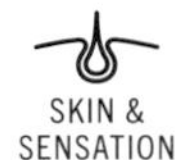
SKIN & SENSATION
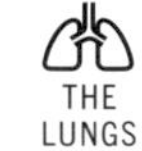
THE LUNGS
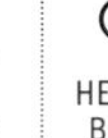
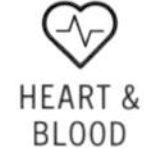
HEART & BLOOD
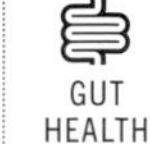
GUT HEALTH
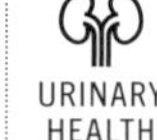
URINARY HEALTH
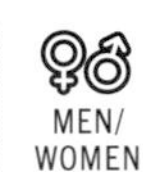
MEN/ WOMEN

QUORN 5-SPICE STIR-FRY

This vegetarian protein comes with a longevity-friendly, low-fat, high-fiber content that is filling, offers umami tastes, and protects against cancer.

SERVES **2**

Ingredients

4oz (120g) raw buckwheat (soba) noodles
1 tbsp sunflower oil
1–2 garlic cloves, finely chopped
4in (10cm) fresh ginger, peeled and finely chopped
7oz (200g) Quorn, cut into bite-sized pieces
Chinese 5-spice powder, to taste
14oz (400g) package stir-fry vegetables

1 Cook the noodles according to the package instructions, drain, and set aside.

2 Heat the oil in a nonstick frying pan or wok. Gently cook the garlic and ginger for 1 minute until softened.

3 Add the Quorn and the 5-spice powder and cook until lightly browned. Next, add the stir-fry vegetables and cook for 3–4 minutes until the vegetables are softened but still crispy. Toss well with the cooked noodles and serve.

NUTRITION PER SERVING Calories **395** Total fat **10.4g** Saturated fat **2.5g** Cholesterol **0mg** Carbohydrates **49.7g** Dietary fiber **16.2g** Sugars **7.6g** Protein **26.7g** Sodium **402mg**

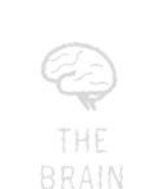
THE BRAIN
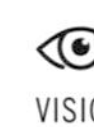
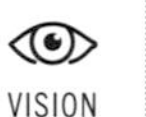
VISION
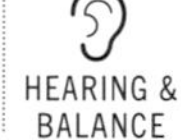
HEARING & BALANCE
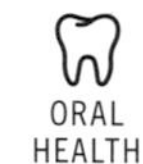
ORAL HEALTH
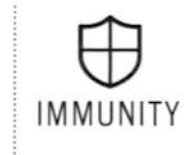
IMMUNITY
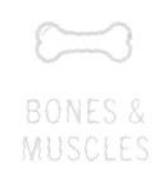
BONES & MUSCLES
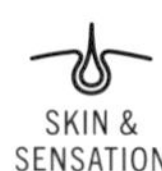
SKIN & SENSATION
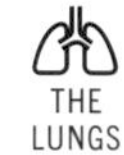
THE LUNGS
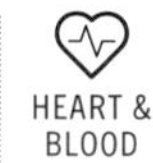
HEART & BLOOD
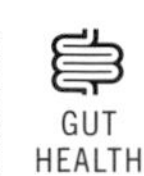
GUT HEALTH
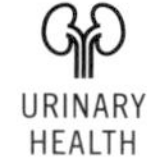
URINARY HEALTH
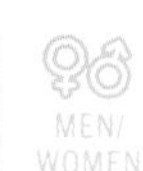
MEN/ WOMEN

-SUPERGROUP-

SPICES

The medicinal and longevity properties of spices have been known about since ancient times. Now scientific studies are providing evidence to back up their potential health benefits, which include cancer protection and improving memory. Plus, they add flavor to food, helping us to slash our salt intake.

WHICH SPICES?

All spices are antioxidant boosters, but different spices have particular benefits.

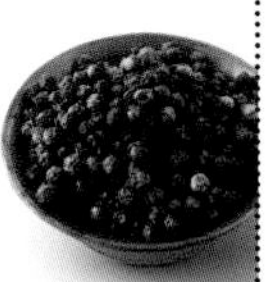

Black pepper

- Is heart-friendly, as it cuts the need for salt
- Contains digestion-boosting piperine

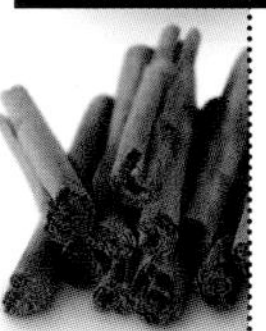

Cinnamon

- May help lower blood sugar levels, so is useful for weight management and those with diabetes

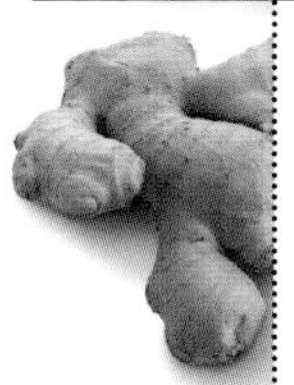

Ginger

- Contains gingerol, an anti-inflammatory that helps ease osteoarthritis pain
- Is known for helping to ease nausea

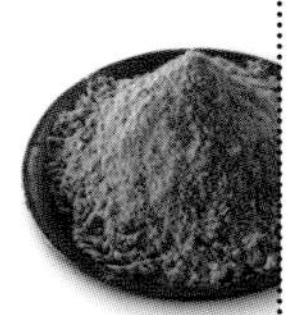

Turmeric

- Is packed with curcumin, which helps relieve long-term inflammation
- May benefit brain health in particular

HOW MUCH?

Add spices liberally to your meals every day for salt-free flavorings.

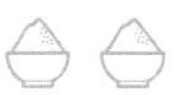

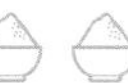
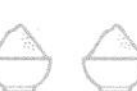

BEST BOUGHT

Buy fresh, dried, or frozen spices. Dried are a more concentrated source of antioxidants. Freezing preserves the antioxidants in fresh spices.

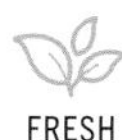

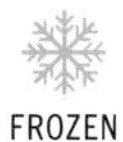

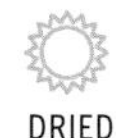

HOW TO STORE

Keep dried spices in a sealed container in a cool, dark place. Store fresh spices in the refrigerator and frozen in the freezer.

RAW OR COOKED?

Use raw or cooked for health benefits.

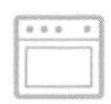

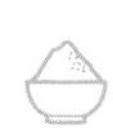

Pain reliever

Ginger's strong anti-inflammatory action may help to relieve pain associated with conditions such as arthritis. A review of five studies found taking ginger reduced pain by nearly a third and disability by 22 percent in people with osteoarthritis. Another study found ginger was just as effective as an anti-inflammatory pain killer at reducing painful periods.

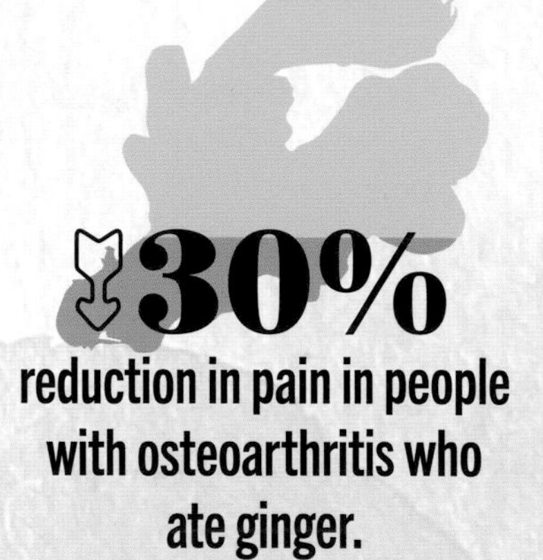

30%

reduction in pain in people with osteoarthritis who ate ginger.

Fights inflammation

Lab-based tests show many spices act as anti-inflammatories, but it's curcumin (in turmeric) and ginger that top the list. Several studies show signs of inflammation are reduced in people when capsules containing these spices are taken. It's good news for fighting aging, as long-term inflammation can lead to health problems such as inflammatory bowel disease, some cancers, dementia, and arthritis.

Protect against cancer

Several spices have been linked to protecting against cancer, including ginger and black pepper. But the strongest evidence so far is for turmeric. Several lab-based studies show curcumin in turmeric seems able to kill cancer cells, particularly in the breast, colon, stomach, and skin, plus it even seems to prevent more from growing.

Brain boosters

Early lab-based studies suggest curcumin, which is found in turmeric, may prevent amyloid-beta plaques forming in the brain—one of the hallmarks of Alzheimer's disease—and may even help break them down. Far more studies are needed to see whether the same beneficial effects are seen in people.

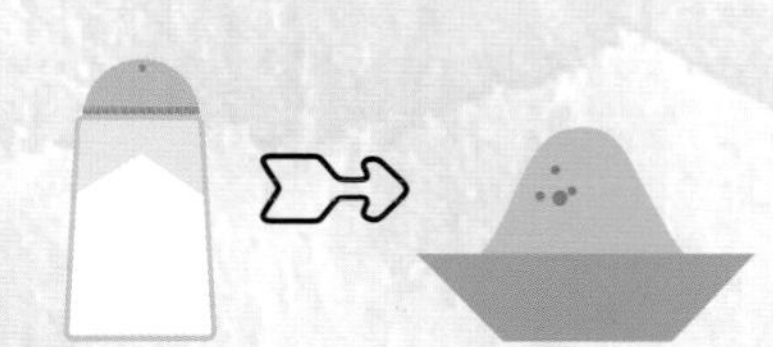

½ tsp

decrease in daily salt intake of adults who learned how to cook with spices instead of salt.

Sodium reducers

Using spices in place of salt means dishes contain less sodium. This replacement of salt offers major health benefits, as high sodium intakes are linked to high blood pressure, a condition that can cause heart disease and may lead to blindness, kidney failure, and cognitive impairment.

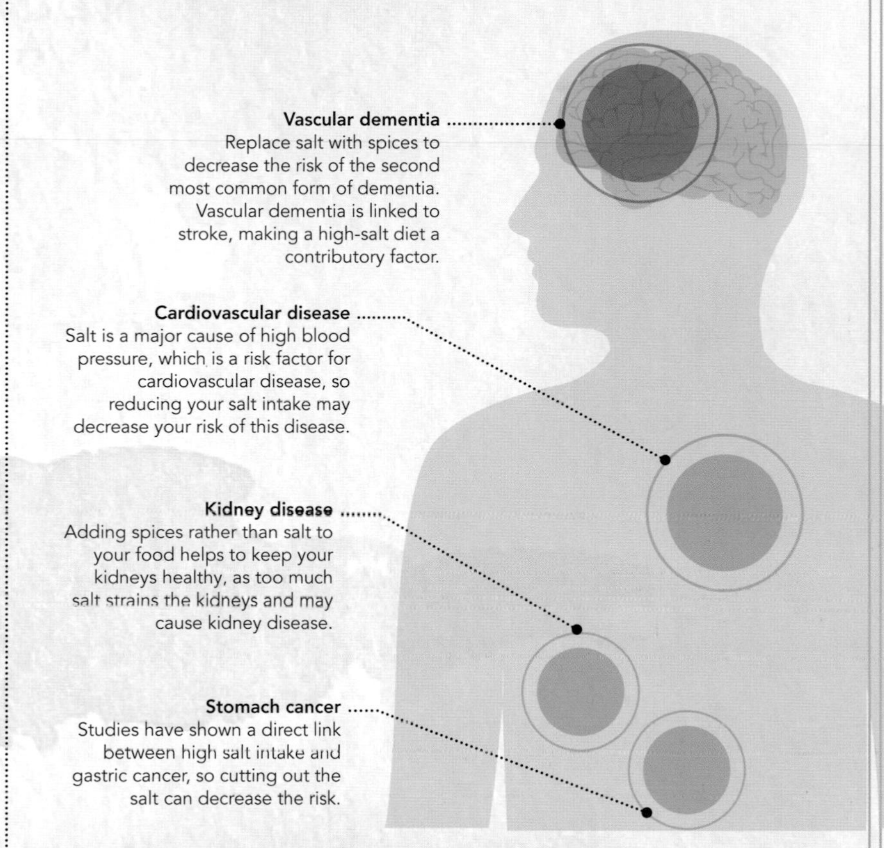

Antioxidant bonus

Spices are full of antioxidants. This is good news for boosting longevity because antioxidants mop up an excess of free radicals, molecules (see also page 11) that are thought to cause many age-related diseases, including cancer and dementia.

Diabetes aid

Many studies show that cinnamon may help to improve insulin sensitivity and beneficially aid blood sugar control. One review of studies found that cinnamon significantly improved fasting blood sugar levels in people with type 2 diabetes.

THE BRAIN | VISION | HEARING & BALANCE | ORAL HEALTH | IMMUNITY | BONES & MUSCLES | SKIN & SENSATION | THE LUNGS | HEART & BLOOD | GUT HEALTH | URINARY HEALTH | WOMEN'S HEALTH

TURKEY STEAK WITH KALE AND SQUASH

A rare meat-containing dinner. Turkey provides just enough fat to help your body absorb the beta-carotene in the squash and the lutein and zeaxanthin in the kale.

SERVES **2**

Ingredients

1 small butternut squash (about 1lb 2oz/500g flesh)

2½ tbsp olive oil

5 garlic cloves, unpeeled

2 quick-cook, thin turkey steaks (about 9oz/250g total)

freshly ground black pepper, to taste

4 tbsp red wine vinegar

1 tbsp whole-grain mustard

1 small red onion, finely chopped

7oz (200g) shredded kale

1 Preheat the oven to 400°F (200°C). Peel and seed the squash, then cut it into ¼in- (5mm-) thick slices. Toss the slices with 1 tablespoon of the oil and 4 garlic cloves. Place the slices on a baking sheet and spread them out so they cook in a single layer (you may need two sheets), then roast in the oven for 20 minutes.

2 Put a griddle pan over medium-high heat. Place the turkey steaks on a plate and rub them with ½ tablespoon of the oil and a halved garlic clove. Season with black pepper and set aside.

3 In a bowl, peel and mash the garlic cloves from the roasting pan into the red wine vinegar, then stir in the mustard and ¼ cup (60ml) water to make a dressing.

4 Heat a large frying pan with 1 tablespoon of oil. Add the red onion to the pan, frying it for 1–2 minutes until it is just starting to cook. Throw in the shredded kale and stir-fry for another minute. Add the mustard "dressing" to the pan. Allow the liquid to bubble, putting a lid on top of the pan and turning the heat to low. Leave to cook down for 2–3 minutes.

5 Place the turkey steaks on the hot griddle, cooking for 2½ minutes on each side. Transfer the steaks to a warmed plate and allow them to rest for 1 minute.

6 To serve, place the roasted squash slices on a plate with a pile of greens. Slice the turkey steak diagonally and arrange on top.

NUTRITION PER SERVING Calories **409** Total fat **17.4g** Saturated fat **2.6g** Cholesterol **71mg** Carbohydrates **25.7g** Dietary fiber **10.8g** Sugars **14.9g** Protein **38g** Sodium **240mg**

Smart swaps

- Use **turkey-leg** meat if you prefer. Although it contains more fat than the breast meat, it has double the vitamin B12 and three times more iron and zinc—all important for a strong immune system.
- Replace the turkey steaks with fresh **tuna steaks** to get three times more iodine, nine times more selenium, and 10 times more vitamin D—all nutrients that many people are low in.

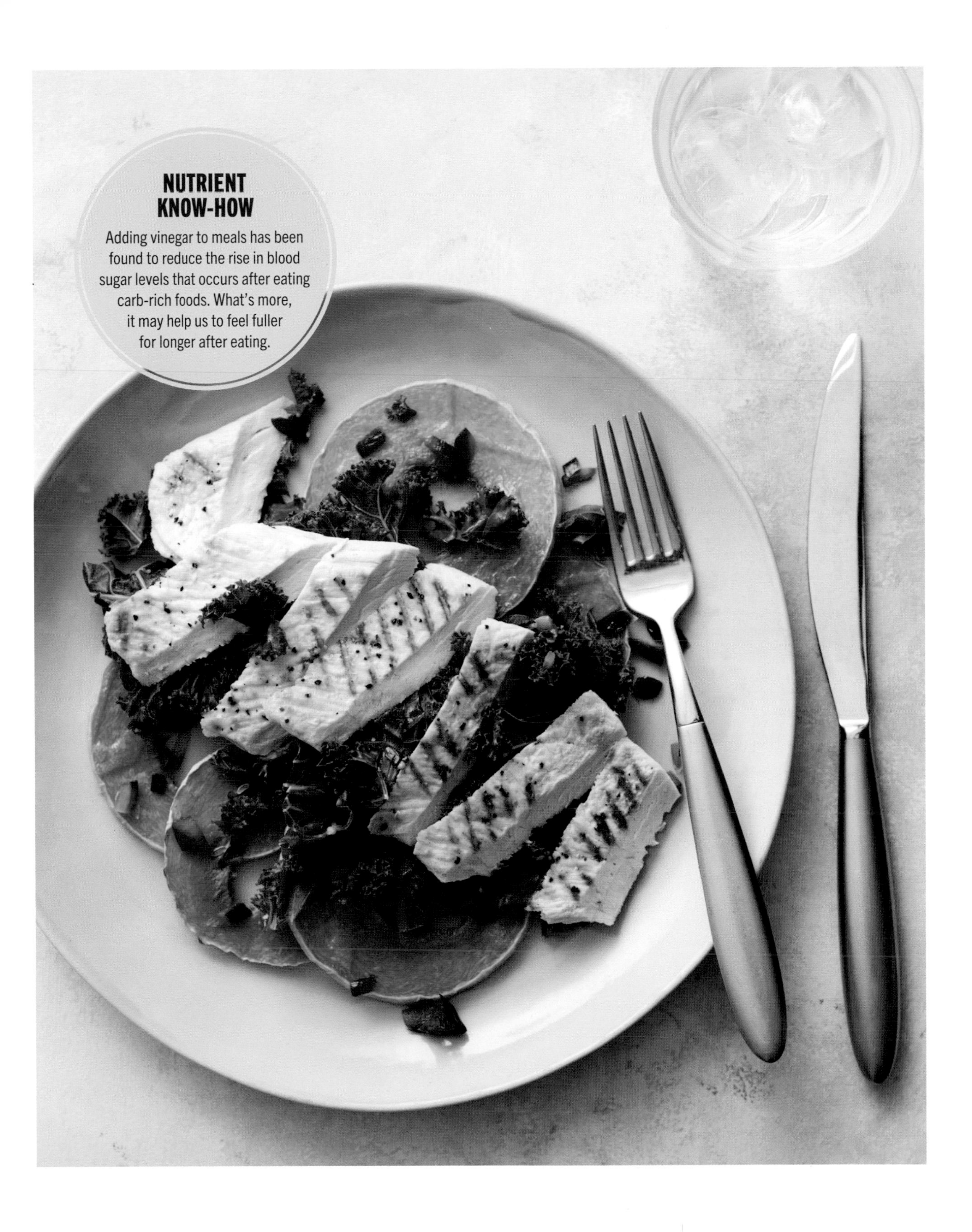
NUTRIENT KNOW-HOW
Adding vinegar to meals has been found to reduce the rise in blood sugar levels that occurs after eating carb-rich foods. What's more, it may help us to feel fuller for longer after eating.

-SUPERGROUP-

SQUASHES

These brightly colored vegetables are especially rich in carotenoids, which have been linked to keeping the eyes healthy, as well as protecting against heart disease and some cancers. All varieties of squashes contain vitamin C and fiber, but the amount and types of carotenoids vary according to color.

WHICH TO CHOOSE?

Enjoy year-round longevity benefits from these commonly eaten squashes. The colors (orange/winter and green/summer) signify different benefits.

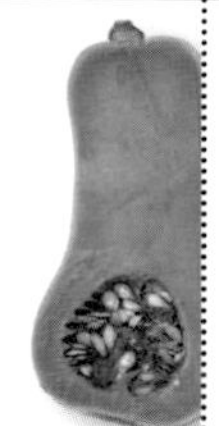

Butternut squash

- Is the best natural plant source of cancer-fighting beta-cryptoxanthin
- Is one of the richest sources of vitamin C in the squash family

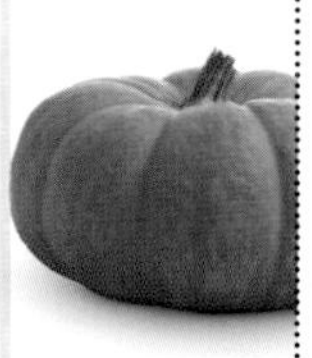

Pumpkin

- Is an excellent source of beta-carotene, a powerful antioxidant that the body uses to make vitamin A
- Seeds contain mood-boosting tryptophan

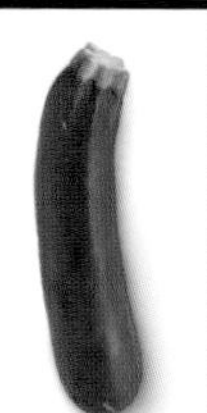

Zucchini

- Are the best providers of zeaxanthin and lutein, essential for good eye health
- Provide a good amount of immune-boosting vitamin C

HOW MUCH?

Eat squashes three times a week.

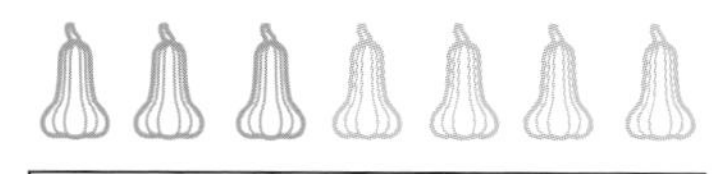

BEST BOUGHT

Buy winter squashes with a dull skin and summer squashes with a glossy skin.

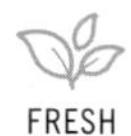

HOW TO STORE

Keep winter squashes in a cool place and summer squashes in the refrigerator.

RAW OR COOKED?

Cook winter squashes. Either eat the skin, peel close to the skin, or bake and then scrape out—the skin and flesh near it is richest in carotenoids. Eat all parts of summer squashes raw or cooked.

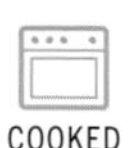

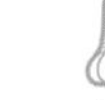

Heart help

Squashes are rich in a number of carotenoids, with butternut squash a particularly good source of beta-cryptoxanthin. Studies have linked good intakes of carotenoids to healthier hearts and a reduced risk of cardiovascular disease and heart attacks. A large part of this protective factor is likely to be due to their powerful antioxidant effect.

33%

less chance of having an acute heart attack for those with the highest versus the lowest blood levels of beta-cryptoxanthin in one study.

Good for lung health

Squashes are full of antioxidant nutrients, including vitamin C and carotenoids, as well as vitamin E in pumpkin and butternut squash. These antioxidants help to protect against the damaging effects of oxidative stress in our airways from airborne pollution and irritants, and numerous studies support the link between antioxidants and good lung health.

Boosts immunity

Beta-carotene in squashes is converted into vitamin A in the body, and this nutrient is vital for a strong immune system. It works its immune magic in many ways, as it is important for healthy skin and eyes, plus the respiratory, gastrointestinal, and genitourinary tracts, all of which act as barriers against infections.

Cancer protection

Good intakes of carotenoids, such as beta-carotene and beta-cryptoxanthin, from food are linked to a lower risk of a number of cancers, including those of the lungs, mouth, pharynx, and larynx. A review of studies found those with the highest intakes of carotenoids had a 21 percent lower risk of developing lung cancer than those with the lowest.

57% less risk of developing cancer of the larynx for people with the highest intakes of beta-carotene.

Eye friendly

Squashes benefit our eyes in many ways—whether it's the retina, cornea, or lens (see below and also pages 162–65). Those with orange skins and flesh are packed with alpha-carotene, beta-carotene, and beta-cryptoxanthin, all of which can be converted into vision-friendly vitamin A and then transformed into the light-sensitive pigment rhodopsin. Green-skinned squash, such as zucchini, are rich in lutein and zeaxanthin, which protect against age-related macular degeneration and cataracts.

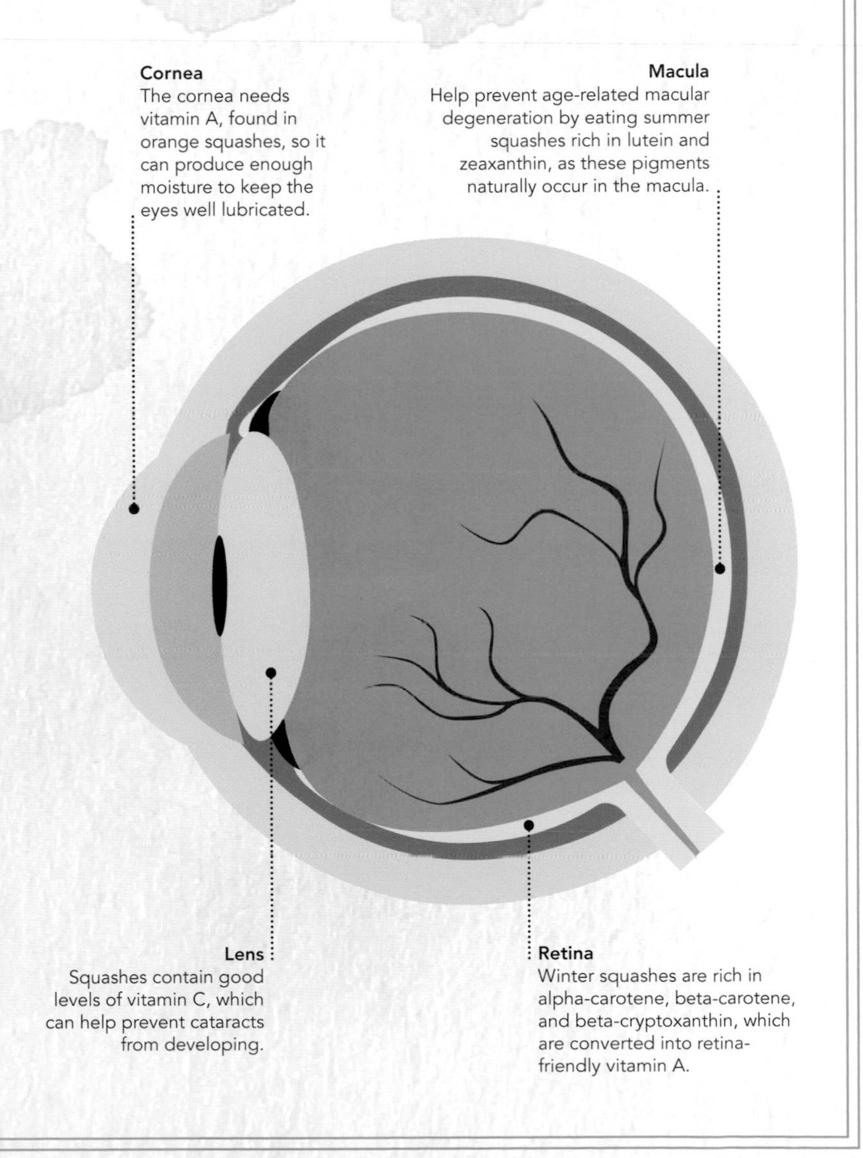

Life beyond the plan

After 4 weeks on the longevity eating plan, you'll be feeling completely rejuvenated. So what's next? You should now feel confident in what eating habits and foods make a positive difference to health. Use the prompts here to continue the good work and reap the rewards of a healthy, happy, and extended life.

6 STEPS TO LIFE-LONG HEALTHY EATING

1} BUILD UP RECIPE RESOURCES

Having successfully followed the plan for a month, you may want to know how to branch out for extra recipe ideas. Use your newfound knowledge to expand your stash of longevity recipes. Simply repeat the 28-day plan, if you've strayed far from the ideal, to get back on track.

2} NEVER SKIP BREAKFAST

We've said it before, but we'll say it again: avoid missing out on breakfast at all costs. Leaving time for a healthy and nutritious breakfast is essential for setting up good eating habits for the day. Plus, skipping a meal makes it really hard to meet daily nutrient needs.

3} MIX AND MATCH

Enjoy using every recipe in the book; make the most of all the dishes, even those from weeks 1 and 2, with a little tweak. Make breakfasts from the first 2 weeks slightly bigger by adding extra fruits or more whole grains. Scale down dinners by cutting portions a little.

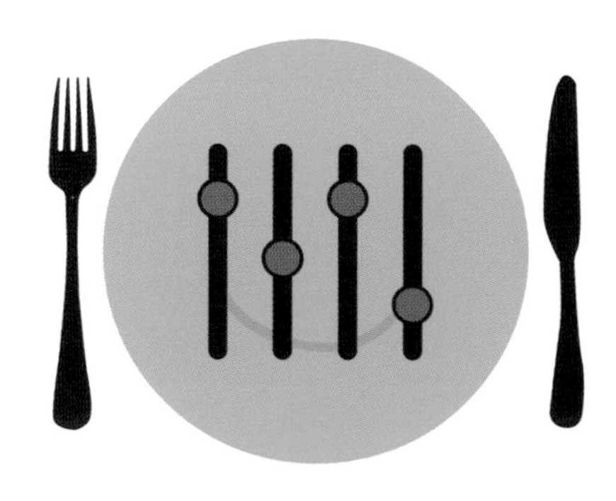

4} GET ORGANIZED

Batch cook and freeze your favorite recipes—that way, you will always have healthy "ready meals" on hand for times when you're tired or pressed for time.

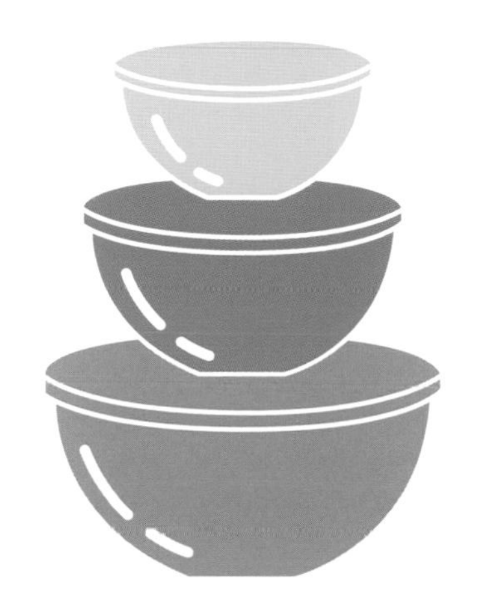

6} SWAP IN NEW INGREDIENTS

Experiment with the plan's recipes. Don't be afraid to adapt the recipes—not only will that add variety to your diet, but it will also enable you to take advantage of seasonal ingredients. For example, swap pasta for buckwheat noodles, rice for whole-wheat couscous, tuna for salmon, clams for mussels, or cherries for blackberries.

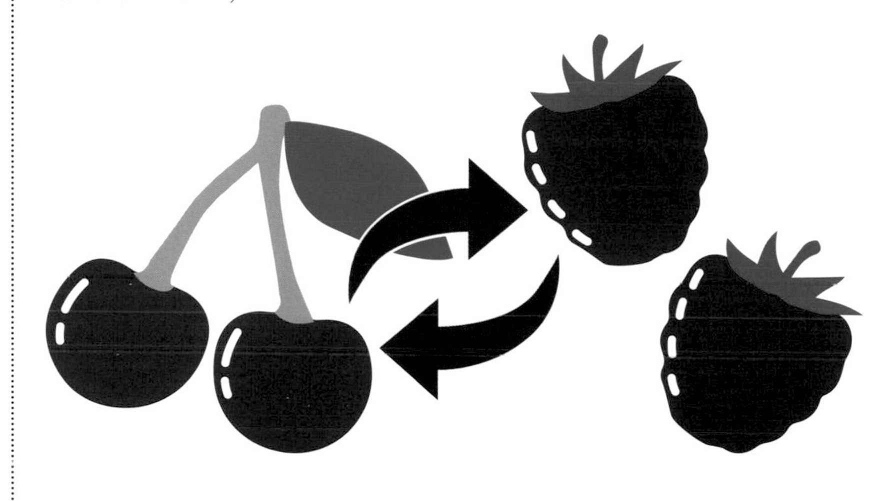

5} WRITE A WEEKLY MENU

Plan your meals each week, then write a shopping list to ensure you have all the ingredients you need. If a trip to the supermarket ends up with lots of impulse purchasing (how did that chocolate pudding get in there?), then perhaps start shopping for groceries online.

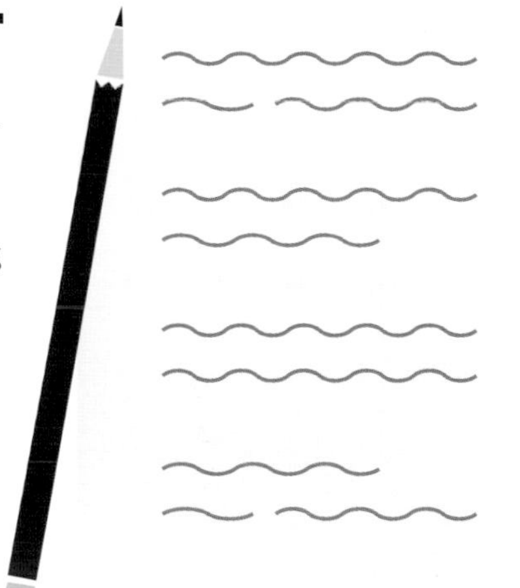

Build a longevity pantry

While following the plan, you'll have started to buy new ingredients. Build on this revitalized pantry and add to this weekly (with a novel whole grain or some frozen edamame), so that your kitchen cabinets and freezer soon contain a stash of the right foods to create healthy meals when time is short or you've run out of fresh ingredients.

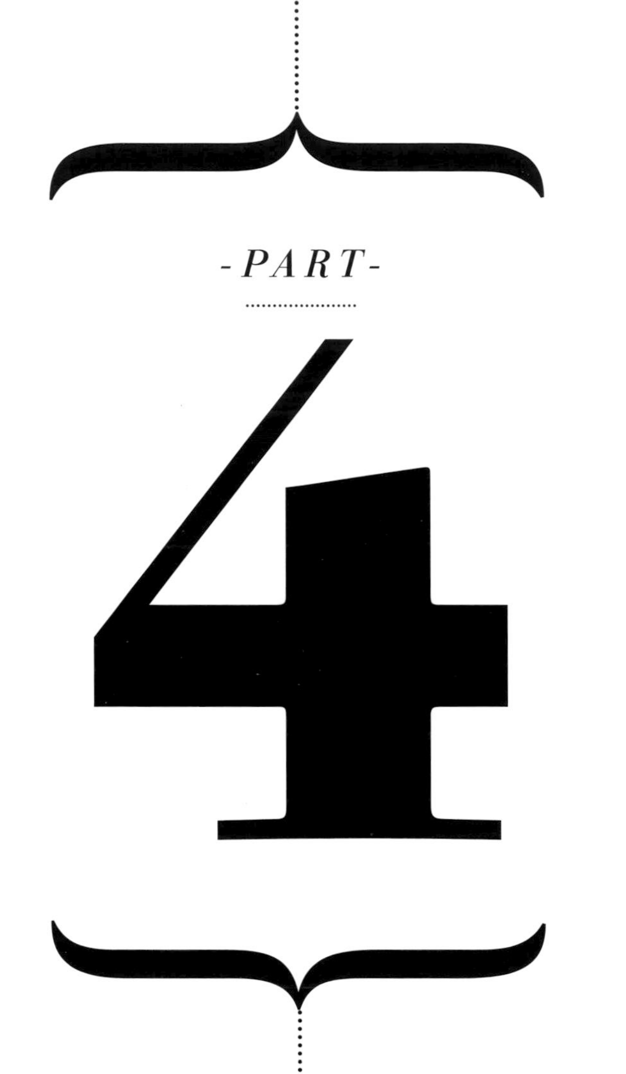
-PART-
4

How the body changes with age

Find out how foods can counteract age-related physical changes, along with the foods to eat for optimal health and for prevention of disease.

THE BRAIN

We can't reverse all the brain changes that come with getting older. But as we find out about how aging affects the brain, research offers up new food solutions to slow cognitive decline, boost mood, improve memory, and protect against dementia and stroke.

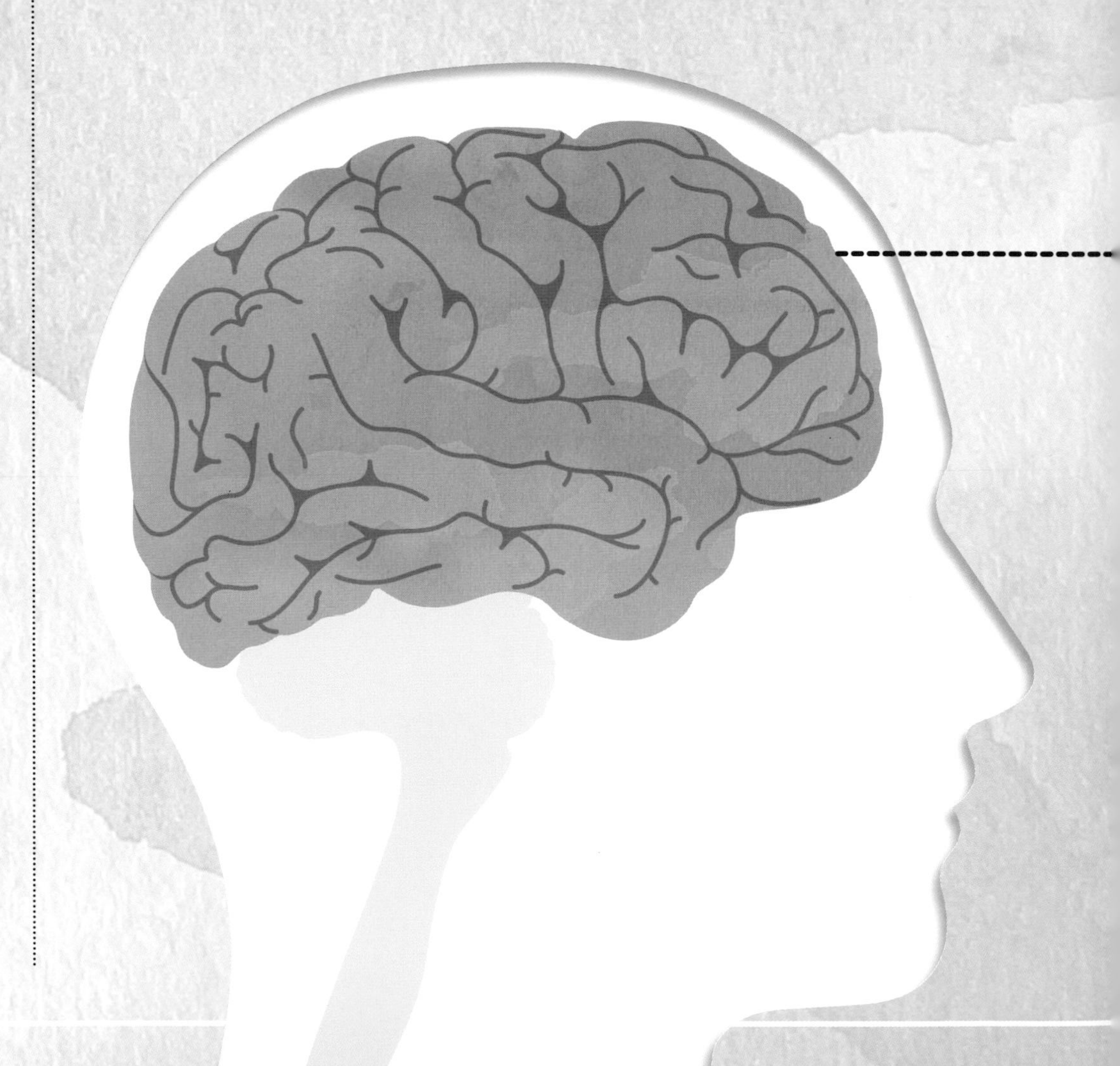

AS WE AGE ...

Our life experiences continue to shape our brains alongside a sequence of physical and chemical changes. Discover how what you eat can help right the balance of age-related changes.

New brain cells are made

An adult brain has about 100 billion nerve cells—or neurons. As we get older, these numbers decrease, and this decline tends to start in our 20s. But it's reassuring to know that certain parts of our brain continue to create new neurons via the process of neurogenesis. The hippocampus (a part of the brain that's key in learning and memory formation) is one such center. And by the age of 50, all the neurons in the hippocampus we were born with will have been replaced by new ones. Research shows that we can influence neurogenesis with our lifestyle (via physical activity and dealing with stress), as well as through what we eat (with berries being heralded for their neurogenetic benefits).

The brain shrinks

The brain is super-organized: the cell bodies of neurons occupy its gray matter, while its white matter is home to the connecting fibers between neurons. From young adulthood, the brain's white matter is diminishing—about 15 percent across a lifetime—and this white matter plays an important role in mood, walking, and balance. Information processing, thinking, and memory are functions that reside within the gray matter. The volume of gray matter also diminishes with age, but it's not until significant reductions are seen that cognitive decline and dementia arise. Foods can counteract age-related reductions in cognitive powers; turn to pages 158–59 to find out how.

Age-related brain shrinkage is not necessarily a sign of cognitive decline.

Sleep patterns can change

The body's master clock, which sits in the brain's hypothalamus, controls the production of various hormones, including those that influence sleep—melatonin and serotonin. The rhythm of changing levels of these hormones gives us our sleep/wake cycle. Many people believe that as you get older you need less sleep, but this isn't true: adults continue to need about 7–9 hours of sleep a night. Many healthy older adults report few sleep problems, but some experience a shift in their cycles that causes them to wake up in the early hours of the morning. If your sleep patterns are changing, take a look at what you're eating to see how it can make a difference (see page 161).

CONTINUED

FOODS FOR THE BRAIN

The brain receives a soup of chemicals via the bloodstream that enable it to function. Find out which foods provide key brain-healthy nutrients, which of the recipes are super-healthy for the brain, and what foods you'll need to avoid to lower the risk of disease.

EGGS

Eggs are a rich source of choline (see also page 70), which is vital for the production of one of the brain's neurotransmitters, acetylcholine. What's more, a study has shown that proteins similar to those found in egg whites stimulate brain cells that help us stay awake and alert.

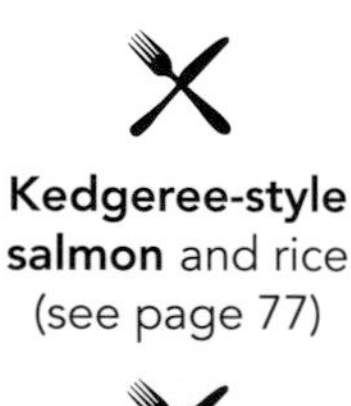

Kedgeree-style salmon and rice (see page 77)

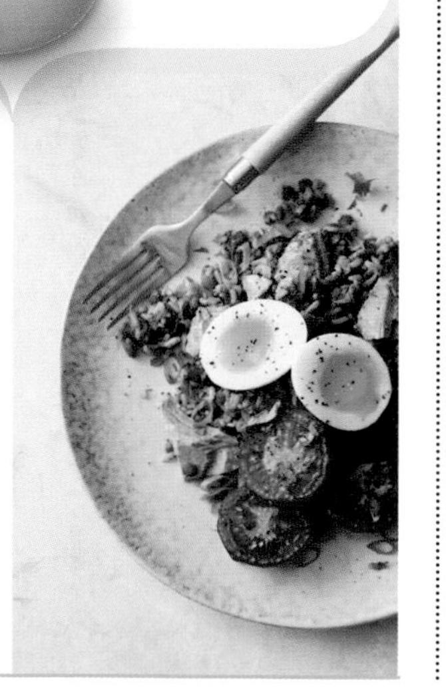

BERRIES

A review of studies published in 2017 found that eating anthocyanin-rich foods improves verbal learning and memory. Previous studies have shown that eating two servings of berries a week can slow down age-related cognitive decline. All red and blue berries contain anthocyanins—they're responsible for their color (see also pages 38 and 60).

Cinnamon toast with blueberry compote (see page 63)

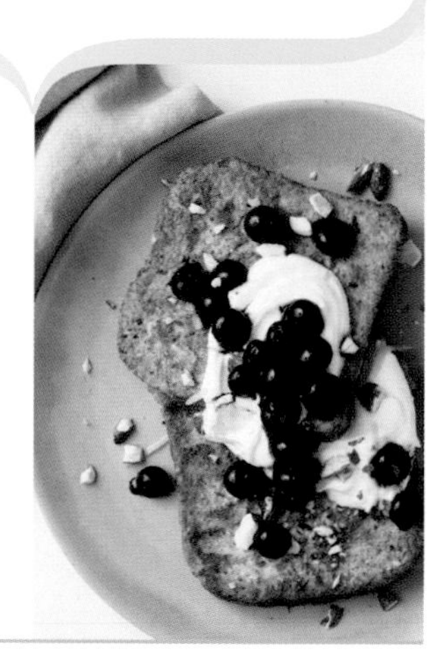

TEA AND COFFEE

Research links a higher intake of caffeine (present in tea and coffee) to a lower risk of dementia. One study found that women with high caffeine intakes had less cognitive decline over 4 years than those consuming low amounts.

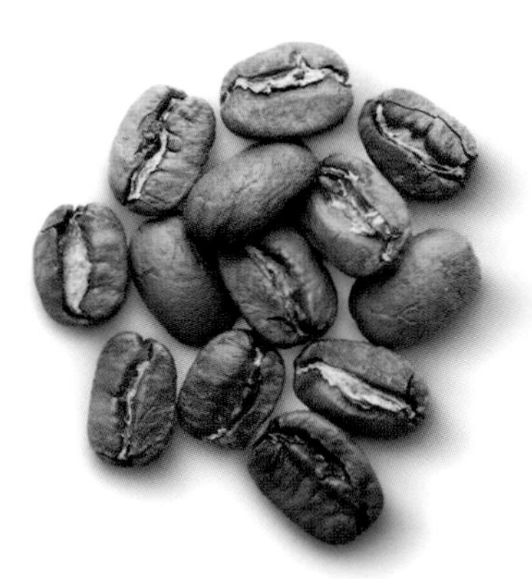

LEAFY GREENS

Folate is a B vitamin that's vital for brain function and emotional well-being. A study found a supplement of folate reduced brain shrinkage in adults at risk of dementia. Spinach, brussels sprouts, and kale top the folate list.

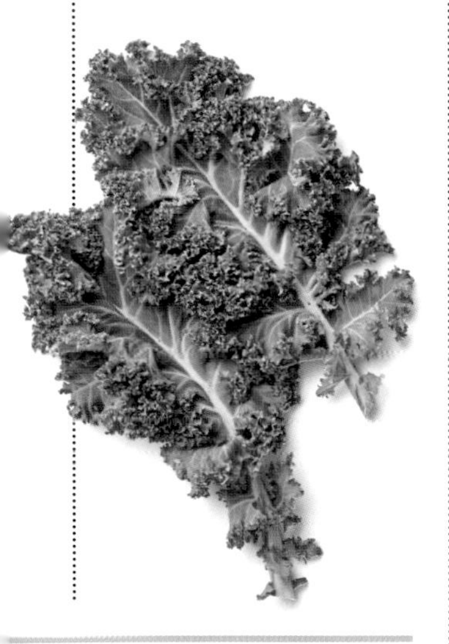

CURRY POWDER

Turmeric is often singled out for its potential protection against dementia via the chemical curcumin. But curry powder (with extra chili, ginger, coriander, cumin, and pepper) may offer even more brain function benefits.

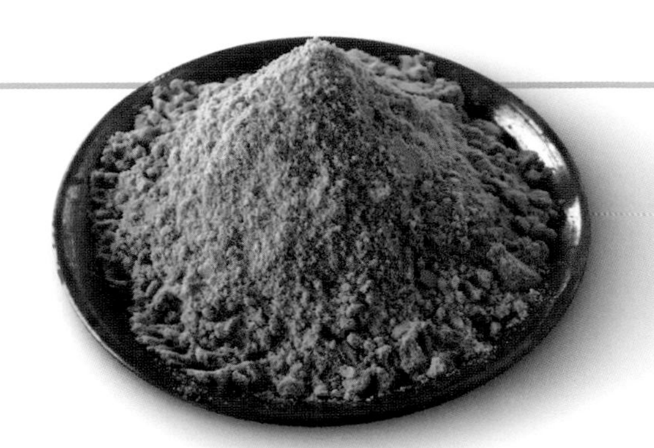

A study found that adults aged 60–93 who ate curry at least once a month performed the best in cognitive tests.

FISH

One of the omega-3 fats found naturally in fish—DHA—is vital for brain function throughout life (see also page 112). All fish, including whitefish and shellfish, contain this omega-3 fat, but oily fish are the richest source, with mackerel ranking at the top.

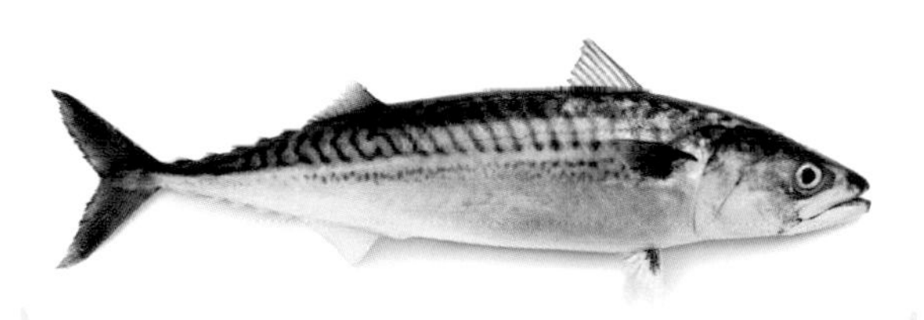

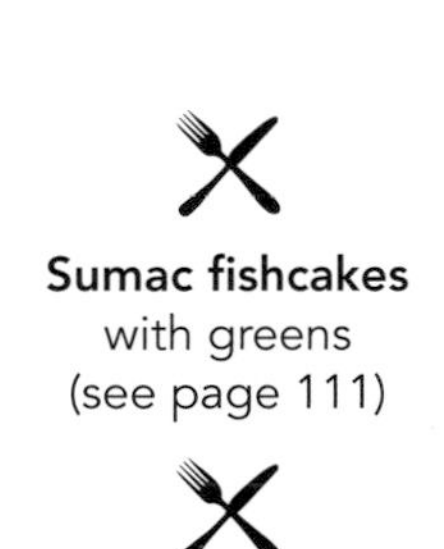

Sumac fishcakes with greens (see page 111)

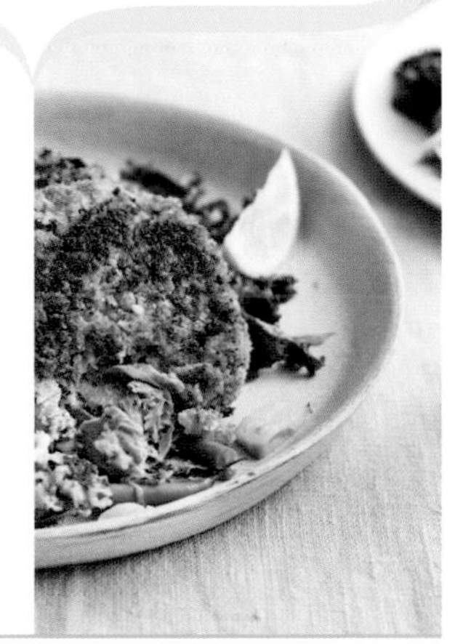

26%

drop in risk of dementia with daily caffeine intakes of two mugs of coffee or three mugs of tea.

Foods to avoid

Evidence suggests risk factors for Alzheimer's disease and dementia are similar to those for heart disease, so a heart-friendly diet (see page 192) that limits sodium and saturated and trans fats (see page 34) is also brain friendly.

- **Sodium** High sodium intake increases the risk of high blood pressure, which in turn increases the risk of having a stroke. Don't add salt during cooking or to meals, limit processed foods, and choose lower-sodium options wherever possible.
- **"Bad" fats** Several, although not all studies, indicate negative relationships between saturated and trans fat intake and risk of cognitive problems. One study showed high intakes of saturated fat (26g a day) were linked to double the risk of developing Alzheimer's disease as those eating 13g a day.

CONTINUED

BRAIN AND MENTAL HEALTH CONDITIONS

The brain is highly responsive to chemical intervention, whether that's through medicines or via foods. Here, we cover common age-related conditions that significantly affect health and how these can be addressed through adapting the foods that you eat.

DEMENTIA

With our aging population, dementia has become a much more familiar term in everyday parlance. But dementia isn't a disease as such; it's an umbrella term for various symptoms, such as memory loss, confusion, and personality changes.

Don't let worries over not being able to remember a name or where you put your to-do list lead you to a self-diagnosis of dementia. The brain's functions—especially in the memory-forming areas—are affected by age, but individuals are affected very differently. That said, keeping mentally sharp can compensate for age-related declines.

A 2016 study found that DHA (an omega-3 fat in fish) boosts the cognitive effects of B vitamins in greens.

Alzheimer's disease is the most common cause of dementia (40–70 percent), followed by vascular dementia (15–30 percent), and a minority with other types. The parts of the brain most affected by Alzheimer's disease are the hippocampus and the amygdala.

While many people with dementia are over 65, dementia is not an inevitable part of aging, though the likelihood of developing dementia does increase with age. Symptoms of dehydration can be confused with dementia; what's more, dehydration can cause and aggravate dementia. So be sure to keep yourself well hydrated (see page 40).

Several studies suggest that "oxidative stress" (see page 10) may play a role in the changes that cause Alzheimer's disease. Such free-radical attacks of brain cells can lead to damage similar to that seen in those with Alzheimer's disease. Since antioxidants counter the effects of free radicals, researchers propose that foods rich in antioxidants can help reduce the likelihood of Alzheimer's disease. A diet rich in fresh fruits and vegetables (and thus antioxidants) also reduces free-radical damage in the blood supply to the brain, which cuts the risk of a stroke (see below).

+ EAT PLENTY
Fresh fruits and vegetables (particularly berries, red bell peppers, leafy greens), fish and shellfish, olive oil, spices

− LIMIT
Processed foods, sodium, saturates

STROKE AND MINI-STROKE

You can think of a stroke as a "brain attack"; similar to a heart attack, in a stroke the blood supply to the brain is cut off suddenly. The exact consequences of a stroke or a mini-stroke (TIA, or transient ischemic attack) depends on where exactly the event happens and for how long the event persisted (and so deprived the brain of vital oxygen and nutrients). To protect your brain against a stroke, you need to look after your heart (see also page 192). Since stroke and heart conditions are major causes of death, all recipes in the longevity eating plan has been designed with these in mind. In essence, to minimize your risk of stroke, eat plenty of antioxidant-rich foods, and avoid salt and refined foods.

EAT PLENTY
Fresh fruits and vegetables (particularly berries, beets, garlic, tomatoes), fish and shellfish, oilive oil

LIMIT
Processed foods, sodium

INSOMNIA

Insomnia—difficulty falling asleep or staying asleep—can have many causes, but improvements in sleep quality and quantity can be linked to diet. Sleep deprivation spells disaster for heart and brain health.

Studies have shown that food can directly affect how well we sleep. Key mineral deficiencies, such as calcium and magnesium, may be linked to sleep disorders. Boost calcium intake via reduced-fat dairy products and muscle-relaxing magnesium by eating whole grains, leafy greens, nuts, and seeds. Foods such as fish, eggs, and beans are rich in tryptophan, which helps to boost serotonin levels, which in turn is converted into sleep-inducing melatonin. Finally, avoid eating large meals late at night—indigestion interferes with sleep quality.

EAT PLENTY
Yogurt, eggs, whole grains, legumes, leafy greens, fish, nuts and seeds

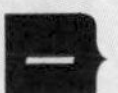
LIMIT
Caffeinated drinks after midday

DEPRESSION

Everyone has times when they feel down, which is normal, but not wanting to get out of bed, feeling hopeless, or being persistently sad for weeks at a time could be depression. The causes of depression are many and complex: research suggests that depression isn't just a simple chemical imbalance, but could also include genetic vulnerability, medications, and faulty mood regulation.

Luckily, what we eat may help to protect against depression. First and foremost, eat regularly and choose starchy, fiber-rich foods to prevent low blood sugar levels, which can leave us feeling irritable and miserable. Include plenty of foods rich in tryptophan (see Insomnia, left) to boost levels of feel-good serotonin. Low blood levels of vitamin D have also been linked to depression, so eat foods high in vitamin D (see page 36). Seafood has been linked to a better mood in several studies, possibly thanks to its brain-friendly omega-3 fats. A review of 26 studies found adults who ate the most fish were 17 percent less likely to become depressed than those what ate the least.

A 2017 study showed that a Mediterranean-style diet cut symptoms of depression by 32 percent.

A study in 2017 looked specifically at the impact of diet on depression. It concluded that a Mediterranean-style diet can treat depression. In the study, symptoms were reduced by 32.3 percent.

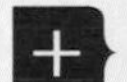
EAT PLENTY
Bananas, eggs, whole grains, lentils, beets, leafy greens, fish, nuts, seeds

LIMIT
Alcohol, caffeine, processed foods

VISION

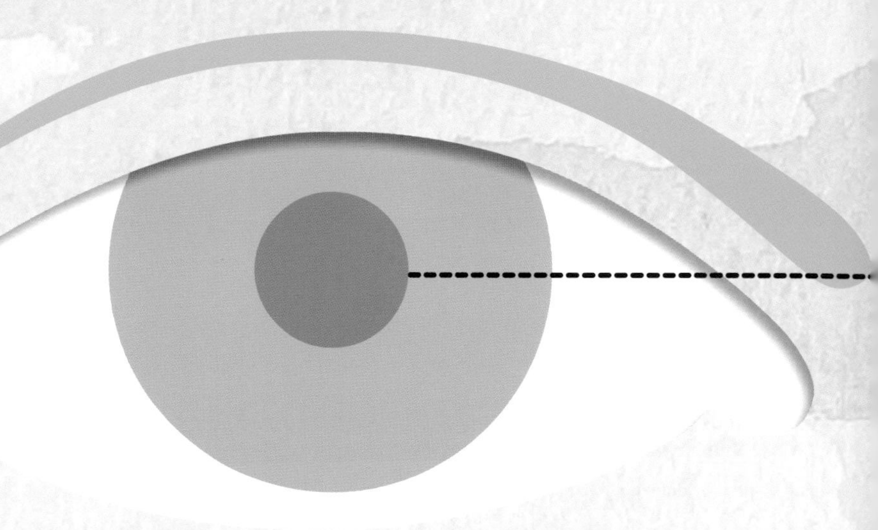

Our vision may require adjustment throughout life, but universally we become more farsighted in older age. Despite such inevitable changes, key nutrients in particular foods can help to promote eye health, as well as ward off age-related macular degeneration and cataracts.

AS WE AGE ...

The need for reading glasses comes to us all in older age, but there are other changes going on in your eyes. Find out what else is happening and how foods can lessen their impact.

We become farsighted

The lens, supported by ciliary muscles in the eye, changes its shape so that we can adapt our focus from near to far and back. Over time, the lens thickens and hardens, losing its flexibility—a normal and inevitable part of aging known as presbyopia, or farsightedness. The consequences are that usually by our mid-40s, we struggle to read in dim light or decipher close-up text. Foods rich in antioxidants can play a key role in supporting lens health (see page 164).

Eyes become drier

Moisture is essential for our eyes to function. Each time we blink, a film of tears spreads across the surface of the eye, protecting it and keeping it from drying out. Once we're into our 50s, tear production slows, and the tears we do produce may not be enough to cover the eye evenly or efficiently, leaving eyes feeling scratchy and tired. Rather than reaching for drops, look at how foods can help rehydrate and calm your eyes. Omega-3 fats (see page 164) boost the microcirculation in the tiny blood vessels around the eyes, which helps to reduce the inflammation that accompanies dryness and keep the eyes moist and irritant-free.

The world we see shrinks

Our field of focus may narrow with age. By our 80s, we can have lost as much as 30 percent of our peripheral vision. The ability to see objects outside of our central field of vision, in our periphery, is controlled by cells on the retina called rods; these are super-sensitive to light and movement. Foods rich in a range of vitamins and minerals—particularly lutein, zeaxanthin, zinc, and selenium—deliver nutrients to make light-sensitive pigments (see page 164).

Our eyes need three times as much light for reading in our 60s as in our 20s.

Reaction to light slows

The tiny muscles that control the pupils weaken with age, and our pupils constrict. Consequently, our eyes react more slowly when we move between areas of light and dark, so that it can be tricky to focus when entering a dark room, and bright light can be dazzling. Beta-carotene-rich foods (see page 164) bring up levels of vitamin A, essential for the production of rhodopsin, a pigment that works in dim light conditions.

CONTINUED

FOODS FOR VISION

For vision, it's good to think "ACE"—vitamins A, C, and E are all especially beneficial for eyes, though other micronutrients come into play, too. Below, discover what foods—and meals—best benefit your eyesight and what foods to avoid for the sake of your vision.

OILY FISH

DHA, one of the omega-3 fats in oily fish, is vital for eye development and a functioning retina. A deficiency in omega-3 fats has been linked to dry eye syndrome.

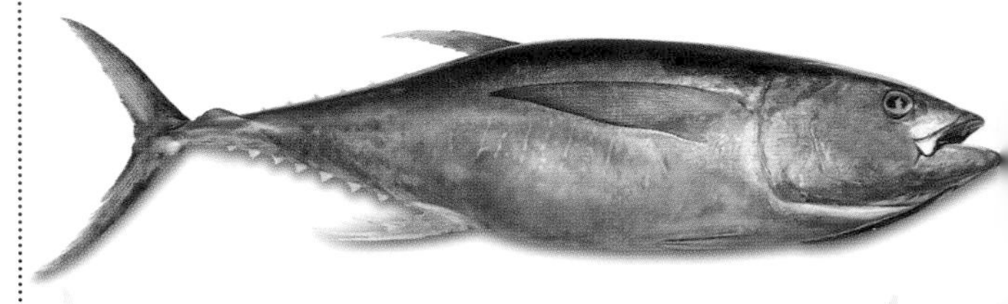

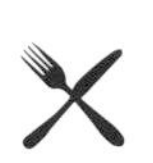

Asian-style tuna salad (see page 99)

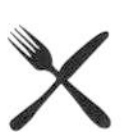

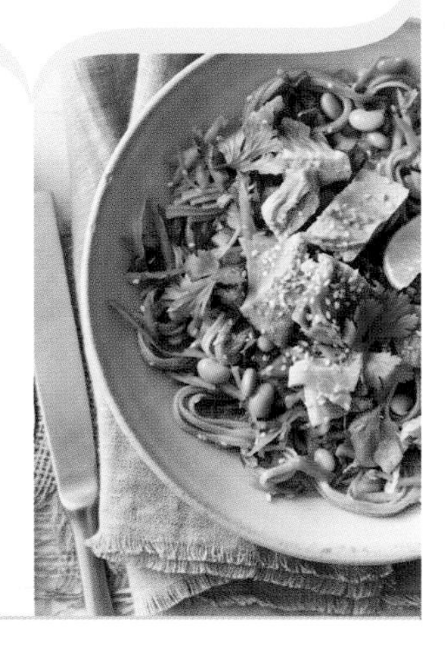

SHELLFISH

Zinc is a crucial nutrient for eye health, and shellfish provide it in abundance (see page 112). Zinc is found mostly in the eye's retina and choroid; low intakes are linked to cataracts and poor night vision.

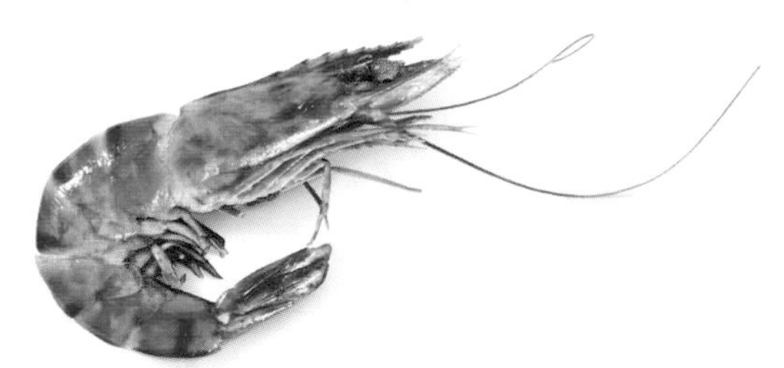

LEAFY GREENS

With a perfect combination of lutein, zeaxanthin, and vitamins C and E, these vegetables help protect against age-related macular degeneration, a leading cause of blindness.

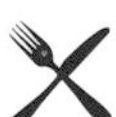

Turkey steak with kale and squash (see page 148)

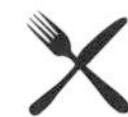

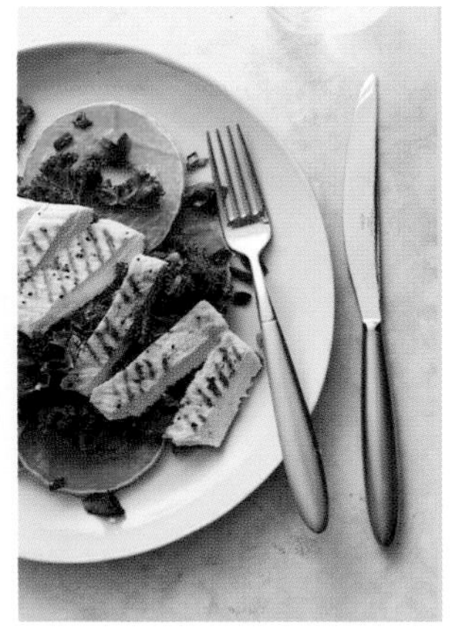

SWEET POTATOES

The body converts the beta-carotene in sweet potatoes into vitamin A, which is further transformed into rhodopsin—a pigment in the retina that helps with vision in low light.

BELL PEPPERS

All bell peppers are loaded with vitamin C, which helps keep the eyes' blood vessels healthy and cuts the risk of cataracts. One study showed that a daily supplement of 300mg vitamin C seems to prevent cataracts; one bell pepper contains about 240mg.

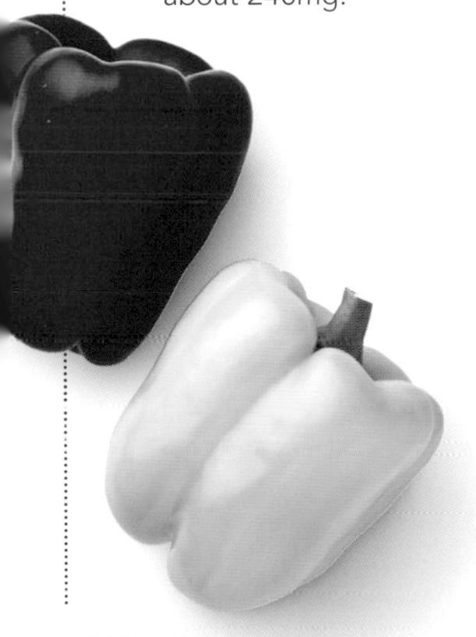

Foods to avoid

- **High-calorie, processed, and sugary foods—** These can lead to weight gain. Obesity increases the risk of developing several conditions with dire visual consequences, including type 2 diabetes (such as cataracts and diabetic retinopathy).

VISION CONDITIONS

Certain conditions respond favorably to dietary intervention. Discover how foods—whether boosting portions or cutting them out—can help protect your eyesight.

CATARACTS

It's common to find that vision becomes misty and colors more faded as we get older. The lens consists largely of water and protein. When proteins start to clump together, they affect the passage of light through the lens, creating a cloudy area that makes vision less sharp. This clouding over is known as a cataract and affects many of us in old age. Cataracts can start to form in our 50s and enlarge over time, so vision slowly deteriorates. Thankfully, cataracts are easily treated with simple surgery. A plant-rich (meat-free) diet is one of the best ways to protect against cataracts.

EAT PLENTY
Berries, avocados, bell peppers, leafy greens, shellfish, orange fruits and vegetables, citrus fruits

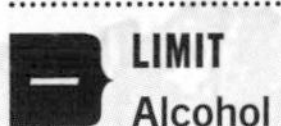

LIMIT
Alcohol

GLAUCOMA

When pressure builds up in the fluid inside the eye, it can damage the optic nerve, causing glaucoma. Regular eye tests are vital so an optician can check eye pressure, as the condition has few symptoms. When caught early enough, eye drops can help to prevent sight loss from glaucoma. As with other vision-related conditions, regularly eating foods that contain antioxidants can help to protect against further damage.

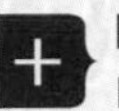

EAT PLENTY
Fresh fruits and vegetables

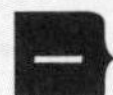

LIMIT
Sodium, processed foods, caffeine

AGE-RELATED MACULAR DEGENERATION (AMD)

The macula at the center of the retina is densely packed with specialized light-receptive cells. These cells fire messages via the optic nerve to the brain's visual cortex, where they are interpreted as images. If the cells are damaged, central vision can become distorted, and a partial loss of sight, or macular degeneration, results. It's most common in people over 60. Straight lines may appear wavy, it can be hard to focus on faces, and dark areas may appear. AMD can be "dry" or "wet," though both result in blindness. So protect your eyesight with proven food solutions, such as leafy greens and zinc-rich foods (see opposite and also pages 112–113), to lower your risk of AMD.

EAT PLENTY
Eggs, avocados, leafy greens, oily fish and shellfish, orange fruits and vegetables

HEARING AND BALANCE

A lifetime's exposure to loud noises can take its toll on our hearing, in tandem with age-related changes in the inner ear's balance system. But research shows that particular nutrients can help prevent or lessen the effects of age-related hearing loss, tinnitus, and balance problems.

AS WE AGE ...

Whether you're turning up the volume or finding yourself oddly unsteady, physical changes alter your hearing and balance as you age. Learn how the power of foods can reduce their effects.

Sensitivity is lost

Nestled inside the cochlea—the hearing vessel of the inner ear—are thousands of tiny hair cells. These sensory cells convert sound vibrations from the outside world into nerve signals that travel to the auditory cortex in the brain to be processed into sounds. When loud sounds strike these delicate hair cells, they bend and break; once broken, the hair cells don't grow back, which impacts on hearing in later years. Such "sensorineural" hearing loss arises from cumulative damage to the sensory hair cells in the inner ear or from damage to the nerve pathways. In addition, there are "conductive" issues that interfere with sounds traveling into the inner ear, caused by factors such as an accumulation of wax in the ear canal, an infection in the middle ear, or damage from a perforated eardrum.

Magnesium, for instance, helps to counter the effects of damaging free radicals on the inner ear hair cells. Studies also show that antioxidant vitamins A, C, and E work with magnesium to help protect against noise-induced trauma. Higher intakes of omega-3 fats from fish have been linked to protecting against hearing loss, too. And folate can help to break down homocysteine, an inflammatory compound, that, in turn, boosts circulation to the inner ear hair cells. See page 168 for foods that support hearing.

Sounds over 85 decibels (equal to heavy traffic noise) creates free radicals that damage hearing.

Balance starts to waiver

Our sense of where we are in space, which enables us to balance, is controlled by the vestibular system in the inner ear, a network of tiny, fluid-filled tubes with specialized nerve endings that send signals to the brain's balance center. From the age of 55 or so, we start to lose cells in this system, which may cause us to feel dizzy and a bit unsteady.

In a healthy ear, electrolyte-containing fluid is kept at a constant volume, and changes in this volume can cause symptoms such as tinnitus and dizziness (see page 169). Dehydration exacerbates dizziness, so keeping hydrated with the right drinks (see page 40) and foods (fresh fruits and vegetables are rich in water) will enhance the function of the vestibular system by helping to balance electrolytes in the inner ear fluid.

CONTINUED

FOODS FOR HEARING AND BALANCE

Nutritional studies offer up a basketful of micronutrients that support the vital functions of hearing and balance. As well as eating plenty of these foods, it's also good to know which foods can promote disease so you can avoid those.

ORANGE VEGETABLES

Such vegetables are rich in beta-carotene, which forms vitamin A. Adults with the highest vitamin A intakes were 47 percent less likely to suffer hearing loss than those with the lowest intakes, in one study.

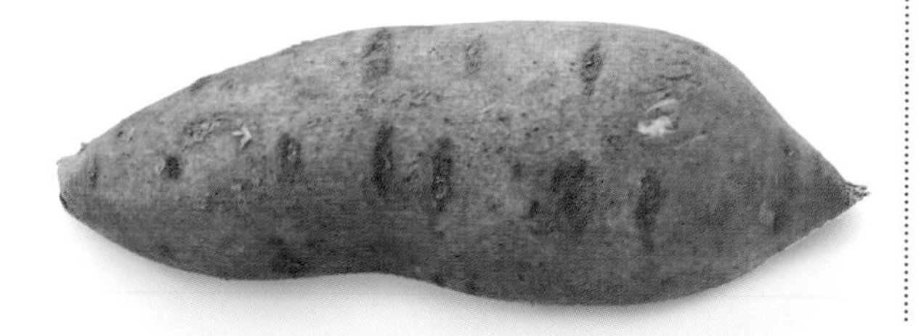

LEAFY GREENS

Green leafy vegetables are rich in folate, which is great news for hearing, since good intakes of this B vitamin have been linked to lower rates of hearing loss. Top choices for folate are spinach, kale, and Brussels sprouts.

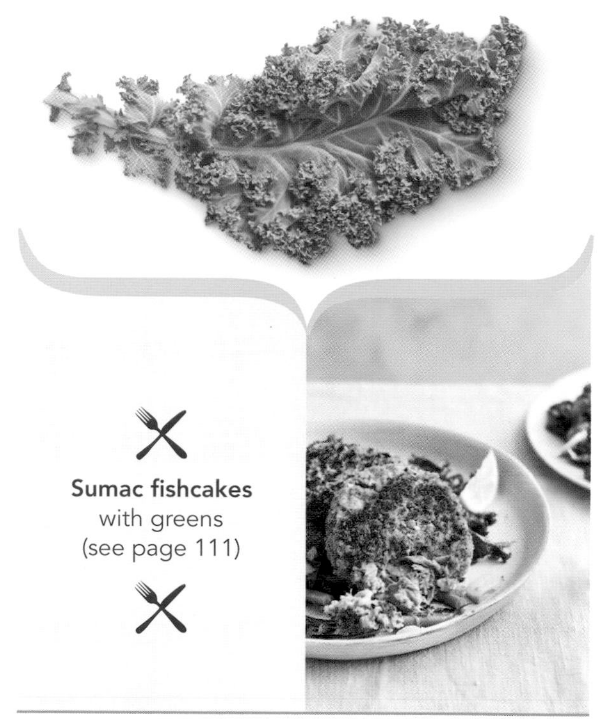

Sumac fishcakes with greens (see page 111)

NUTS AND SEEDS

Nuts and seeds are rich in magnesium, a mineral that may help reduce noise-induced hearing loss. Brazil nuts are the richest source, followed by sunflower seeds, sesame seeds, and almonds.

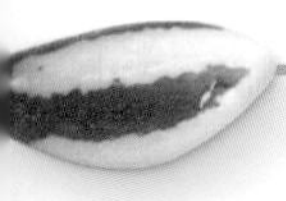

Freekeh with roasted veggies and greens (see page 93)

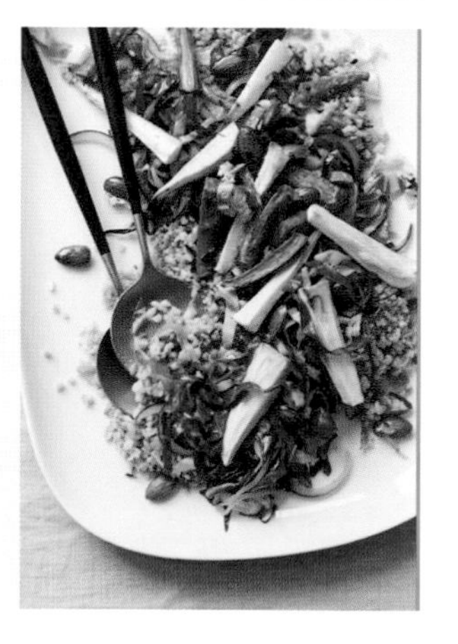

COFFEE

Research from 2014 suggests caffeine may help to protect against tinnitus. In a large study, women who had the daily caffeine equivalent of four to six mugs of coffee were 15 percent less likely to have tinnitus, compared with those who drank only one to two mugs.

FISH

Eating fish at least once a week was found to cut the risk of tinnitus in one study. Another study found that people eating two or more servings a week were 42 percent less likely to develop age-related hearing loss than those eating less than one serving a week. Another study found the highest intakes of omega-3 fats cut the risk of hearing loss by 22 percent.

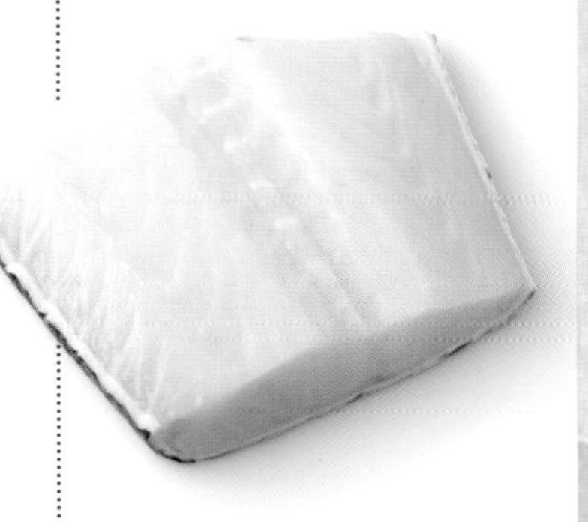

Foods to avoid

- **Sugar-rich and processed carbs**—Studies of older adults show that those eating diets with a high glycemic load (high in refined sugars) have an increased risk of hearing loss—by 76 percent in a 2010 study.

HEARING AND BALANCE CONDITIONS

Studies show that certain nutrients can protect against hearing loss and tinnitus, as well as balance problems. Find out which foods to dig into and which to shun.

AGE-RELATED HEARING LOSS

A degree of hearing loss can set in as early as middle age, though it often goes unnoticed. But after the age of 75, more than half of people have significant hearing loss and can find it hard to pick out high-frequency sounds and soft consonants such as "s" and "f." Whether the age-related hearing loss is due to problems with sound traveling into the inner ear or cumulative damage to the sensory hairs, foods offer potential solutions or preventive approaches. Certain nutrients, such as beta-carotene and folate (see opposite), have been shown to have protective effects.

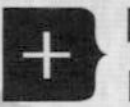

EAT PLENTY
Bell peppers, leafy greens, tomatoes, oranges, squash

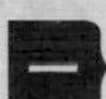

LIMIT
Sodium, monosodium glutamate

TINNITUS

This particularly distressing hearing problem, where ringing, buzzing, or humming is heard in the ear, is a symptom rather than a disease in itself. Its causes are still not fully understood, and though it can affect many ages, it often accompanies age-related hearing loss and can be more severe in the elderly. Tinnitus can come and go, but if the noise is continuous, it can cause anxiety. Nutritional research has shown that particular foods can impact this condition in a positive way, including coffee and fish (see opposite).

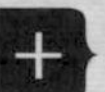

EAT PLENTY
Fish, caffeine (tea and coffee)

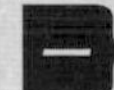

LIMIT
Sodium

PROBLEMS WITH BALANCE

The vestibular system in the inner ear plays an important role in balance. It contains three structures—the semicircular canals—that are positioned at right angles to each other and which detect changes in movement, such as moving our head up and down or from side to side. This system interacts with other areas in the body to maintain balance, and problems elsewhere may affect the vestibular system and cause us to lose our footing. Hydration is key, so drink plenty of fluids (see page 40) and always report to your doctor any dizziness or sensations of spinning.

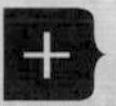

EAT PLENTY
Fresh fruits and vegetables, fluids

LIMIT
Sodium, sugar, processed foods

ORAL HEALTH

A combination of age-related changes means it's more important than ever to look after oral health as we age. There are food strategies to deploy to keep the mouth healthy, to prevent gum disease and tooth decay, and to counteract a reduction in saliva.

AS WE AGE ...

Gradual and significant changes occur in your mouth, gums, teeth, and jaw with advancing years. Discover how to employ foods to boost oral health and maintain it for the future.

Saliva production slows

Our saliva, produced in three pairs of salivary glands, is 99 percent water, but it also contains a host of key chemicals that are essential to health, such as electrolytes, mucus, and digestive enzymes. Without saliva, we wouldn't be able to chew, taste, or swallow food; saliva also keeps the mouth moist between meals. With age, the production of saliva can decline, which can affect how we taste foods, as well as our general oral health. Saliva helps to keep teeth clean, which protects them against decay, so lower levels of saliva can mean less protection. Certain foods can promote saliva production (see page 172).

The sense of taste subsides

While you may not be able to see the taste buds on your tongue, they are there in the thousands. The little bumps you do see on your tongue are called papillae, and it's on top of these tiny projections that the taste buds reside. Taste buds are groups of taste receptors that detect the chemicals dissolved in saliva, which your brain interprets as different flavors. Numbers of taste buds fall with age, which can mean a diminished sense of taste. So use citrus zests, fresh herbs, and spices to stimulate your taste buds and boost the flavors of foods, rather than adding salt.

Our 9,000 taste buds start to decline in number from age 50, then they shrink from age 60.

The jaw is remodeled

Your bones are in a constant state of flux, being broken down and rebuilt to allow for growth and repair throughout life. Bone is made of specialized cells and protein fibers. Bone-making cells (osteoblasts) calcify bone as it forms; osteocytes maintain healthy bone structure; and osteoclasts absorb bone tissue where it is degenerating or not needed. As you get older, the jaw bone in particular suffers with being dissolved more than it's rebuilt, and the shape changes over time. This remodeling may lead to gum problems and tooth loss. So feed your body with a steady stream of bone-building nutrients (see page 172).

Teeth are wearing out

Teeth are designed to last a long time if you look after them. But a lifetime of biting, chewing, and grinding can wear away the enamel and the flat surfaces of certain teeth. What's more, acidic foods and drinks can damage the enamel coating, so reduce exposure to such items throughout the day.

CONTINUED

FOODS FOR ORAL HEALTH

When it comes to eating with oral health in mind, first up is avoiding sugary foods and limiting acidic foods. Then, focus on choosing tooth- and gum-friendly foods packed with vitamin C, calcium, phosphorus, and fluoride that promote health and prevent decay.

EGGS

These vitamin D–rich foods help the body absorb calcium and phosphorus for strong and healthy teeth. Eggs also contain vitamin B12, low levels of which have been linked with gum disease.

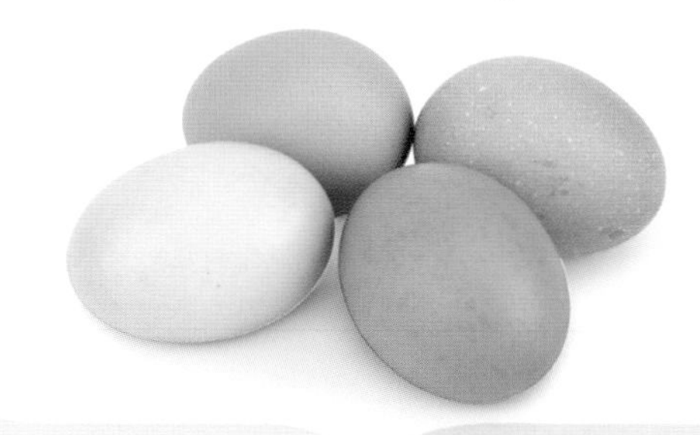

Cinnamon toast with blueberry compote (see page 63)

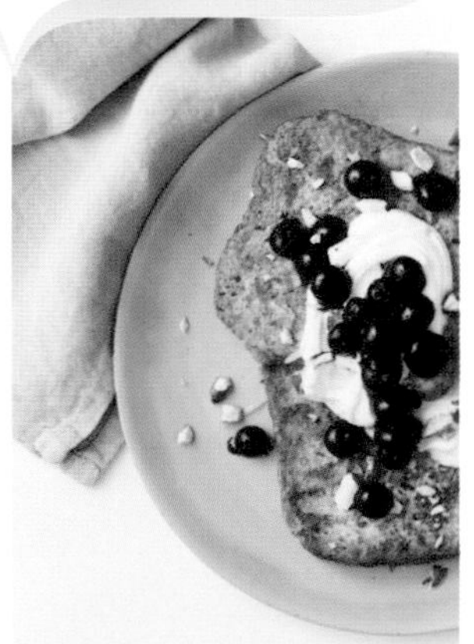

BELL PEPPERS

All bell peppers are rich in vitamin C, a nutrient that's vital for making collagen. Collagen is the main component of connective tissue, which holds the teeth in place in the gums. Bell peppers are also low in sugars and acids, and their crunchiness promotes saliva production.

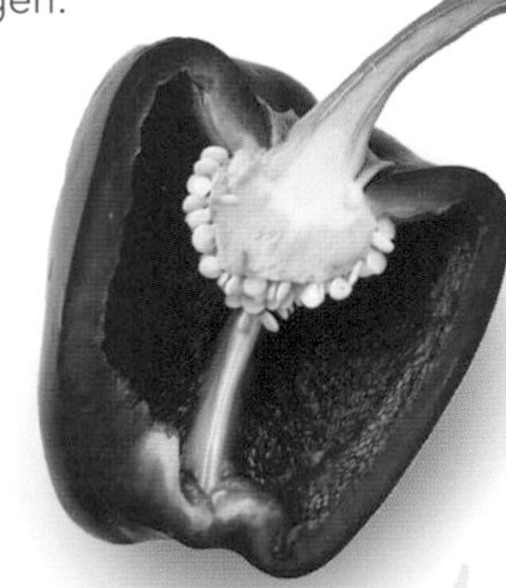

Roasted haddock with a herby crumb (see page 115)

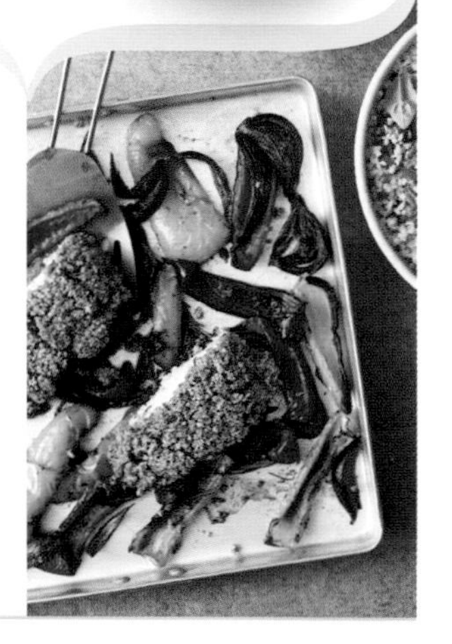

YOGURT

Yogurt is packed with tooth-friendly calcium and phosphorus—both of which help to protect and rebuild tooth enamel after an acid attack. Research also suggests probiotics in yogurt may be beneficial for oral health and for fighting bad breath.

NUTS AND SEEDS

Crunchy foods, such as nuts and seeds, stimulate saliva production. Saliva helps to wash away food debris left in the teeth and neutralize harmful acids in the mouth. What's more, nuts and seeds come packed with tooth-friendly nutrients.

TEA

Tea is rich in fluoride, which strengthens tooth enamel, reduces plaque acids, and cuts decay. Fluoride levels can vary greatly with tea type and water; brew tea for longer to increase its fluoride content.

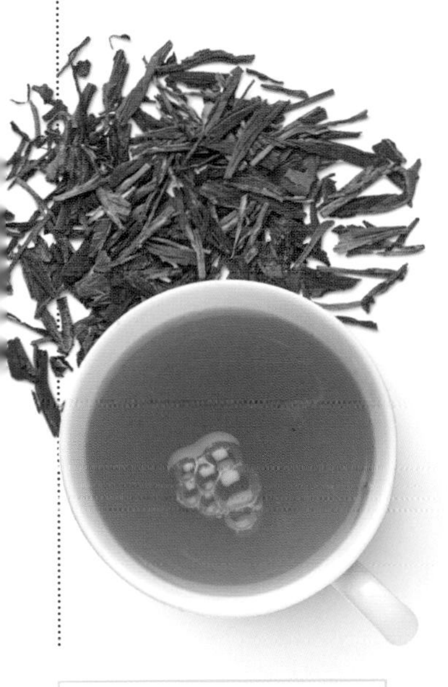

Foods to avoid

- **Sugary foods and drinks**—It's the frequency rather than the quantity that's harmful to teeth. Every time sugary foods or drinks are consumed, teeth are exposed to acid attack, which in the long term causes tooth decay. Sipping sugary drinks, sucking on hard candy, or eating foods such as toffee or dried fruit that stick to teeth means teeth are bathed in sugar.

ORAL HEALTH CONDITIONS

There's more to oral health than brushing your teeth. Find out which foods positively influence the health of your teeth and gums, and which foods should be left on the shelf.

DRY MOUTH

Having a dry mouth (also known as xerostomia) from a lack of saliva can be beyond irritating and actually make it hard to eat or talk—it feels as if your mouth is full of cotton and is often partnered by dry lips and bad breath. Such a lack of saliva can take its toll on your oral health, promoting gum disease and tooth decay. Some strategies to try to quench a dry mouth are: drinking plenty of water throughout the day, sucking on ice cubes, and chewing gum (choose sugar-free versions).

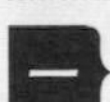

EAT PLENTY
Yogurt, unsweetened drinks, fresh juicy fruits (such as oranges and melons)

LIMIT
Sodium, dry foods, caffeine, alcohol

GUM DISEASE

Inflammation of the gums is known as gingivitis and is the result of plaque build-up around the base of the teeth. Toxins produced by plaque bacteria irritate the gums, causing them to become infected, swollen, tender, and red. This condition, if caught early enough, can be corrected and prevented by good oral hygiene. Regular dental check-ups and dentist visits should go hand in hand with your own cleaning regime. Vitamin C–rich foods are good for gums; crunchy and hard-to-chew foods, such as celery and seeds, are abrasive and "brush" the teeth, removing bacteria and debris.

EAT PLENTY
Yogurt, fresh fruits and vegetables (particularly bell peppers and leafy greens), crunchy foods (nuts and seeds)

LIMIT
Sugary drinks, sugary foods

TOOTH DECAY

A lowered production of saliva can mean that cavities are more common as you age; you may even need a filling at a dental visit. Tooth decay and periodontitis (where gum disease has spread to the outer layers of the teeth and supporting bone) are the leading causes of tooth loss in older adults, but these conditions are mostly preventable. As well as undertaking good oral hygiene, choose tooth- and gum-friendly foods (see opposite) to slow the effects of the jaw bone remodeling.

EAT PLENTY
Crunchy foods (nuts and seeds), sugar-free gum

LIMIT
Sugary foods and drinks, unsweetened fruit juice

IMMUNITY

The immune system regulates inflammation and responses to infection. With advancing age comes a rise in infections. Look to probiotics and key nutrients to help fight germs and manage autoimmune conditions.

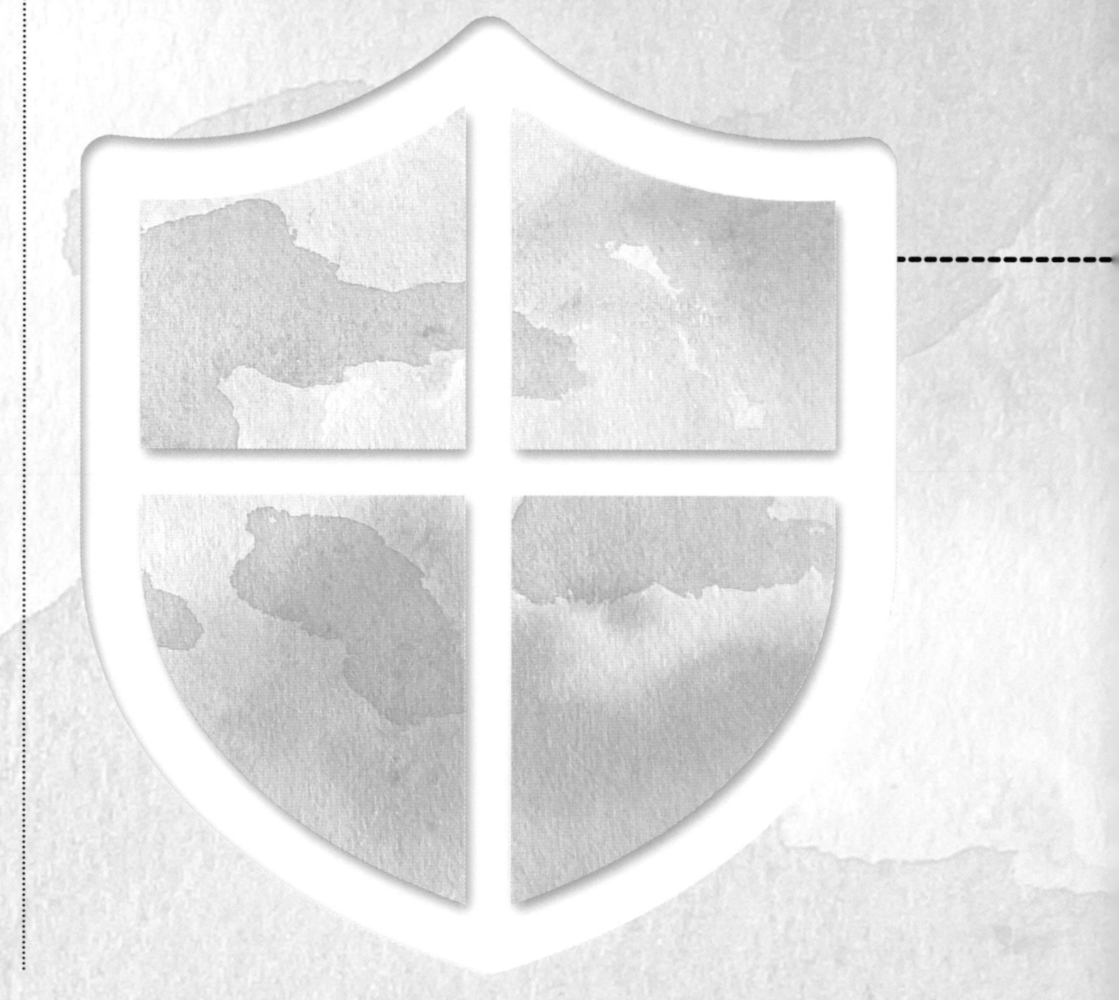

AS WE AGE ...

Notice that you're getting more colds and bugs than you used to? Discover how else age affects the immune system and what foods can help to redress the imbalance.

We need more "friendly" microbes

Bacteria and other micro-organisms make up over half the cells in our bodies. These "friendly" microbes help on three fronts: they crowd out potential pathogens; they secrete substances that kill potentially dangerous invaders; and they regulate the inflammatory part of the immune response. In the developed world, years of antibiotic overuse and an abundance of antibacterial products have resulted in a potential mismatch between the once-symbiotic relationship between microbes and immunity, leading to a rise in autoimmune diseases. Probiotics offer a food solution to promote good immunity. Foods such as yogurt and miso are loaded with probiotics, which inject beneficial bacteria and yeasts into the body and can help conditions such as inflammatory bowel disease (see page 177).

Cancer is more common

Macrophages are white blood cells that patrol the body; when they meet a foreign invader, they engulf, ingest, and destroy it (whether it's a bacterium or a cancer cell). With age, these cells seem to function more slowly, which may be why cancer is more common among older people. See below for immune-supporting micronutrients and page 176 for immune-boosting foods.

Vaccinations are not as effective in older people, but they still lower the risk of serious diseases.

Defenses weaken

The immune system is a complex network of cells, tissues, and organs. Together, these defend your body against foreign invaders, such as toxins, bacteria, and viruses. White blood cells are pivotal: they're responsible for identifying microbes, targeting them, and destroying and removing them. As we get older, the number of certain immune cells called T-cells declines, which is why we can find it harder to recover from infections and can succumb more easily than we once did. It's proven that a wide range of micronutrients play a part in keeping our immune system strong and healthy, including iron; zinc; selenium; copper; folate; and vitamins A, B6, B12, C, and D. Unfortunately, as we grow older, our bodies become less efficient at absorbing certain micronutrients, and the immune system may not get all the nutrients it needs to stay in tip-top shape. See page 176 for plenty of foods to support immune health, whatever your age.

CONTINUED

FOODS FOR IMMUNITY

An optimally functioning immune system needs access to many micronutrients and omega-3 fats. What's more, a healthy dose of "friendly" bacteria goes a long way to supporting immunity and keeping you free of disease for longer.

MUSHROOMS

Most mushrooms contain good amounts of copper, a deficiency of which is associated with low levels of white blood cells, potentially increasing susceptibility to infection. Mushrooms are also a prebiotic and so provide food for probiotic gut bacteria, keeping the digestive tract healthy and immunity strong.

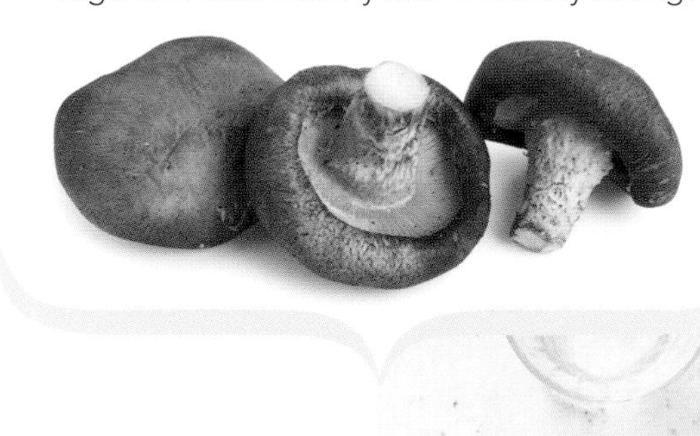

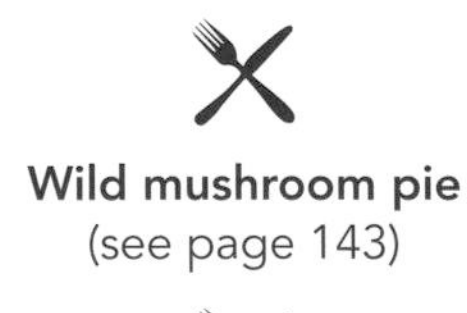

Wild mushroom pie
(see page 143)

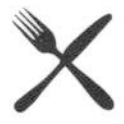

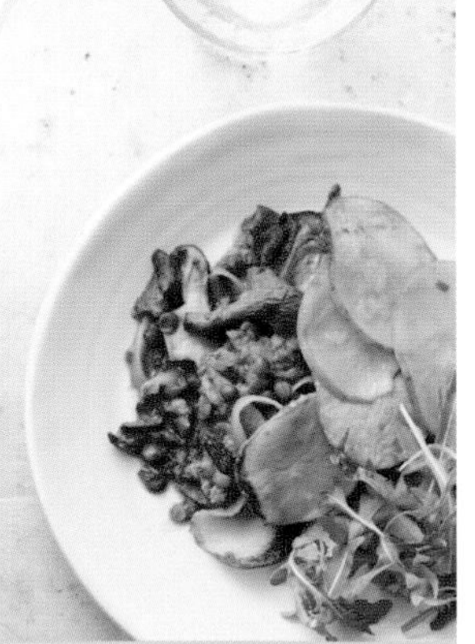

SQUASHES

Squashes are rich in vitamin C and beta-carotene (a precursor of vitamin A). Vitamin A promotes the health of the body's main barriers to the world—skin, eyes, lungs, and urinary and digestive tracts.

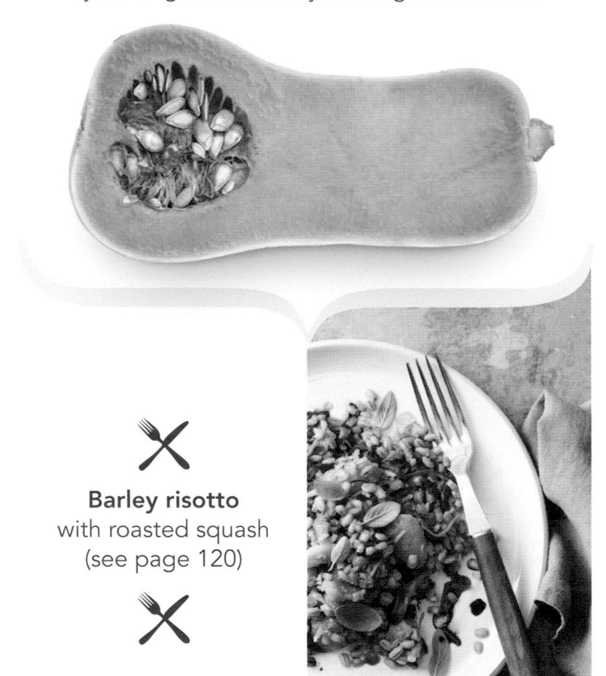

Barley risotto
with roasted squash
(see page 120)

YOGURT

Eating fermented foods such as yogurt helps to boost "friendly" probiotic bacteria in the gut. About 70 percent of our immunity resides in the digestive system, and the microflora living in the intestines play an important part in keeping it healthy.

OILY FISH

Omega-3 fats are increasingly thought to benefit the immune system, and oily fish has these in abundance. Low levels of vitamin D (oily fish are rich in this vitamin) have also been linked to autoimmune conditions, such as lupus and rheumatoid arthritis.

CITRUS FRUITS

These fruits are rich in vitamin C, a vital nutrient for keeping the immune system in tip-top shape. Several immune cells need vitamin C to perform their tasks, including T-cells and phagocytes (such as macrophages, see page 175). Vitamin C also aids the absorption of iron, a nutrient needed for immunity and wound healing.

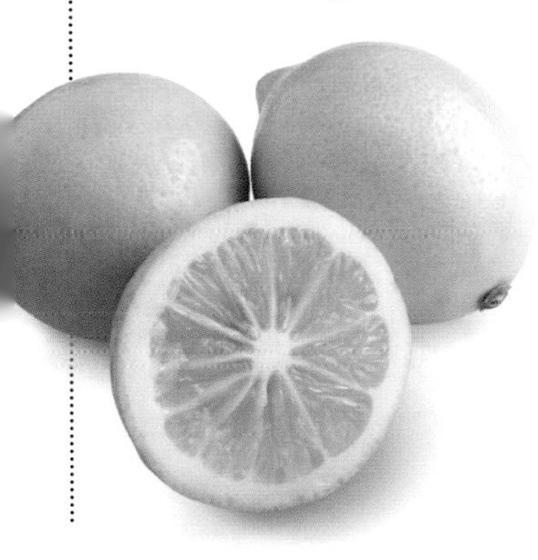

Foods to avoid

- **High-fat and high-sugar foods**—Being overweight or obese can inhibit immunity. A higher body mass index has been linked to an increased susceptibility to infection. One study found obesity associated with a higher risk of skin infections, cystitis, and respiratory infections. Obese people were also much more likely to receive hospital treatment for an infection.

IMMUNE CONDITIONS

Good nutrition can benefit all parts of the immune system. Find out how foods—eating more or cutting down—can help lessen the impact of these conditions that increase with age.

RESPIRATORY TRACT INFECTIONS

Respiratory tract infections are any infection of the sinuses, throat, airways, or lungs. Upper respiratory tract infections include colds, tonsillitis, sinusitis, and flu; lower respiratory tract infections include bronchitis and pneumonia. In a lifetime, we probably suffer from about 200 colds, with their associated coughs, sore throats, and congestion. Most of these infections are caused by viruses, though sometimes they can be bacterial. Eating plenty of vitamin A– and vitamin C–rich foods and those rich in omega-3 fats ensures immunity is working optimally to fight off invading microbes. Scientific communities are still divided on the idea that large doses of vitamin C as a supplement can prevent colds; research continues.

+ EAT PLENTY
Fresh fruits and vegetables, oily fish, nuts, seeds

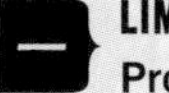

LIMIT
Processed and sugary foods

INFLAMMATORY BOWEL DISEASE

Inflammatory bowel disease covers a group of diseases that cause sores and inflammation in the digestive tract. The two most common conditions are ulcerative colitis and Crohn's disease. Symptoms include diarrhea, stomach pain, loss of appetite, bloody stools, and weight loss. Some people find that certain foods trigger symptoms or make them worse, but this can vary from person to person. Keeping a food diary can help to identify if there's a link between food and your symptoms. Always make changes to your diet in conjunction with a dietitian to ensure your diet remains nutritionally balanced.

LUPUS

In this autoimmune condition, people develop antibodies against their own tissues all around the body, resulting in inflammation and pain. Lupus is more prevalent in women and can be diagnosed by a butterfly-shaped rash on the face, along with other symptoms of fatigue, fever, joint pain, and photosensitivity. A healthy, balanced diet—such as the longevity eating plan—is suitable for many lupus sufferers, but always consult a dietitian before making significant changes to your diet.

+ EAT PLENTY
Fresh fruits and vegetables, whole grains, legumes

− LIMIT
Alfalfa sprouts, processed foods, saturated and trans fats, high-sugar foods, high-sodium foods

BONES, MUSCLES, AND JOINTS

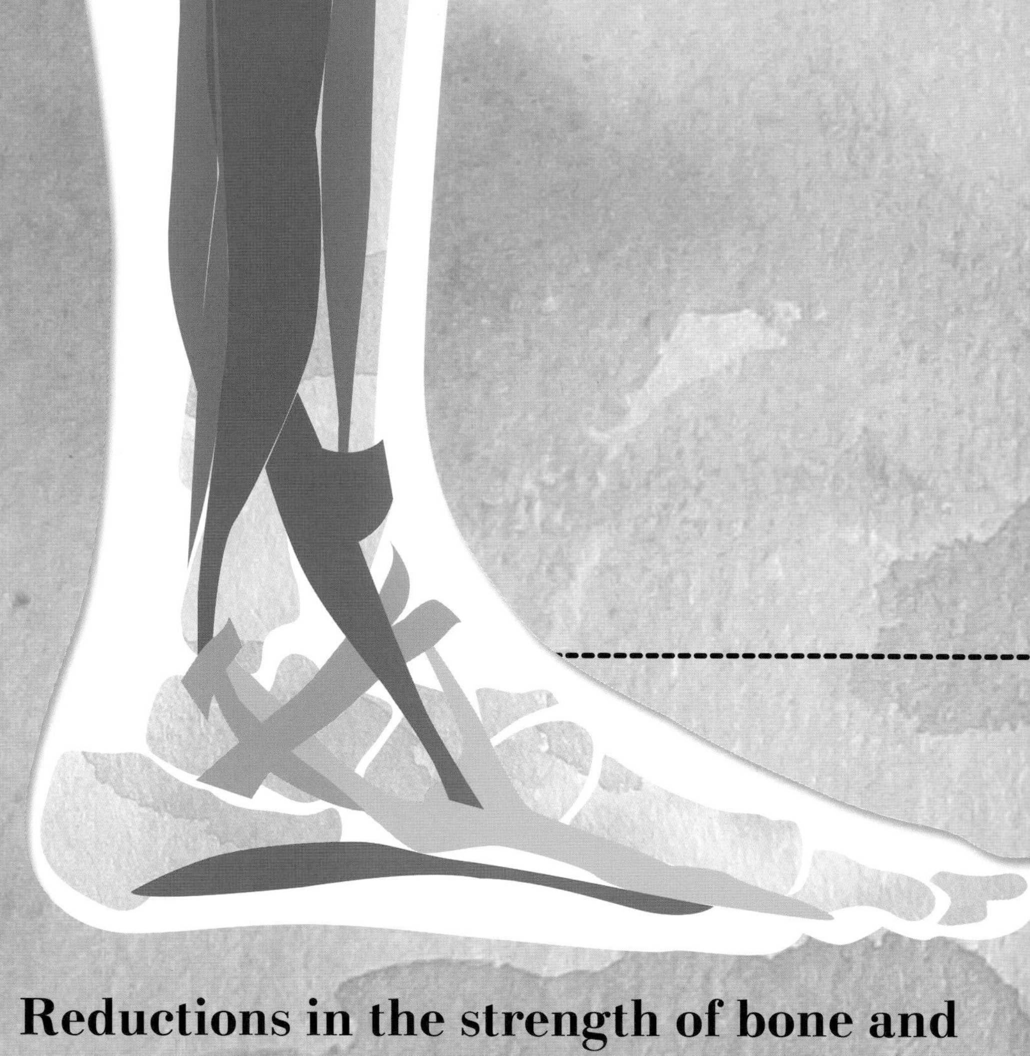

Reductions in the strength of bone and muscle are a natural consequence of aging, but there are plentiful food solutions to slow the decline. Good nutrition helps maintain bone density, keeps muscles strong, supports joints, reduces inflammation, and protects against osteoporosis and arthritis.

AS WE AGE ...

Bones weaken, joints stiffen, and muscle mass declines as we age, but nutrients in foods can make a positive difference for a strong and healthy musculoskeletal system.

Bones lose density

By the age of 35, our bones are at their strongest. From this point, they steadily lose density at a rate of about 1 percent a year, although in women this can accelerate to 20 percent in the years after menopause. As the minerals in bone are constantly replaced, dietary sources are vital to keep bones healthy and strong. A well-balanced diet can deliver plenty of bone-friendly nutrients—calcium, protein, phosphorus, magnesium, and vitamins D and K (see page 180)—whatever your age.

Muscles get weaker

At around the age of 30, muscle mass starts to diminish—in fact, without lifestyle measures, 8 percent of muscle mass can be lost each decade from the age of 40. Such muscle loss can be earlier for men and a little later for women; this loss correlates with reduced strength; ebbing energy levels; and changes to movement, balance, and posture. When related to aging, this condition is called sarcopenia and can accelerate between the ages of 65 and 75. The good news is this decline isn't inevitable—muscle strength can be maintained and the decline slowed down with resistance exercises and the right diet. Our muscles need slightly more muscle-building protein the older we get, but this is easily achieved, even if we follow a vegetarian or vegan diet (see page 30). Healthy proteins help the body to obtain essential amino acids such as leucine (good sources are animal foods, nuts, legumes, and soy), which is vital for strong muscles. Vitamin D also helps maintain healthy muscles (see page 36).

Bones become more brittle with age, and our spinal vertebrae can be squashed—we actually shrink a little.

Joints become less flexible

We can move thanks to a system of joints—where bones connect and where cartilage and synovial fluid provide cushioning and prevent friction. As we age, a reduction in fluid and depleting levels of cartilage can restrict movement, and abnormal calcium deposits can harden tissues. Cartilage isn't constantly replaced, so it wears out, and inflammation can increase stiffness. Dietary essential fatty acids can help to reduce inflammation and stiffness, allowing the joints to move more freely. Vitamin E may help prevent joint degeneration, and curcumin and gingerol in certain spices (see page 146) may have anti-inflammatory effects.

CONTINUED

FOODS FOR BONES, MUSCLES, AND JOINTS

There's more to the musculoskeletal system than calcium for bones. All manner of nutrients are needed for the healthy production of connective tissues and for easing inflammation, which makes moving pain-free and easy.

CITRUS FRUITS

Citrus fruits are rich in vitamin C, which is needed in the formation of collagen—the connective protein vital for the strength and flexibility of muscles, tendons, ligaments, bones, and cartilage. Vitamin C's antioxidant powers can mop up free radicals to avoid affecting bone strength.

YOGURT

Yogurt provides the bone- and muscle-building combination of protein and calcium. Yogurt also contains potassium, which regulates muscle activity. A new area of research suggests probiotics found in yogurt may be beneficial for bones, helping to maintain and even increase their strength.

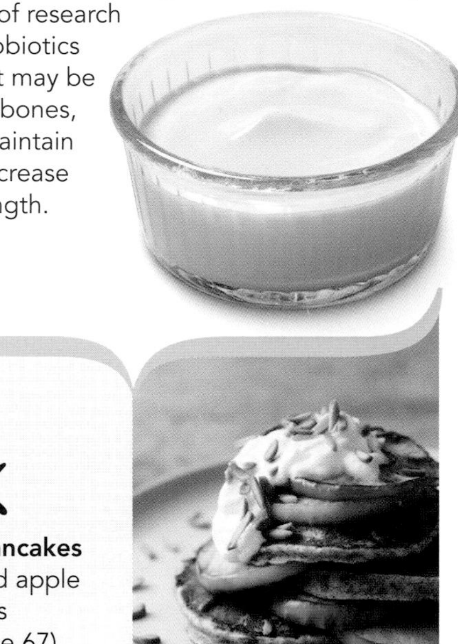

Banana pancakes with spiced apple rings (see page 67)

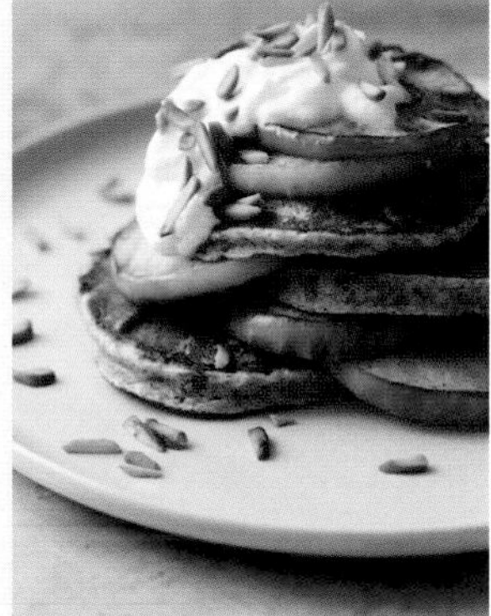

SOY

Some (but not all) studies show that isoflavones in soy may help slow the bone loss that occurs around the time of menopause. Soy products also provide a fabulous source of protein and calcium.

Japanese-style noodle soup (see page 139)

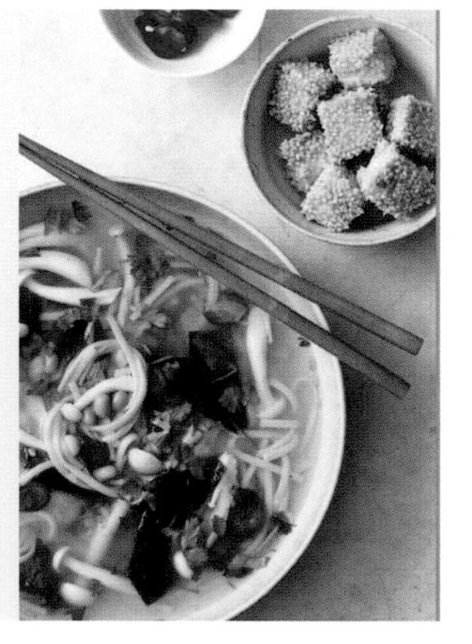

OILY FISH

All fish are rich in bone- and muscle-building protein, but oily fish are also a rich dietary source of vitamin D, which helps the body absorb calcium. Oily fish are rich in omega-3 fats, which have been shown to ease inflammation in rheumatoid arthritis.

NUTS AND SEEDS

Nuts and seeds are rich in protein, zinc, manganese, and magnesium, all of which are important for healthy bones. Magnesium helps muscles contract normally. Nuts and seeds are also rich in copper, which is used to make connective tissue.

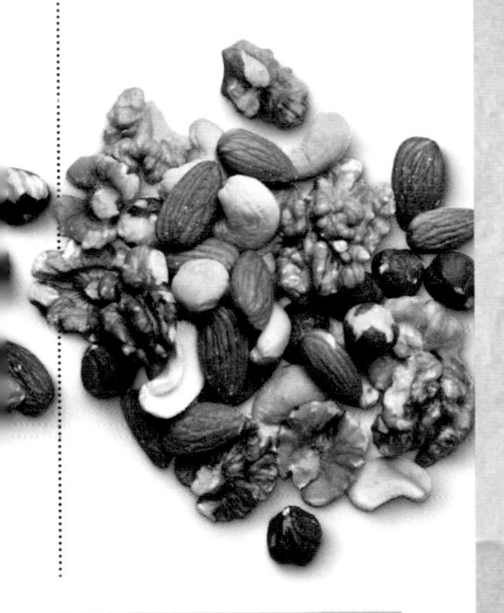

Foods to avoid

- **Vitamin A–rich foods**—A high intake of vitamin A (more than 1.5mg a day) over many years increases the risk of osteoporosis. If you're taking any supplements, check their vitamin A content, too.
- **Drinks**—The high level of phosphoric acid in soda is known to cause bone loss. Excessive amounts of alcohol seem to slow bone building.

BONE, MUSCLE, AND JOINT CONDITIONS

Certain conditions respond favorably to nutrition-based therapies, many of which can also be preventive. Discover what to eat and what to avoid for the sake of your skeleton.

OSTEOPOROSIS

Bones have a tough outer covering and an inner "honeycomb" mesh. Bone tissue is in constant flux, which keeps bones strong and resilient. After the age of 35, tissue loss outpaces bone renewal: the mesh gets bigger and bones become more porous and more vulnerable to fractures; a minor fall or bump can break a bone. Both sexes can suffer, but postmenopausal women are particularly vulnerable (see page 207). As well as bone-friendly phosphorus, protein, calcium, magnesium, zinc, manganese, and vitamin D, it's vital to get vitamin K. Some studies link low levels of vitamin K to lower bone mineral density and more fractures.

EAT PLENTY
Yogurt, eggs, whole grains, soy, leafy greens, oily fish, citrus fruits, nuts

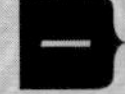

LIMIT
Caffeine, sodium, soft drinks

OSTEOARTHRITIS

Some wear and tear of joints and tissues is inevitable as we age. But if cartilage wears down excessively, bones grate against each other, causing tissues to flare up and bits of cartilage and bone to break off. Osteoarthritis is a painful condition, but it can be relieved via exercise, shedding excess weight, and diet. There's emerging research that lutein (in leafy greens) may support cartilage. There's evidence that omega-6 fats (found in large amounts in certain vegetable oils) may increase inflammation in the body, while omega-3 fats reduce it.

EAT PLENTY
Berries, leafy greens, oily fish and shellfish, onions, citrus fruits, nuts, spices

LIMIT
Safflower, sunflower, and corn oils

RHEUMATOID ARTHRITIS

In rheumatoid arthritis, the immune system mistakenly attacks healthy tissues in the lining of joints, leading to inflammation and pain. It can happen at any age, but it's most common between 40 and 60 in women, a bit later in men. Today, treatment options include diet. One recent study found that swelling and tenderness in joints was reduced after following a Mediterranean diet for 3 months.

EAT PLENTY
Berries, whole grains, avocados, leafy greens, oily fish, olive oil, nuts

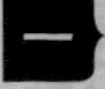

LIMIT
Meat, processed foods

SKIN AND SENSATION

Our skin, the body's largest organ, is a true multitasker: protecting us from the world at large and allowing us to experience it through sensation. Key nutrients in foods can help support the skin against its biggest foe—the sun—as well as prevent common age-related conditions.

AS WE AGE ...

Signs of aging are often first noticeable on our skin, as changes beneath its surface lead to wrinkles. Discover how foods can help support skin health and combat age-related changes.

Skin's strength and suppleness fade

Our skin is supple and strong thanks to stretchy elastin fibers and the gluelike protein collagen, made up of a fibrous matrix that provides the scaffold for skin tissues. From the age of 20, we lose 1 percent of our collagen each year and elastin fibers gradually decrease, paving the way for wrinkles and fine lines. The sun's UVA and UVB rays hasten the natural breakdown of collagen and elastin. Applying a minimum SPF15 sunscreen is the first line of defense, but foods can also protect skin (see page 184).

Pigmentation declines

Our skin contains the protective pigment melanin. This gives skin its color and acts as an absorbent filter of the sun's UV rays, helping to block damage from UVA and UVB light. Melanin is produced by cells called melanocytes, and the number of these tails off as we age, making our skin more susceptible to sun damage. Age spots are your skin's way of trying to defend against further sun damage. Foods rich in antioxidants, such as vitamin C, can offer help with sun protection (see page 184).

A plentiful supply of essential fats has been shown to reduce the chance of dry skin by 25 percent.

Skin becomes more fragile

The part of your skin that's visible is the epidermis—the thin, protective outer layer. Beneath this, the thicker dermis houses sweat and oil glands; then a subcutaneous layer of fat insulates the body. Aging occurs across all layers. The epidermal and fat layers thin, so skin is more vulnerable to the harmful effects of UV rays and less effective at locking in warmth. In the dermis, blood vessels become more fragile, which is why we bruise more easily, and the glands secrete less oil, leading to dry, itchy skin. Staying well hydrated, as well as eating skin-friendly foods, supports your skin (see page 184).

Sensation diminishes

Our skin is home to an extensive network of nerve endings and receptors that relay messages to the brain, so we experience a whole range of sensations. We lose sensory receptors as we age, but it's not really until around the age of 70 that some people experience a noticeable loss in sensitivity. Vitamin B12 helps to boost nerve health, so regularly eating sources (such as salmon, cod, milk, and eggs) is one way to help keep your nerve endings receptive.

CONTINUED

FOODS FOR SKIN AND SENSATION

In addition to good hydration (which is vital for healthy skin), the skin benefits from a host of foods packed with healthy fats and antioxidant phytochemicals. Discover, too, which foods you'll need to give a wide berth for the sake of your skin's health and function.

OILY FISH AND SHELLFISH

The omega-3 fats in oily fish help to reduce inflammation in the body, and their vitamin D helps to address the decreasing ability to make this vital micronutrient with age. Shellfish are packed with zinc for wound healing and copper for skin pigmentation.

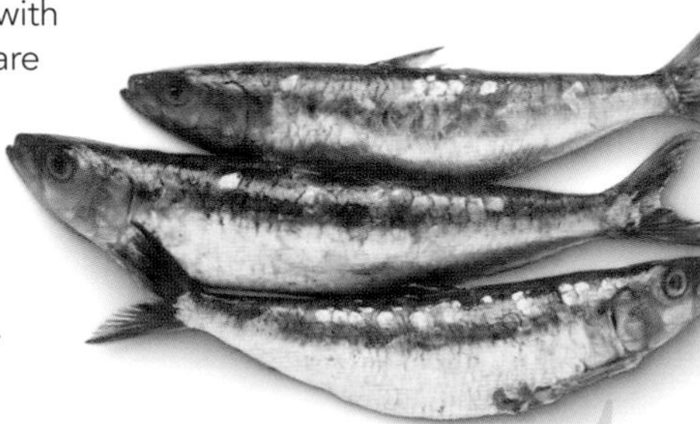

Whole-wheat pasta salad with sardines (see page 103)

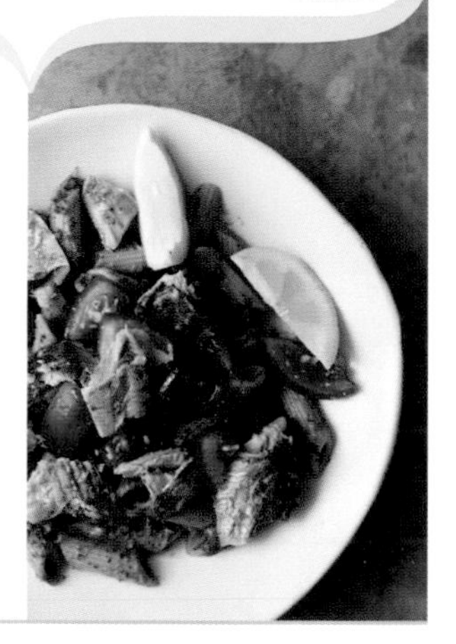

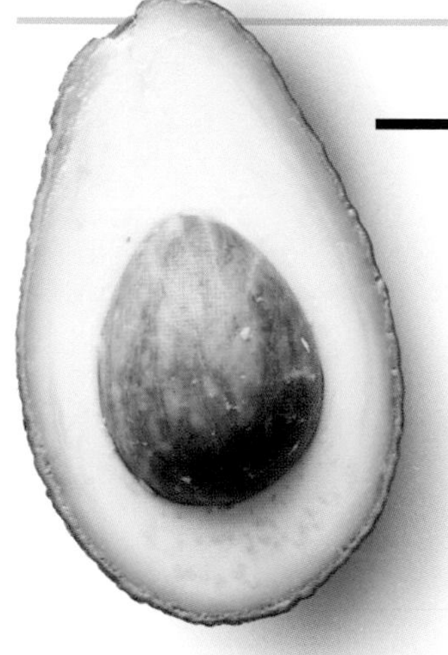

AVOCADOS

Avocados are rich in skin-healthy monounsaturated fat and vitamin E. In a study, high intakes of monounsaturated fat were found to protect against wrinkles caused by sun damage.

ORANGE VEGGIES

Orange vegetables are rich in beta-carotene, a nutrient that the body uses to make vitamin A—which is vital for the growth and repair of skin tissue and for wound healing. This vitamin has also been linked to a reduced risk of skin cancer.

Freekeh with roasted veggies and greens (see page 93)

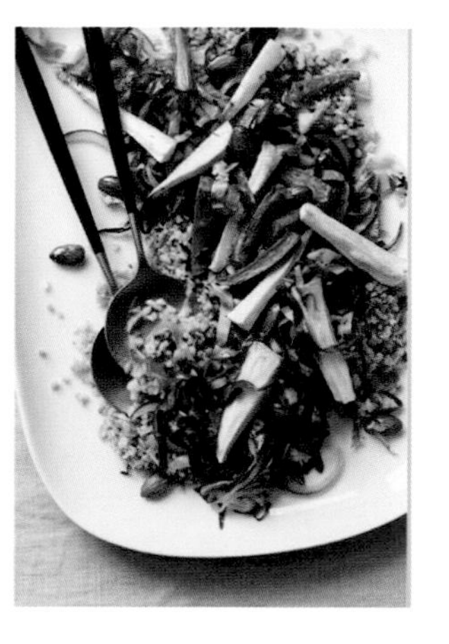

TOMATOES

In addition to their skin-friendly beta-carotene, tomatoes are rich in lycopene, which studies show may protect against sunburn. One study showed that those eating more lycopene (via tomato purée) had 33 percent more protection against the sun.

CITRUS FRUITS

The vitamin C in citrus fruits offers dual benefits. First, it's essential for the production of collagen, a protein that gives skin its structure. Second, vitamin C within the skin's epidermis protects against the free-radical damage from the sun's UV rays.

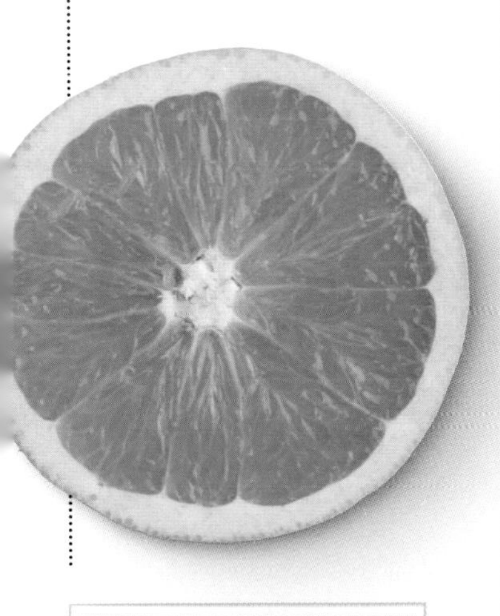

Foods to avoid

- **Sugary foods**—High intakes of sugar can affect the skin via a process called glycation, where sugar molecules attach themselves to collagen, causing it to stiffen and become inflexible, resulting in wrinkles.
- **Excessive alcohol**—High intakes have been linked to an increased risk of melanoma skin cancer.

SKIN CONDITIONS

The decline in certain glands, along with the fragility and increased vulnerability of the skin with age, lead to some common conditions—and food has a proven part to play.

DRY, ITCHY SKIN

The sebaceous glands produce sebum (oil), which helps to keep skin moisturized, but this protection diminishes with age as these glands shrink. Men fare better than women, enjoying a healthy production into old age; for women, sebum levels start to drop off with menopause, making skin more prone to dryness, flaking, and itching. Reintroducing moisture from within is a good way to counter dryness. Avoid foods that prompt skin reactions and eat those that help—essential fatty acids work to reduce skin inflammation, and vitamins A and C have potent antioxidant powers.

+ EAT PLENTY
Fresh fruits and vegetables (particularly avocados, orange vegetables, tomatoes, and citrus fruits), oily fish and shellfish, olive oil, nuts, seeds

BRUISING AND WOUND HEALING

Extra bumps and bruises are often put down to clumsiness, and while an escalation in clumsiness shouldn't be ignored, changes in our aging skin are the most likely cause of injury and slow healing. With age, padding provided by our subcutaneous fat layer diminishes, and the epidermis thins to leave us more susceptible to damage. And, once hurt, lower levels of collagen and increasingly fragile blood vessels mean that wounds and bruising take longer to heal. Foods rich in vitamin C and zinc play a role in both collagen synthesis and wound healing. Vitamin K is key to blood clotting; eating plenty of leafy greens will ensure you get a good supply.

+ EAT PLENTY
Berries, leafy greens, oily fish and shellfish, tomatoes, citrus fruits, squash

− LIMIT
Processed foods

SKIN CANCER

Repeated exposure to sunlight over time or severe episodes of sunburn can cause long-term skin damage that leads to skin cancer. Both UVA and UVB rays are harmful to skin—UVA penetrates the skin, while UVB rays burn the surface. Sunburn early in life increases the risk of melanoma; later and repeated exposure to sun over time leads to other types of skin cancer. Sun protection is key to preventing skin cancer. Many foods have cancer-preventive powers, including antioxidant-rich fruits and vegetables and omega-3 fatty acids.

+ EAT PLENTY
Leafy greens, oily fish, tomatoes, orange vegetables

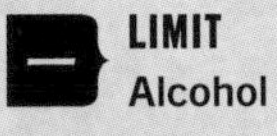

− LIMIT
Alcohol

THE LUNGS

A combination of physical changes mean that breathing can become more difficult and less efficient. But lung-boosting nutrients can help lower the risk of serious conditions, such as asthma and even lung cancer.

AS WE AGE ...

We may give breathing little thought, but as we get older, natural changes lead to functional decline. Use the power of food to help counteract events within your body and improve respiratory health.

Air sacs become less efficient

The air sacs—or alveoli—in the lungs are where inhaled oxygen passes into tiny capillaries to be distributed around the body, and carbon dioxide and waste products pass back into the lungs for exhalation. These sacs lose elasticity from our mid-30s, becoming less efficient at exchanging gases. If waste isn't exhaled fully, harmful toxins can clog up the lung tissues, and further damage by free radicals is likely. Luckily, antioxidants help fight the damage caused by free radicals from toxins harbored in lung tissue. In particular, nutrients such as vitamins A, C, and E, together with carotenoids, such as beta-cryptoxanthin and lycopene—all of which have antioxidant actions—have been implicated in helping to prevent an array of lung problems (see page 188).

Lung function declines

Natural aging changes in muscles and bones (see also page 179) have an indirect effect on lung capacity. Bones lose minerals and thin with age, which alters the shape of the ribcage, making it harder for the lungs to expand and contract. The diaphragm, which helps to draw air into and out of the lungs, weakens as we age, so it becomes harder for air to move in and out efficiently. Support the airways and respiratory muscles with magnesium-rich foods, such as whole grains, nuts, seeds, and green leafy vegetables. Foods containing theophylline, such as coffee (see page 189), dilate the airways and make breathing easier.

Infections can become problematic

Each part of the respiratory system—from the trachea to the bronchial tubes and tiny terminal air sacs in the lungs—can become inflamed when infected. With age, the body finds it increasingly hard to fight off infections (see page 174) and reduce inflammation in lung tissue. More serious infections can result, including influenza and pneumonia; in some countries, older adults are offered flu vaccinations every year to prevent serious illness. A wide range of micronutrients support the body's immune system, including iron; zinc; selenium; copper; vitamins A, B6, B12, C, and D; and folate. The 28-day longevity eating plan (see page 44) ensures you get enough of all of these nutrients.

Nerves that trigger coughing become less sensitive. Germs may collect in the lungs and be hard to cough up.

CONTINUED

FOODS FOR THE LUNGS

The lungs and respiratory tract respond well to support from nutrition—in fact, eating across the rainbow will give your body plenty of the nutrients it needs to promote good lung health. It's also important to know which foods to limit to lower the risk of respiratory conditions.

SQUASH

Butternut squash is the richest dietary source of beta-cryptoxanthin, a nutrient that seems to protect against lung cancer. In one study, higher blood levels of this carotenoid were linked to a lower risk of mortality from lung cancer.

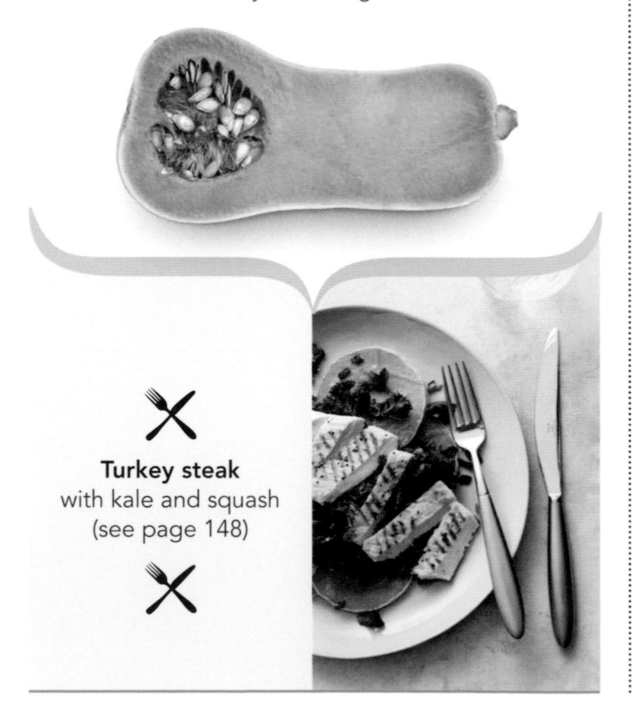

Turkey steak with kale and squash (see page 148)

TOMATOES

Lycopene in tomatoes may help protect against respiratory conditions. In a small study of people with asthma, 45mg of lycopene a day (about 12 sun-dried tomatoes) reduced inflammation of the airways.

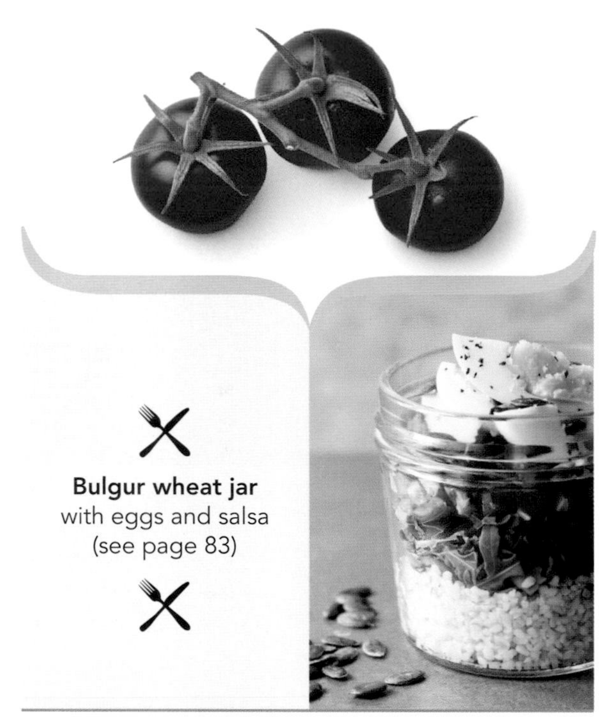

Bulgur wheat jar with eggs and salsa (see page 83)

OILY FISH

As well as omega-3 fats having anti-inflammatory action in the lungs, oily fish are rich in vitamin D, which seems to protect against susceptibility to and severity of respiratory infections.

AVOCADOS

Avocados are rich in vitamin E, a nutrient that keeps lungs healthy. A review of studies found the risk of lung cancer was cut by 5 percent for every daily 2mg increase in dietary vitamin E. A small avocado (3½oz/100g) contains 3.2mg of vitamin E.

LEAFY GREENS

Green leafy vegetables provide vitamins C and E, both of which have been shown to reduce the effects of pollution on lungs, especially in those with respiratory conditions. Kale and broccoli contain the most of both of these vitamins.

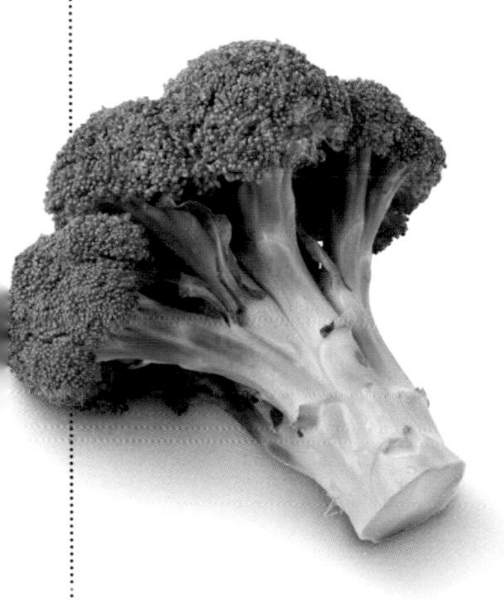

Foods to avoid

Although not a food as such, it's important to be aware that smokers should not take supplements of beta-carotene, as it may actually increase the risk of lung cancer. When eaten in foods, however, beta-carotene doesn't have this potentially harmful effect and may even be protective.

LUNG CONDITIONS

Studies show that nutrients offer significant support in the fight against common but life-changing or life-threatening lung conditions—whether that's in their prevention or as part of their treatment.

ASTHMA

Commonly thought of as a disease of childhood, asthma can persist into adulthood or be diagnosed later in life. Environmental irritants inflame the airways and tighten muscles, leading to the characteristic wheeze. After the age of 55, reduced lung function can make symptoms more severe and harder to manage. Encouraging studies reveal that eating plenty of antioxidant-rich fruits can markedly improve lung function. Omega-3 fatty acids have inflammatory properties to help improve breathing, and chemicals in coffee can dilate airways.

+ EAT PLENTY
Whole grains, leafy greens, oily fish, tomatoes, coffee (in moderate amounts)

– LIMIT
Omega-6 oils, such as sunflower oil

CHRONIC OBSTRUCTIVE PULMONARY DISEASE (COPD)

After the age of 35, our risk for lung conditions, such as COPD, increases, especially if we've smoked in the past. In COPD, airways become narrowed and partially obstructed, breathing is difficult, and breathlessness occurs on mild exertion. A 2010 study found the incidence of breathlessness and COPD was considerably lower in those with higher folate intakes.

There's mounting evidence to suggest whole grains (see pages 74–75) and foods rich in beta-carotene and vitamin C can improve lung function or keep respiratory disease at bay.

+ EAT PLENTY
Whole grains, bell peppers, leafy greens, oily fish, tomatoes, orange vegetables

– LIMIT
Processed meat, dairy products, sodium, fried foods

LUNG CANCER

Most commonly caused by smoking, lung cancer has a range of serious effects. If caught early, the disease can be treated, but what's more, there are ways to help prevent it. Not smoking, or stopping smoking, is key, but what you eat can actively promote healthy lungs. A study showed antioxidant carotenoids found in brightly colored fresh produce can significantly improve lung health. Smokers should be wary of supplements (see box, left). Beta-cryptoxanthin, in particular, together with lutein and zeaxanthin, are also thought to offer protection.

+ EAT PLENTY
Soy, avocados, leafy greens, orange vegetables, Brazil nuts

– LIMIT
Pickles, preserved foods

THE HEART AND BLOOD

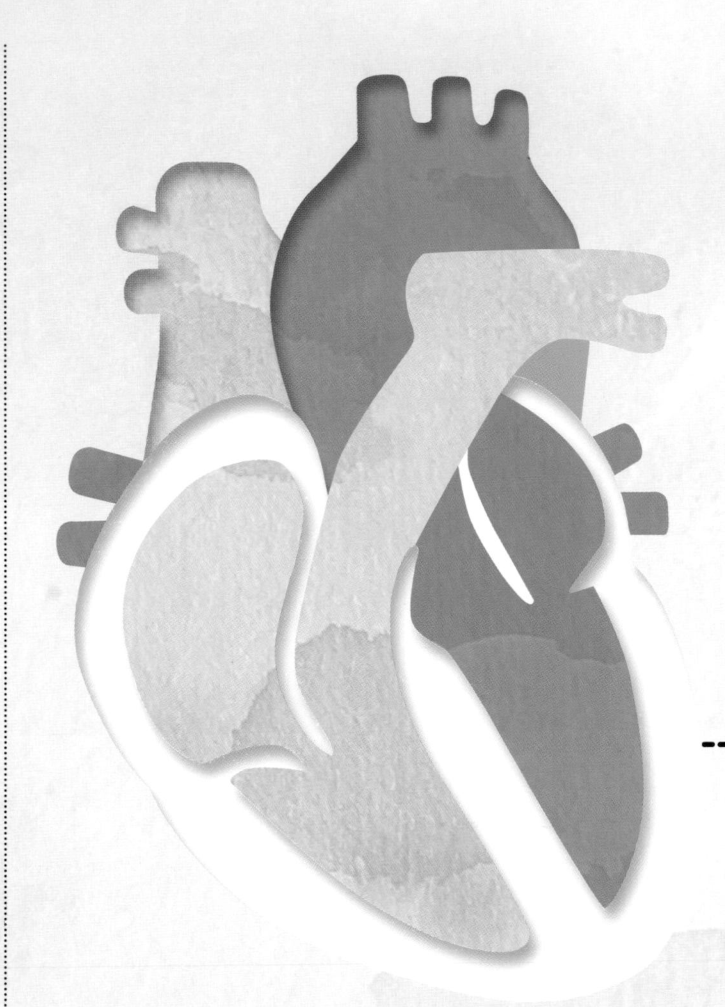

Blood is the body's life force, delivering oxygen and nutrients to cells and removing waste, and the heart is the pump that keeps blood flowing. Any disruption to the flow can be life changing, but nutrition can help maintain heart health into old age.

AS WE AGE ...

With over 100,000 beats a day on average, the heart is a super-hard worker. Discover how foods can counter the subtle but serious changes that occur to the heart and its vessels over time.

The heart's rhythm slows

Your heartbeat is generated automatically by the heart's built-in pacemaker. Electrical signals coordinate the movements involved in a heartbeat and their rhythm. As we get older, there's a reduction in the number of cells in this pacemaker, and the heartbeat slows slightly. Nutrients such as potassium, calcium, and magnesium are vital for muscle contractions to keep the heart functioning optimally. Omega-3 fatty acids, known for lowering blood pressure (see page 192), are also being studied for their potential effects on the heart's rhythm.

Arteries become stiffer

A "hardening" of the arteries is known to accompany old age; it's caused by the process of atherosclerosis (deposits of fatty plaques within the arteries) and the loss of elasticity in these vessels. When the heart has to work against the resistance offered by stiffer arteries, it cannot pump as much blood with each beat. Such stiffening also affects blood pressure, so that it's higher during contraction. The best approach is to reduce the likelihood of atherosclerosis in the first place by maintaining a healthy weight and keeping blood cholesterol levels within healthy limits. Foods that promote vasodilation (the widening of blood vessels), such as the nitrates in beets and vitamin D in oily fish (see page 192), can help keep blood flowing smoothly and arteries relaxed.

A lack of vitamin D has been linked with stiffer arteries and an inability of blood vessels to relax.

Blood's make-up changes

Blood is 50–55 percent plasma (the liquid-only portion) and 45–50 percent blood cells. Plasma is 90 percent water; as we get older, it's harder for the body to retain fluids and to stay hydrated (see pages 40 and 203), and there is a gradual reduction in total body water. Staying hydrated with plenty of fluids and eating lots of water-rich fruits and vegetables can boost total body water.

The body produces over 200 billion new red blood cells every day. To do this efficiently, bone marrow needs vital ingredients—iron and copper (for hemoglobin production), vitamin A (for stem cell activity), and various B vitamins (vitamins B6, B12, and folate for hemoglobin manufacture). A varied diet will provide all the essential micronutrients for making red blood cells.

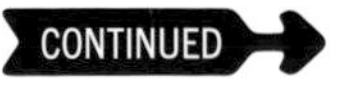

FOODS FOR THE HEART AND BLOOD

The longevity eating plan is designed with the heart and blood firmly in mind, since they're pivotal to life and health. Discover the top heart-friendly foods, along with those that you need to cut down on or avoid altogether.

LEGUMES

Legumes are rich in soluble fiber, which forms a gel inside the digestive tract. The gel binds to cholesterol and reduce its absorption by the body. One review of studies concluded that eating a daily serving of legumes (4½oz/130g) lowers LDL (bad) cholesterol by 5 percent, with the benefits being greater in men than in women.

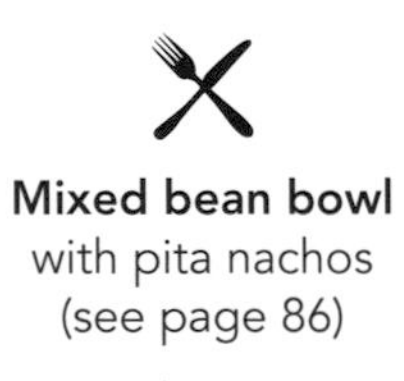

Mixed bean bowl with pita nachos (see page 86)

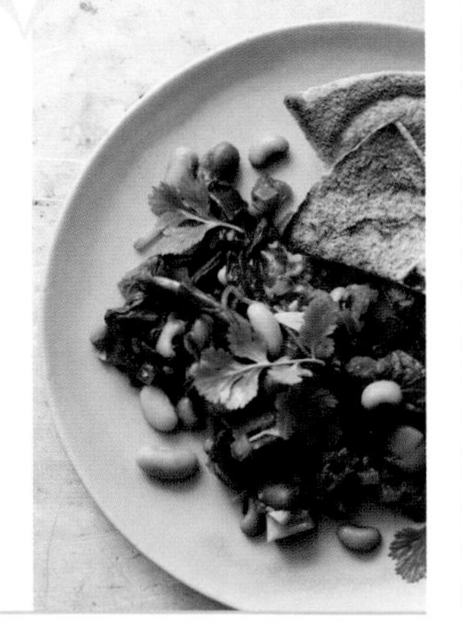

WHOLE GRAINS

Every daily serving of whole grains has been estimated to lower the risk of death from cardiovascular disease by 9 percent. While all whole grains keep the heart healthy, oats are particularly good: their beta-glucans help to lower cholesterol.

Whole-wheat pasta salad with sardines (see page 103)

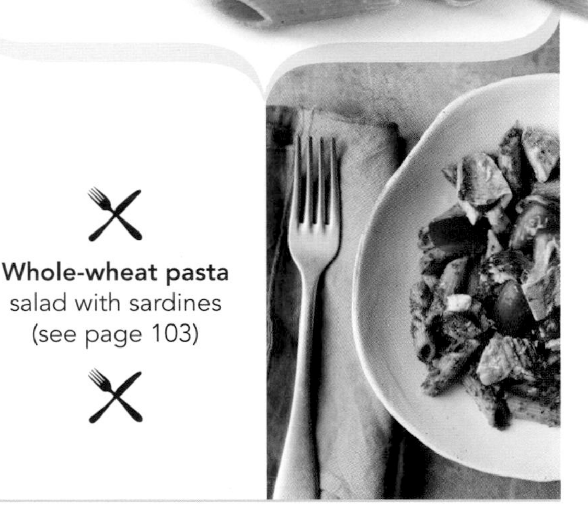

FRUITS AND VEGETABLES

All fruits and vegetables provide a combination of nutrients that keep the heart healthy: they're rich in fiber, which lowers cholesterol; they contain potassium for blood pressure control; and they provide myriad antioxidants that help protect against free-radical damage. The more you eat, the better.

OLIVE OIL

Olive oil is rich in monounsaturated fat, particularly oleic acid, which can help lower blood cholesterol. Lab studies show that the polyphenols in olive oil, such as oleuropein and hydroxytyrosol, may also help to keep the heart healthy thanks to their potent antioxidant powers.

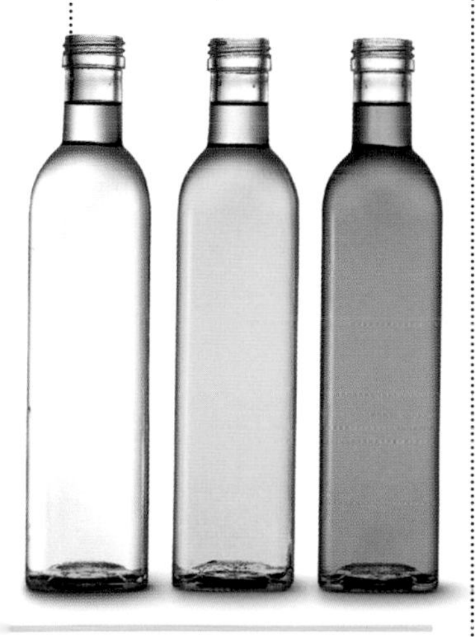

FISH

Omega-3 fats are a star heart health nutrient, but fish contain other valuable nutrients: potassium and vitamins B6 and B12. A review of studies found that eating four or more portions of fish a week was associated with a 21 percent reduced risk of having a heart attack.

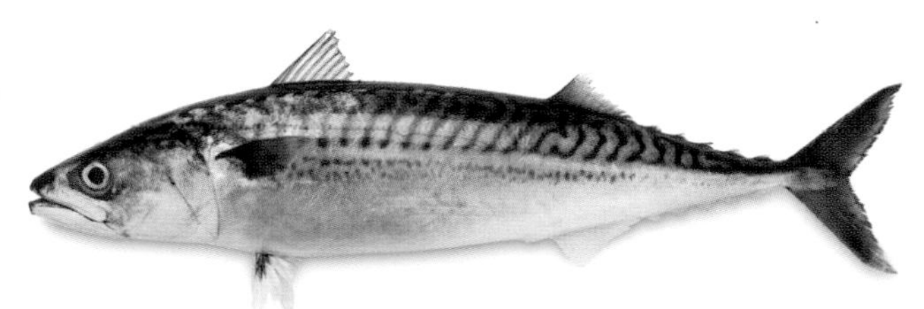

One study found that eating 10oz (300g) of fish a week protected against abnormal heart rhythms by improving the electrical properties of the heart cells.

NUTS

Nuts contain heart-friendly ingredients, including fiber, monounsaturated fat, vitamin E, plant sterols, and the plant-based form of omega-3 fats. Numerous studies confirm that eating nuts helps to lower LDL (bad) cholesterol and raises HDL (good) cholesterol.

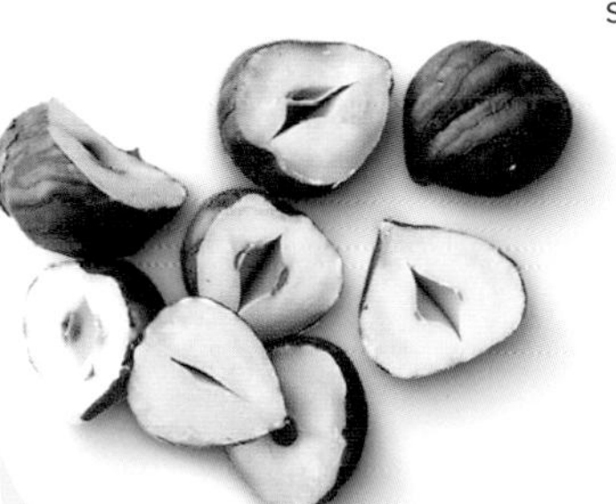

Foods to avoid

- **Salt**—High intakes of salt are linked to high blood pressure, a key risk factor for stroke. The World Health Organization recommends adults have less than 2,300mg sodium a day. Don't add salt when cooking or to meals, and limit processed foods.
- **Saturated and trans fats**—Although the impact of saturated fat on heart disease has recently been questioned, for now, health organizations around the world continue to recommend a reduction in saturated fat. Moving toward a more plant-based diet is the easiest way to achieve this. Follow a diet that minimizes processed foods and, in turn, avoids artificial trans fats.

28% reduction in the risk of heart disease from eating 10 servings of fruits and veggies a day.

Buckwheat and oat porridge (see page 59)

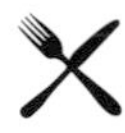

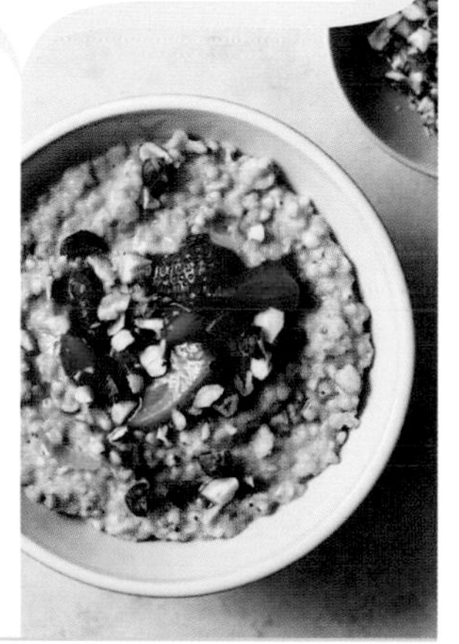

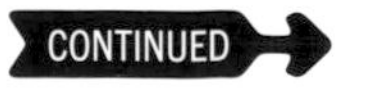

HEART AND BLOOD CONDITIONS

Many studies have been done on food and heart conditions, since the heart's so vital to life. Discover how nutrients can help cut the risk of certain diseases that become more common with age.

HEART DISEASE

Given the heart's never-ending activity, it's no surprise that this fist-sized muscular organ requires a constant supply of blood. The most common problem causing a narrowing of the arteries is atherosclerosis—where cholesterol-rich plaques build up on the insides of artery walls, which can occur anywhere in the body. If a plaque breaks free, it can travel in the blood until it interferes with the flow in a small artery or, worse, becomes lodged, blocking flow entirely and causing a heart attack (see right) or a stroke (see page 160).

Cardiovascular diseases are the number-one cause of death around the world.

Although many people develop some form of cardiovascular disease (a term that groups all diseases affecting the heart and blood vessels) as they get older, it is in no way inevitable. An active lifestyle, including a plant-based diet, goes a long way to preventing cardiovascular disease. Almost every wonderfood in this book has heart-based benefits.

EAT PLENTY
Fresh fruits and vegetables, whole grains, legumes, soy, fish and shellfish, olive oil, nuts, spices

LIMIT
Processed foods, sodium, saturated fat

HIGH BLOOD PRESSURE

To reach all around your body and return to the heart, blood has to be pumped under a certain level of pressure; but too much pressure is bad for the system. Your heart provides the driving force, creating a wave of pressure that passes through all the arteries in the body. Arteries offer a certain and healthy level of resistance when they're elastic and relaxed. However, when arteries become stiff and inflexible, they offer more resistance; this is measurable as high blood pressure, also known as hypertension.

Undiagnosed or untreated, high blood pressure can damage other organs, such as the kidneys and the eyes. There aren't any noticeable symptoms, so it's a good idea to have it measured regularly.

Avoiding sodium is the first line of nutritional defense against high blood pressure, along with eating a plant-based diet rich in fiber and antioxidants.

EAT PLENTY
Yogurt, berries, bananas, root vegetables, avocados, leafy greens, fish and shellfish, mushrooms, tomatoes, olive oil, spices, squashes

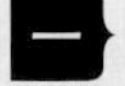

LIMIT
Sodium, alcohol

HIGH CHOLESTEROL LEVELS

Cholesterol is a waxy substance made in the liver. Although it has a bad reputation, you need a certain amount of cholesterol for healthy cell membranes and to make bile acids, vitamin D, and steroid hormones such as estrogen and testosterone. The body packages cholesterol in two main forms: as low-density lipoprotein (LDL) and high-density lipoprotein (HDL).

LDL cholesterol forms tiny, light particles that are associated with hardening and furring up of the arteries, whereas HDL cholesterol forms large, heavy particles that are too big to seep into artery walls. HDL is referred to as "good" cholesterol (LDL is "bad"), as it stays in the blood and transports the cholesterol away from your arteries and to the liver for processing.

Diet can influence blood cholesterol levels significantly, and many of the wonderfoods offer cholesterol-lowering benefits, as does the longevity eating plan.

EAT PLENTY
Fresh fruits and vegetables, whole grains (particularly oats and barley), legumes, soy, fish and shellfish, olive oil, nuts

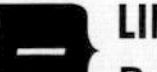

LIMIT
Processed foods, sodium, saturated fat

HEART ATTACK

Your heart has its own network of arteries—the coronary arteries—that supply its hard-working muscle cells with oxygen-rich blood. These fine vessels ensure the heart can pump 70 times or so each and every minute. If this blood supply fails due to narrowed or blocked arteries, you will experience heart muscle pain known as angina. But if the blood supply is compromised more severely—for example, by a blood clot or arterial spasm—then a heart attack occurs as heart muscle cells are deprived of oxygen and die. Emergency medical attention is required to treat a heart attack, but you can do a lot to prevent heart attacks by adjusting what you eat; the longevity eating plan has heart health at its core (see page 44).

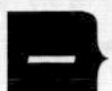

EAT PLENTY
Fresh fruits and vegetables, whole grains, legumes, soy, fish and shellfish, olive oil, nuts, spices

LIMIT
Processed foods, sodium, saturated fat

HEART FAILURE

As we age, our heart gradually declines in its ability to pump blood around the body. The heart doesn't stop pumping, but it can no longer get blood to the peripheral parts of the body, and this comes with consequences. Heart failure most often is caused by one or a combination of the following: heart disease, high blood pressure, cardiomyopathy, or a valve or rhythm disorder.

Heart failure occurs 10 times more often in people over 75 than in younger adults.

Most cases of heart failure occur in people over 80, although its prevalence starts rising from the age of 60. Treatment will depend on the cause, but diet has a part to play. Since the heart is a big muscle, a diet high in potassium-rich foods, such as fruits and vegetables, can be beneficial for muscle contractions.

EAT PLENTY
Fresh fruits and vegetables, yogurt

LIMIT
Sodium, saturated fat, sugar, alcohol

GUT HEALTH

It's good to discover that food can actually help promote the health of your gut, whatever your age. Find out how adjusting what you eat can cut the risk of certain diseases, such as type 2 diabetes and colon cancer.

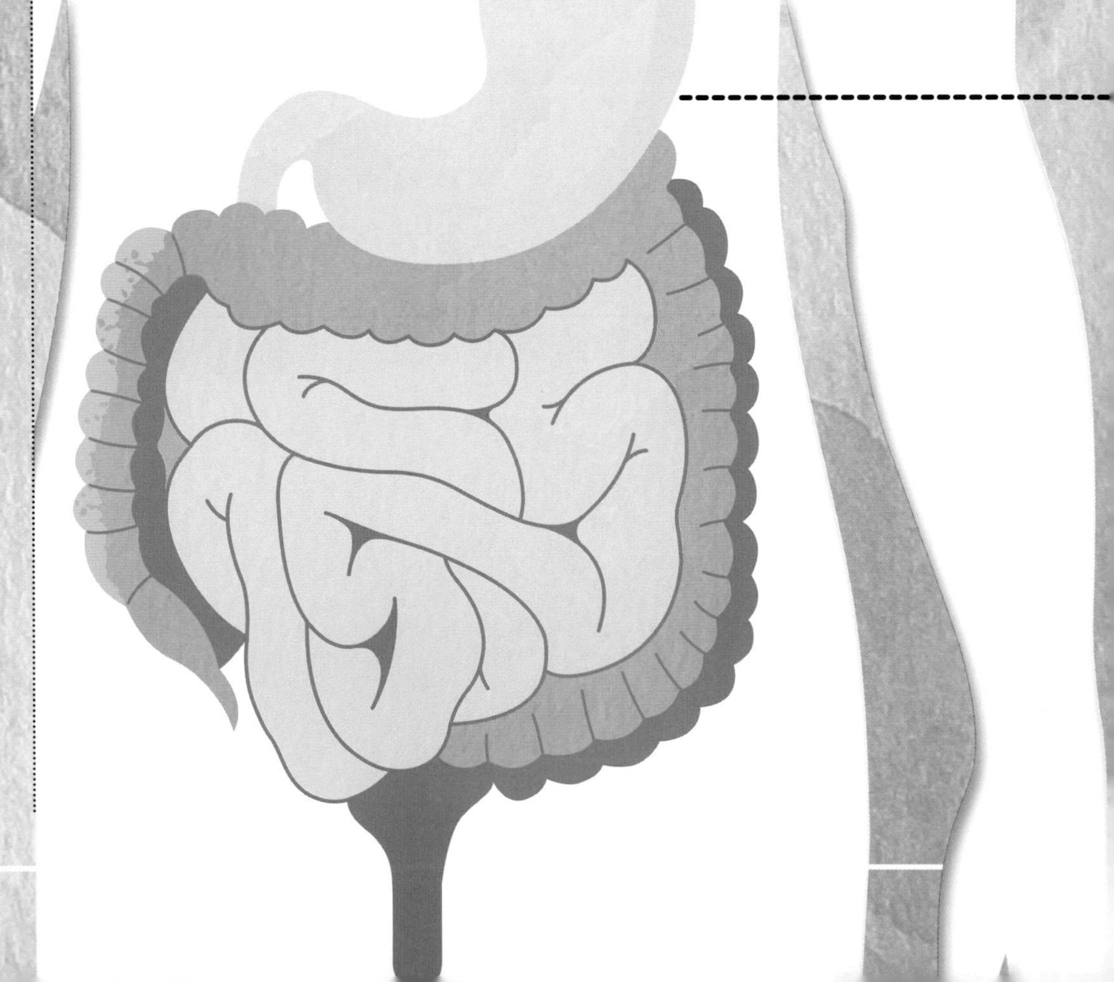

AS WE AGE ...

The digestive tract is basically a long elastic and muscular tube that stretches to fit food in and move it through its length. All manner of changes occur with age, but you can address these via your diet.

Digestive movements slow

The smooth transit of food through the digestive tract is aided by rhythmic wavelike contractions (peristalsis) that squeeze food through the esophagus, small intestine, and colon. We don't need to think about controlling such contractions, as the part of our nervous system not under conscious control automatically takes care of them. But a natural drop in neuron numbers with age, together with slower impulses and a loss in muscle tone, slows down peristalsis and makes digestion increasingly sluggish, making constipation more likely. Eat fiber daily to keep the digestive system functioning smoothly.

Gut flora changes

The digestive tract is teeming with over 100 trillion micro-organisms, which affects not only gut health but many aspects of our well-being, including our immune system (see page 175). As we age, the composition of gut bacteria becomes less diverse. Just one of the side effects is potential digestive complaints, such as constipation and bloating. Eating more prebiotic and probiotic foods (see page 198) helps to promote healthy and diverse gut flora.

It's harder to digest and absorb key nutrients

The right level of stomach acidity is vital to destroy bacteria in food, but also to enable digestive enzymes to work effectively. However, once we reach our 50s, the stomach lining becomes less active and the production of acid can fall. Less acidic conditions can make it harder for the body to absorb several nutrients, including iron, folate, zinc, calcium, and vitamin B12. Eat gut-friendly foods (see page 198) and follow the longevity eating plan (see page 44), which provides all micronutrients in plentiful amounts.

Nearly 40 percent of older adults have one or more age-related digestive symptoms each year.

Stomach capacity declines

The stomach lining loses elasticity with age, so it is less able to accommodate large amounts of food. Food takes longer to move into the small intestine, too, so the stomach feels fuller for longer; as a result, appetite may wane. A poor appetite can result in poor nutrient intake. Eating small amounts regularly, rather than a few big meals, can help to ensure enough food is eaten to meet nutritional needs.

CONTINUED

FOODS FOR GUT HEALTH

The digestive tract—all 29½ft (9m) of it—is designed to extract all the goodness from our diet. Each part of the gut is functionally different and responds better to certain foods. Fiber-rich foods and probiotics promote gut health, while refined foods are linked to disease.

BANANAS

Bananas are an excellent source of prebiotics—nondigestible carbohydrates that make their way into the large intestine to feed good bacteria. One study of overweight women found that eating two bananas a day as a snack increased levels of bifidobacteria (good bacteria) in the gut after 30 days.

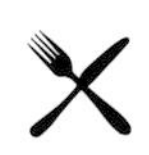

Banana pancakes with spiced apple rings (see page 67)

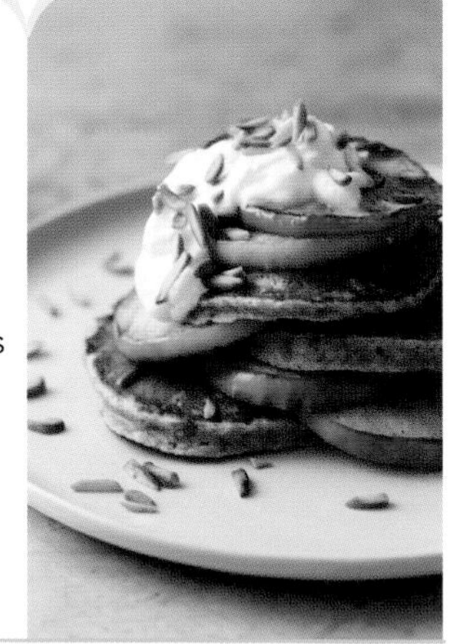

WHOLE GRAINS

Whole grains are packed with fiber, which is essential for healthy digestion and preventing constipation. Studies also show that cereal fiber and whole grains offer the greatest protection against colon cancer—one study found three daily servings of whole grains reduced the risk by 17 percent.

Mushrooms stuffed with tomato couscous (see page 125)

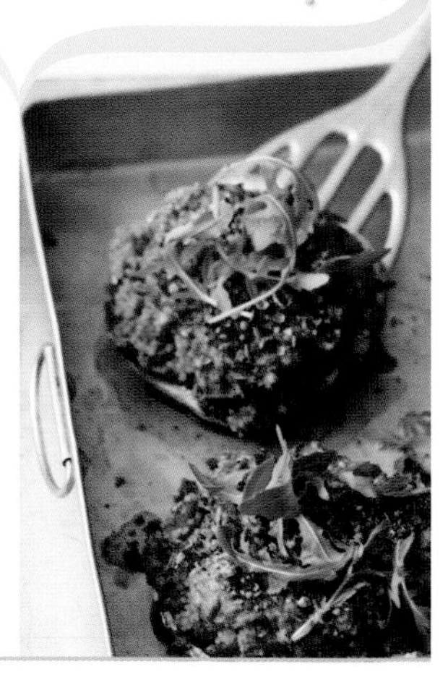

NUTS

Studies show that people who eat nuts find it easier to control their weight, possibly because nuts are satiating. Research also shows some of the nuts' fat passes into the gut undigested, so fewer calories than would be expected are absorbed. Studies also show that those who eat at least 1oz (28g) of nuts five times a week had a 25–30 percent lower risk of gallstones.

GINGER

Studies show ginger fights nausea, stimulates bile production, relieves stomach discomfort, and speeds transit through the digestive tract. It also helps to break up and dispel intestinal gas, to counter bloating.

LEGUMES

Beans, lentils, and chickpeas are high in fiber and protein, helping us stay fuller for longer. Their soluble fiber aids blood sugar control, while insoluble fiber is filling and helps to keep waste moving, guarding against constipation.

33% lower risk of colon cancer by eating legumes at least three times a week.

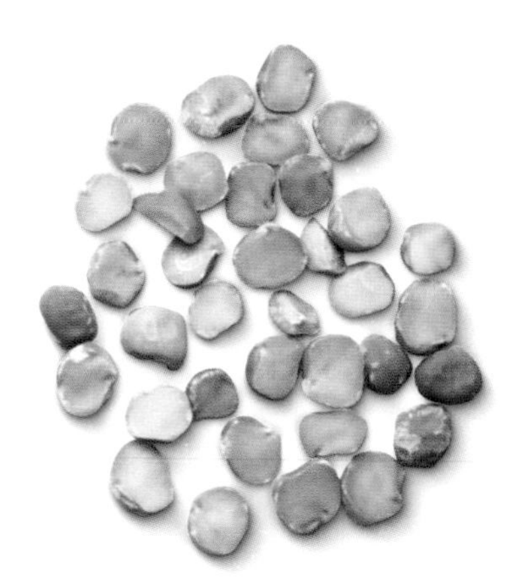

YOGURT

Yogurt is packed with probiotic bacteria, which may protect against constipation and ulcerative colitis. Eating yogurt has been linked to having lower body weight, less body fat, and smaller waists.

Good intakes of yogurt are linked to a reduced risk of type 2 diabetes and a lower body mass index.

FRUITS AND VEGETABLES

All fruits and vegetables have positive effects on the digestive system. Their fiber intake helps to control blood sugar and adds bulk to stools, helping to prevent constipation. Some fiber feeds gut bacteria, helping them to flourish.

Beet, pepper, and chunky hummus wrap (see page 96)

Foods to avoid

- **Meat**—Limit red meat to no more than 1lb 2oz (500g/cooked weight) a week and avoid processed meat altogether. Both are linked to a higher risk of colon cancer. Processed meat has also been shown to increase the risk of stomach cancer.
- **Refined foods**—Skip white, processed carbs (pasta, bread, and rice), as they're low in most nutrients and take the place of fiber-packed and nutrient-rich whole grains.
- **Sugary and soft drinks**—Sugar-sweetened drinks increase the risk of type 2 diabetes. Soft drinks and products containing artificial sweeteners (such as sorbitol, mannitol, or xylitol) can have a laxative effect.
- **Alcohol**—Excessive amounts of alcohol increases the risk of several digestive cancers, including those of the esophagus and colon.

CONTINUED

GUT HEALTH CONDITIONS

When it's working well, we rarely register our gut, but when something goes awry, it can become hard to ignore. Below are common age-related conditions that significantly affect gut health and how these can be addressed through diet.

CONSTIPATION

Even if you are failing to pass a stool every day, this doesn't mean you're constipated. Chronic constipation is defined as having fewer than three bowel movements a week for at least 3 months. Physiological changes make constipation more likely with age. Bowel contractions weaken, so waste moves more slowly and more water is absorbed en route, making stools harder and more difficult to pass. Eat whole-grain foods and a range of fruits and vegetables every day to boost fiber, and increase your intake of fluids. If constipation doesn't ease, visit your doctor.

Drinking plenty of fluids is one of the simplest ways to avoid constipation and keep things moving.

EAT PLENTY
Fresh fruits and vegetables, whole grains, legumes, fluids

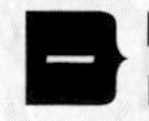
LIMIT
Processed foods, refined carbs

OBESITY

Doctors use body mass index, or BMI, to assess whether a person's weight is healthy for their height and to identify if they are under- or overweight or obese. A BMI of 25 to 29.9 means you're above your ideal weight, and a BMI of 30 or above is obese. Obesity can exacerbate the natural changes that occur with aging, these changes increase the risks of many conditions, such as heart disease, type 2 diabetes, and certain cancers. Being active and eating a diet such as the longevity eating plan (see page 44, with its high intake of fruits and vegetables, fiber-rich food, and monounsaturated fats) helps to keep weight at a healthy level.

EAT PLENTY
Fresh fruits and vegetables, whole grains, legumes

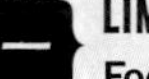
LIMIT
Foods high in saturated fat, processed foods

TYPE 2 DIABETES

The hormone insulin plays a crucial role in keeping blood sugar levels under control. It's responsible for allowing glucose into cells for conversion to fuel, which is either used immediately or stored as glycogen for later use. When insulin isn't working as it should, diabetes can result. Type 1 diabetes is an autoimmune condition that destroys insulin-producing cells. In type 2 diabetes, cells no longer respond properly to insulin; this type of diabetes has a close correlation with obesity and age. As we age, the body also becomes less efficient at using glucose, so our diabetes risk increases. However, this type of diabetes has a close correlation with lifestyle and age, and is far more likely to develop in people who are overweight or obese.

Diabetes can have a cumulative effect on health overall and accelerate aging, especially if it's undiagnosed or poorly controlled, contributing to eye and joint problems and affecting kidney function. Type 2 diabetes is largely preventable.

Several large-scale studies have shown that making targeted lifestyle changes can slash the chances of developing diabetes by as much as 50 percent in at-risk individuals. Building periods of activity or exercise into each day is essential, and following a balanced healthy eating regime, such as the longevity eating plan (see page 44), can help control weight.

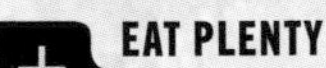
EAT PLENTY
Yogurt, fresh fruits and vegetables, whole grains, legumes, spices

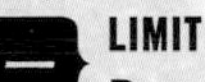
LIMIT
Processed foods, sugary foods

GALLSTONES

The gallbladder stores bile, a substance produced by the liver to help the body digest fats. If there is an imbalance in the chemical make-up of bile, gallstones can form; these can be large or small. As many as one in six of us has these stones; their presence is known only when a stone becomes stuck in one of the bile ducts and causes pain. If this happens, doctors may remove the gallbladder via keyhole surgery. Obesity is a contributing risk factor, so being a healthy weight reduces your risk. If you need to lose weight, aim to achieve this slowly, since studies show that rapid weight loss increases the risk of developing gallstones.

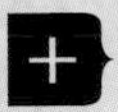
EAT PLENTY
Fresh fruits and vegetables, legumes, nuts

LIMIT
Processed meats, fatty foods

DIVERTICULAR DISEASE

After the age of 50, changes in the large intestinal wall can lead to the formation of small pouches, known as diverticulae. Up to one in three people between 50 and 60 are affected. The condition can have no symptoms, but if waste in the colon gets lodged in a pouch and becomes infected, diverticulitis results. Though common with age, diverticular disease isn't inevitable; being a healthy weight and active reduce the risk of the condition. Research is ongoing into the causes, but it's thought that healthy gut flora may play a part in promoting colon health (see page 198).

EAT PLENTY
Yogurt, fresh fruits and vegetables, whole grains, legumes, nuts, fluids

COLON CANCER

Colon cancer risk rises with age. Most cases develop from polyps, which are stalklike growths in the colon, but not every polyp becomes cancerous. Polyps can usually be removed before they become harmful, so have a check-up if you have a family history of polyps or an inflammatory bowel condition. Eat plenty of high-fiber foods and aim to get most protein from sources such as fish, beans, and soy.

Cancer is a leading cause of death. Colon cancer is the third most common cancer worldwide.

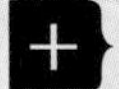
EAT PLENTY
Fresh fruits and vegetables (particularly berries and leafy greens), whole grains, legumes, nuts, spices

LIMIT
Red meat, processed foods

URINARY HEALTH

Your kidneys work tirelessly, filtering all your blood several times a day to remove waste, which exits the body via the bladder in urine. A decline in function and control is coupled with an upsurge in infections—thankfully, all respond well to nutrients in food.

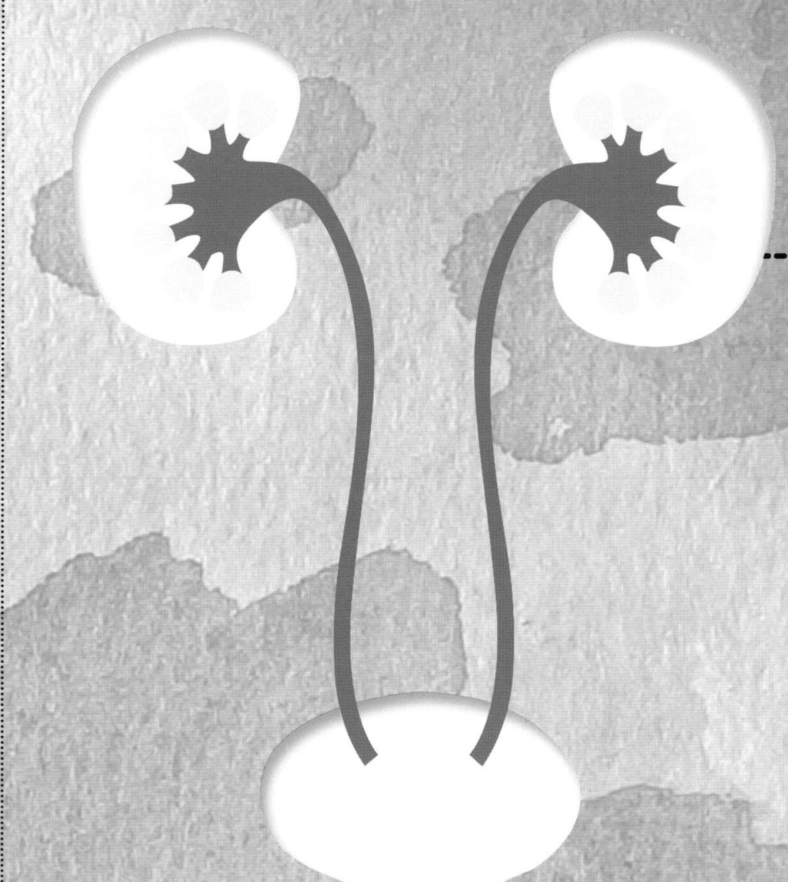

AS WE AGE ...

Gradual physical changes can lead to some commonly experienced urinary conditions, but fluids and foods offer plenty of possible approaches for good urinary health.

Filtration rates fall

The kidneys have a huge blood supply, and ever-narrowing blood vessels channel the blood into microfiltering units called nephrons. The numbers of nephrons and the kidney's filtration rate decline with age. Hardening of blood vessels within the kidney via the process of atherosclerosis means that blood is filtered more slowly. So eating foods that are good for your heart and circulation—such as fruits, vegetables, whole grains, and olive oil (see page 192)—may also benefit your kidneys.

UTIs are more common

Urinary tract infections, or UTIs, are the second most common infection and become more numerous with age; plus, women are more prone to them than men (due to anatomical differences). Studies also show that bladder infections can be directly linked to *E. coli* bacteria. Probiotic foods, such as yogurt (see page 56), are key to promoting healthy bacteria in the gut to cut *E.coli* numbers. Some studies find little evidence for the use of cranberry juice; other studies show that its anti-adhesion powers can stop *E.coli* sticking to the urinary tract walls and reduce UTIs.

Ninety percent of urinary tract infections are caused by *E. coli* bacteria from the gut.

Salt is an issue

High salt or sodium levels in the blood stress the kidneys as they try to retain water to dilute the sodium. As kidney function declines with age, the kidneys have to work even harder to counteract the sodium, resulting in stiffer blood vessels and high blood pressure. Potassium opposes sodium and can help relax vessels, excrete sodium, and lower blood pressure. Limiting salt and eating potassium-rich foods (see page 164) can help the kidneys work better and cut the risk of disease.

Bladder control declines

The tissue in the bladder wall loses its elasticity over time, so the bladder can no longer hold the same volume and empties less completely. With age, it also becomes harder to delay urination after sensing the need to go. Such changes mean older people may urinate more often and suffer more with urinary incontinence. Foods can help: high-fiber foods, such as whole grains (see page 204), keep you regular. (Constipation exacerbates incontinence.) Older people can also suffer from an overactive bladder, which can be irritated by certain foods and drinks.

CONTINUED

FOODS FOR URINARY HEALTH

When it comes to supporting urinary health, fluid intake is of paramount importance, along with reducing sodium intake and eating more potassium-rich foods. What's more, addressing gut bacteria can help dramatically reduce the risk of urinary tract infections.

FRUITS AND VEGGIES

They're rich in water and potassium, which helps to normalize blood pressure when combined with a lower sodium intake. High blood pressure is one of the most common causes of kidney damage. Top choices for potassium include potatoes, parsnips, bananas, avocados, dried fruits, and baby spinach. The World Cancer Research Fund confirms they may protect against bladder cancer, too.

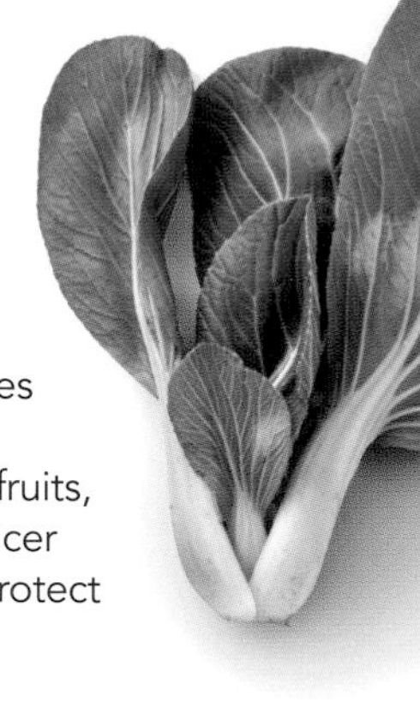

WATER AND TEA

Drinking plenty of fluids helps the kidneys work properly, which lowers the risk of kidney problems such as chronic kidney disease, urinary tract infections, and urinary incontinence. Water is the top choice for hydration. Tea may protect against bladder cancer, according to the World Cancer Research Fund, but caffeine-containing drinks may make incontinence worse by irritating the bladder.

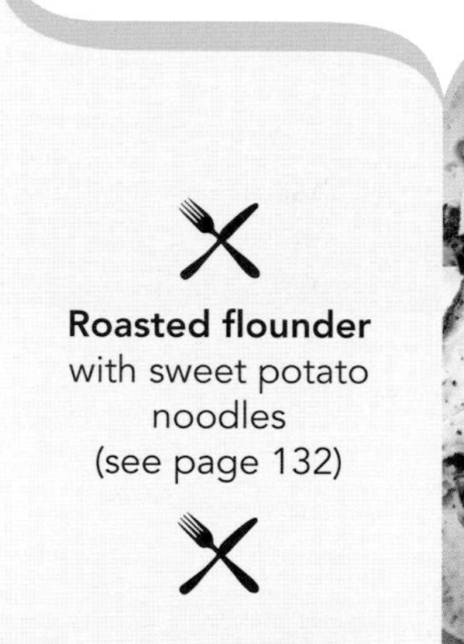

Roasted flounder with sweet potato noodles (see page 132)

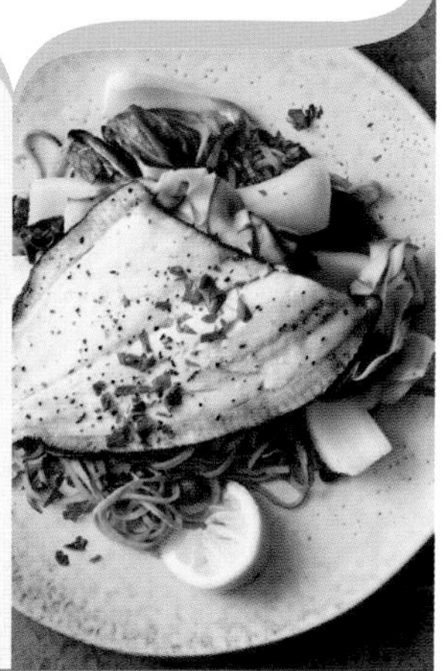

WHOLE GRAINS

A few studies have found that higher intakes of whole grains are linked to improved kidney function. Good intakes also protect against type 2 diabetes, which is a major cause of kidney damage.

Shrimp, pomegranate, and quinoa bowl (see page 80)

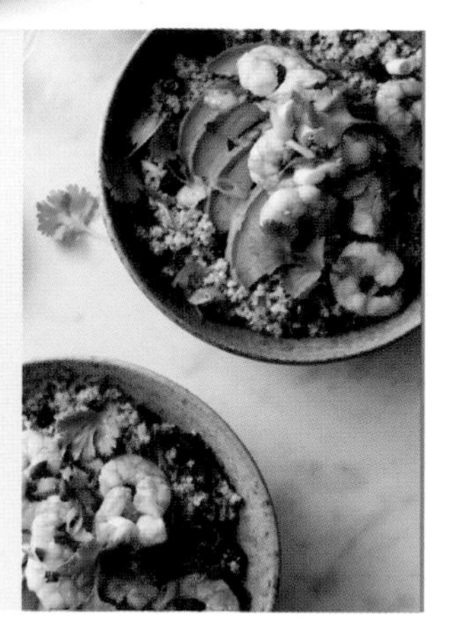

YOGURT

Certain *Lactobacillus* strains (found in yogurt) have been shown to be beneficial against UTIs. In a study, women who consumed fermented milk products at least three times a week cut their odds of UTIs by 79 percent, compared with those eating them less than once a week.

BANANAS

It's not just their high potassium content that makes bananas a great choice for healthy kidneys; they also contain vitamin B6, and some studies show this vitamin may help to reduce levels of oxalate in urine. Oxalate binds with calcium to form the most common type of kidney stones, so keeping oxalate levels down may help to protect against kidney stones.

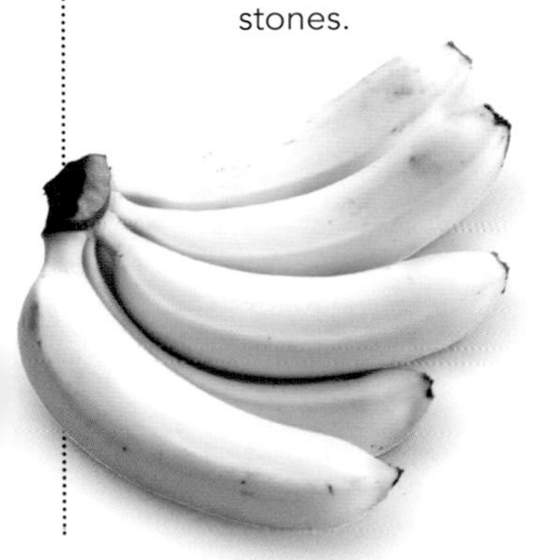

Foods to avoid

- **Salt**—Avoiding salt and limiting salty foods will help to keep high blood pressure under control.
- **High-protein diets**—Excessive amounts of protein can damage the kidneys. A 2017 study found that red and processed meats are linked to an increased risk of developing chronic kidney disease.

URINARY CONDITIONS

Particular nutrients have been shown to help or hinder common age-related urinary conditions. Discover which foods to include and which to exclude.

URINARY INCONTINENCE

Urinary incontinence is a term for any leakage of urine. Stress incontinence is an involuntary leakage of urine when increased pressure "stresses" the valve mechanism that normally keeps the bladder closed; urine leaks on exertion, such as jumping or coughing. In urgency incontinence, an involuntary leakage is accompanied by a sudden need to pass urine that is hard to ignore. This urgency may be associated with an overactive bladder, meaning more frequent toilet trips. Women are twice as likely as men to suffer from incontinence. Drink plenty of fluids, and eat potassium-rich and hydrating foods while avoiding any foods and drinks that could irritate the bladder (see Limit, below).

+ EAT PLENTY
Fresh fruits and vegetables (particularly bananas and avocados), fluids

− LIMIT
Caffeine, alcohol, citrus fruits, spicy foods, sugar

URINARY TRACT INFECTION

Urinary tract infections, or UTIs, are the second most common infection. Postmenopausal women are particularly susceptible because declining estrogen levels make them more vulnerable to infection. Typical symptoms include painful, frequent, and urgent urination along with unpleasant-smelling urine. In mild cases, only one or two symptoms occur, and these may resolve if you drink lots of fluids; if the infection is severe, you will feel very unwell, so visit a doctor. In older people, UTIs can lead to confusion and increase the risk of a fall. Eat foods that promote good bacteria in the gut to help prevent UTIs; keep fluid intake up for healthy kidneys.

+ EAT PLENTY
Yogurt, fresh fruits and veggies, fluids

− LIMIT
Caffeine, alcohol, spicy foods

CHRONIC KIDNEY DISEASE

Anyone can get this common condition that's often associated with getting older, but it's more prevalent in certain ethnic groups, such as African Americans and those of South Asian origin. Many people with kidney disease are able to live long, largely normal lives. Causes include high blood pressure, diabetes, and high cholesterol levels, as well as certain medicines. If you have chronic kidney disease, your doctor may refer you to a dietitian. This person will work with you to devise an eating plan designed to help control your condition while giving you all the nutrients you need to stay in good health.

WOMEN'S HEALTH

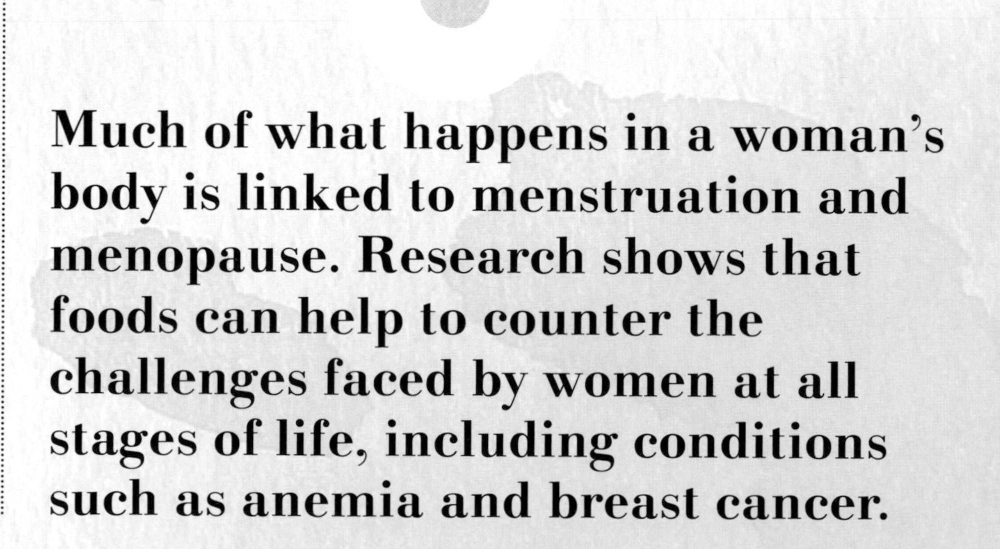

Much of what happens in a woman's body is linked to menstruation and menopause. Research shows that foods can help to counter the challenges faced by women at all stages of life, including conditions such as anemia and breast cancer.

AS WE AGE ...

The end of a woman's reproductive life is a natural part of aging. Most women experience menopause between the ages of 45 and 55, and it can have wide-ranging effects.

Our bodies change shape

Before the age of 40, women tend to have more fat cells in their thighs, hips, and buttocks, so fat accumulates under the skin in those areas. But around menopause, the decline in hormone levels can lead to fat deposits shifting to areas in and around the belly. Known as visceral fat, this fat concentrates around the abdomen and comes with extra health risks related to heart disease and cancers. A diet rich in refined foods, sugars, and saturated fat encourages this "belly fat," so steer clear of those. If you want to shift weight, then fill up on whole grains and fiber-rich legumes (see page 208), eat natural fats in foods (see page 34), and try out the fat-burning power of chilies (see page 90).

Women with waistlines over 35in (88cm) are more likely to die from heart disease and cancer.

Depression may crop up

Menopause sees ovaries cease to release eggs and the end of menstruation, with consequent drops in levels of estrogen and progesterone. Studies have shown that women are at a greater risk of depression compared to men. A study in 2015 discovered that the fluctuations in estrogen levels around menopause make women more susceptible to depression and sensitive to stress. Up to a third of women will develop depression when estrogen levels fall. So it's good to know that food may have a role to play. Certain foods, such as soy, contain plant-based estrogen compounds (phyto-estrogens), and these may mimic the effects of estrogen and help to counter the effects of menopause. Japanese women, for example, who have a diet high in soy appear to suffer fewer menopausal symptoms. Another food solution is omega-3 fats in fish (see page 112), which can improve mood.

Vaginal changes have consequences

As levels of hormones fall at and around menopause, the vaginal walls become thinner, less rigid, and less elastic, while lubrication is produced at lower levels and more slowly than before, all of which can result in irritation, dryness, and discharge. The internal environment of the vagina also becomes more attractive to microbes. Research shows that soy foods (see page 100) can ease vaginal dryness (see page 209), and probiotics (see page 56) may also help avoid infections.

CONTINUED

FOODS FOR WOMEN'S HEALTH

The wide-ranging effects of menopause call for an equally diverse array of foods to oppose the negative effects of declining estrogen levels. Fill up on foods to counteract changes in mood, iron levels, and bone strength, while cutting out or down on alcohol.

OILY FISH

Omega-3 fats help modulate mood swings and depression caused by the hormonal fluctuations associated with menopause. What's more, they're loaded with vitamin D to keep bones strong.

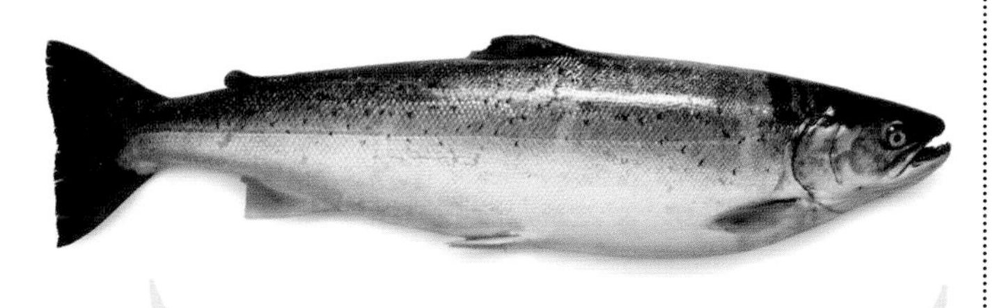

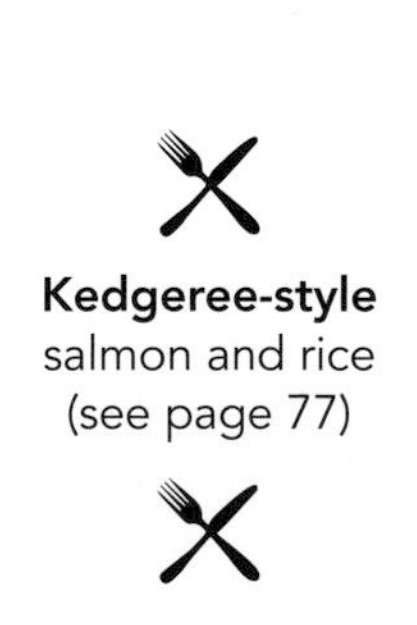

Kedgeree-style salmon and rice (see page 77)

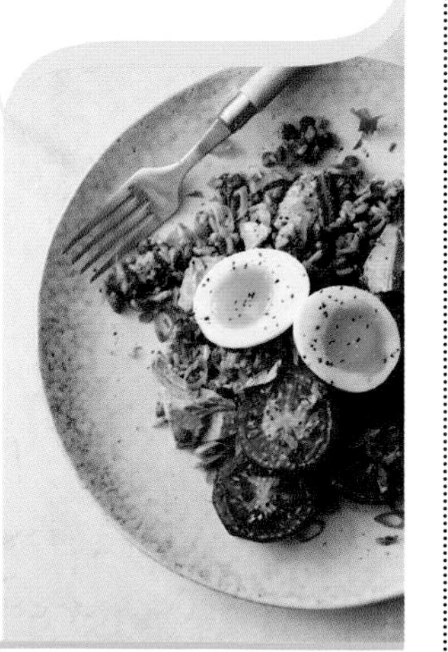

SOY

Research now reveals that soy probably helps to protect against breast cancer. Good intakes of soy may also help to ease menopause-related symptoms, such as hot flashes and vaginal dryness.

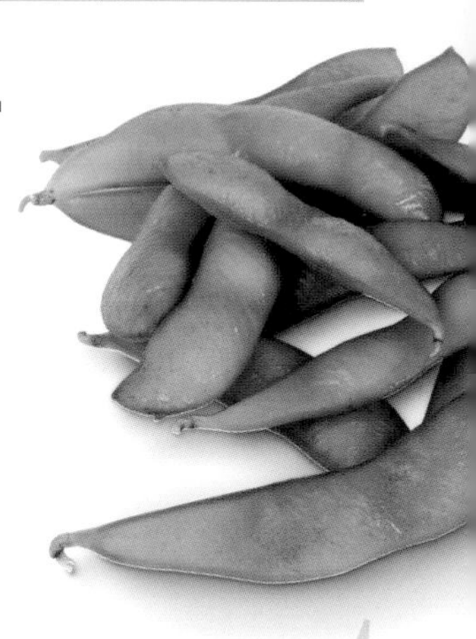

Japanese-style noodle soup (see page 139)

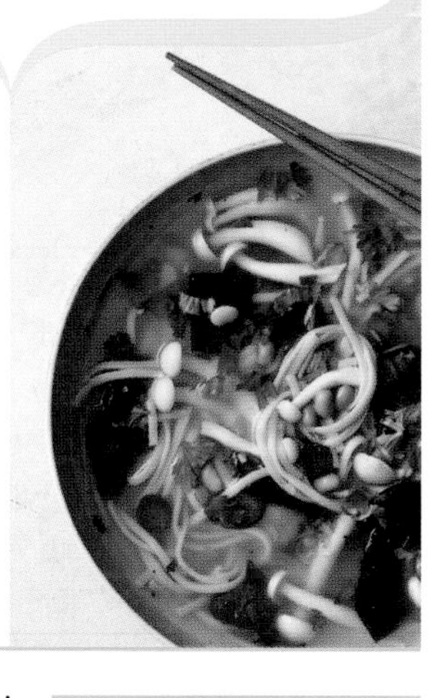

LEGUMES

Nutrient-rich beans, chickpeas, and lentils contain good amounts of phyto-estrogens that help counter both menopausal symptoms and the increased risk of heart disease after menopause.

EGGS

Eggs are naturally rich in vitamin D, which helps the body to absorb calcium and keep bones strong. Plus, eggs are a good vegetarian source of iron, low levels of which can lead to iron-deficiency anemia (see opposite).

YOGURT

Yogurt is rich in three bone-strengthening nutrients—calcium, phosphorus, and protein. Estrogen helps to keep bones strong, so when estrogen levels drop during menopause, bones become weaker. In fact, women lose up to 20 percent of their bone density in the 5 to 7 years after menopause.

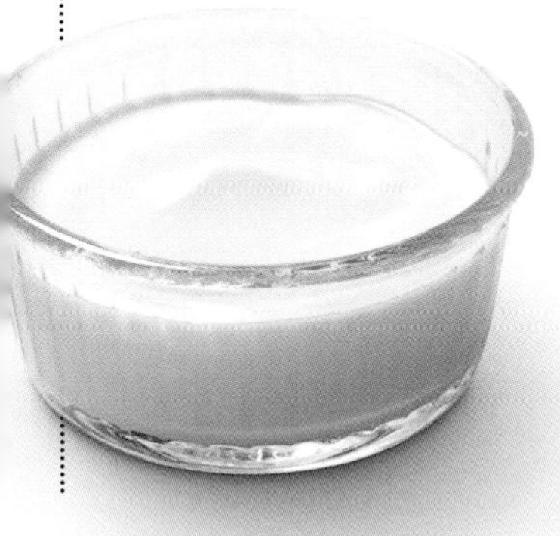

Foods to avoid

- **Alcohol**—Even small amounts of alcohol increase the risk of breast cancer—just one drink a day (about 1.5 units) boosts the risk by 4 percent. This risk increases the more a woman drinks—each additional 1.25 units correlating to a 7–12 percent rise.

WOMEN'S HEALTH CONDITIONS

With menopause comes all manner of body-wide effects. But it's good to know that what you eat can help prevent or reduce the risk of many of these common conditions.

VAGINAL DRYNESS

This common menopausal symptom results from declining levels of estrogen. Up to 40 percent of women may experience such vaginal discomfort, but fewer than 25 percent report it to a doctor. In addition to irritation, vaginal dryness can make sexual intercourse painful and can lead to frequent urinary tract infections (see page 205). Use a water-soluble lubricant to make sex more enjoyable and adjust your diet to include more foods rich in phyto-estrogens (see opposite).

+ EAT PLENTY
Phyto-estrogen-rich foods, such as soy, flaxseeds, whole grains, legumes

IRON-DEFICIENCY ANEMIA

The most common form of anemia, iron-deficiency anemia is a condition where a lack of iron in the body leads to a reduction in the number of red blood cells. Iron is an essential constituent of hemoglobin—the oxygen-carrying pigment within all red blood cells. Fewer red blood cells than normal means your body won't get as much oxygen, which can make you feel breathless, lethargic, and tired; experience heart palpitations; and appear pale. Heavy periods are a common cause of this anemia, so eating plenty of iron-rich foods can help prevent and treat this condition. Calcium can interfere with iron absorption, so be mindful about eating calcium-rich foods.

+ EAT PLENTY
Eggs, brown rice, legumes, tofu, leafy greens, fish, nuts, seeds, dried apricots

– LIMIT
Tea, coffee, calcium-rich foods

BREAST CANCER

A cancerous tumor of the breast almost always affects women; rarely, men can be affected. Breast cancer is the most often diagnosed cancer in women worldwide, with an estimated 1.7 million new cases in 2012. The first sign of cancer is often a painless lump; other symptoms may include nipple discharge or indentation. Mostly, just one breast is affected. Certain foods appear to protect against breast cancer, while others have been shown to increase the risk.

+ EAT PLENTY
Soy, fresh fruits and vegetables (particularly mushrooms and tomatoes), olive oil, spices, green tea

LIMIT
Alcohol, processed foods, red meat

MEN'S HEALTH

Testosterone has a part to play in age-related changes, but it's the prostate gland that can cause the most day-to-day trouble. Luckily, research shows hope for foods to address both erectile function and prostate problems.

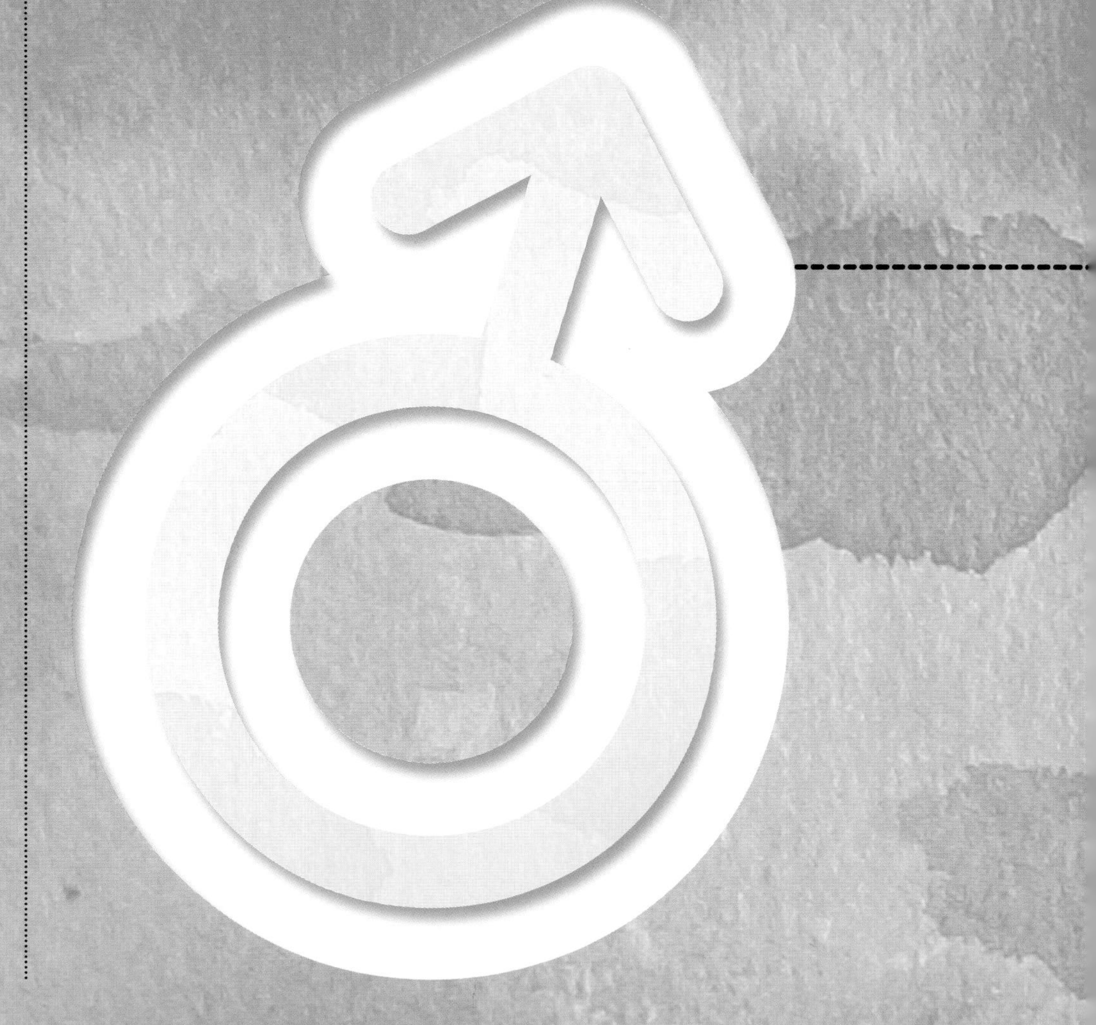

AS WE AGE ...

Small and subtle changes start to make themselves known after the age of 50. Increasingly, there are dietary solutions to lessen the effects of these common age-related changes.

Testosterone levels start to decline

The male hormone testosterone is mostly made in the testes; women do produce testosterone but at much lower levels. Testosterone drives crucial body processes: it regulates sex drive, bone density, fat distribution, muscle mass, and muscle strength, among others. Between the ages of 40 and 60, 1 in 12 men develop symptoms, such as low libido, erectile problems, and mood swings, as a result of low testosterone levels. Some studies suggest that a deficiency in zinc can cause lower testosterone levels, so it's a good idea to address any missing zinc from the diet; see page 212 for zinc-rich foods. There are also reports that men with low levels of vitamin D have lower testosterone levels, so be sure to get enough sunshine (see page 36).

Men's testosterone levels fall by roughly 1 percent every year from the age of 30.

The prostate enlarges

Between early adulthood and the age of 40, a healthy prostate gland is about the size of a walnut. It sits beneath the bladder and surrounds the tube through which urine or sperm exits. The prostate makes secretions, accounting for 30 percent of semen and including enzymes, cholesterol, and fatty acids. After the age of 45, the number of cells in the prostate rises, so the gland grows bigger. An enlarged prostate, or benign prostatic hyperplasia (BPH), can have effects on both urination and erection (see page 213). Thankfully, BPH responds well to dietary intervention—zinc (in shellfish), selenium (in Brazil nuts), and isoflavones (in soy) have been shown to lessen symptoms; see page 212.

Erections diminish

The risk of erectile problems rises with age—half of all men between the ages of 40 and 70 suffer from some degree of erectile dysfunction; in fact, it affects 86 percent of men aged 80 and over. Certain factors increase the likelihood of erectile issues, such as diabetes, heart disease, excess alcohol, and smoking. Nutritional factors also come into play; research has explored the effects of various foods on erectile dysfunction (see page 213). Since blood flow has such a role, enjoying heart-friendly foods (see page 192) also benefits penile function.

CONTINUED

FOODS FOR MEN'S HEALTH

When it comes to men's health, there are myriad multicolored foods with nutrients that support the healthy function of the male reproductive system. And by knowing what to pile on your plate and what to leave off, you can influence your risk of common conditions.

NUTS AND SEEDS

Nuts and seeds offer selenium (Brazil nuts are best), beta-sitosterols (sesame seeds offer a good supply), and zinc (sunflower seeds rank highest). Studies show that men with BPH and prostate cancer tend to have lower zinc levels in their blood and in prostate tissues.

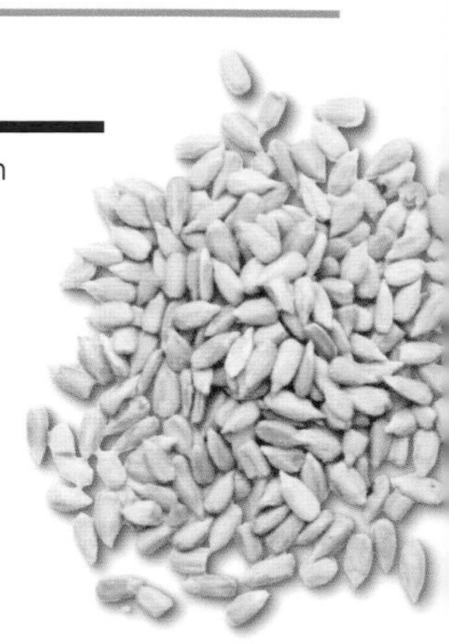

TOMATOES

It's unclear, despite research, if tomatoes or lycopene can prevent prostate cancer. But a review of studies in 2016 found a 14 percent reduction in the risk of prostate cancer in those who ate the most tomatoes.

Plant-based cooked breakfast (see page 68)

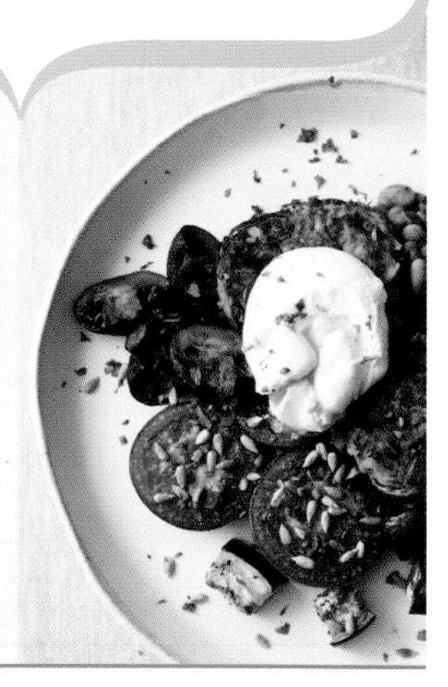

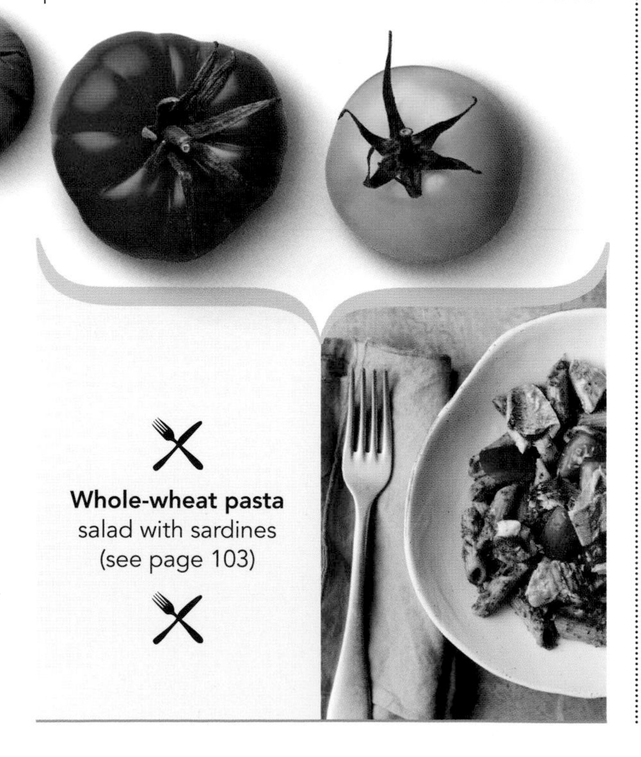

Whole-wheat pasta salad with sardines (see page 103)

FISH

All fish is rich in selenium, which is needed for sperm production. Shellfish (such as shrimp and crab) also contain zinc, which is vital for reproduction and normal levels of testosterone. Some studies also suggest omega-3 fats protect against prostate cancer.

SOY

Some studies suggest soy foods may protect against prostate cancer and benign prostatic hyperplasia. In one study, men who ate two daily servings of soy had lower blood levels of prostate-specific antigen—raised levels of which can indicate prostate problems.

BEETS

Beets are packed with nitrates, which may help with erectile dysfunction. Nitrates relax the muscular lining of all blood vessels, including in those in the penis, which enables the increased blood flow needed for an erection.

Foods to avoid

- **Foods high in saturated fat**—High intakes of saturated fat, such as in red meat and full-fat dairy, have been shown to increase the risk of prostate cancer.
- Since erectile dysfunction is often linked to type 2 diabetes (see page 200), high blood pressure (see page 194), and heart disease (see page 194), avoid foods that contribute to these.

MEN'S HEALTH CONDITIONS

Much research has revealed correlations between certain nutrients and the prevention of common age-related men's health conditions and the lessening of their symptoms.

ERECTILE DYSFUNCTION

A man's inability to have or maintain an erection is known as erectile dysfunction and becomes much more common with age. As well as factors previously mentioned (see page 211), side effects of drugs, nerve damage, and hormone imbalances can also cause erectile dysfunction. Diet has some influence, too; studies have shown that it's relatively uncommon in men eating a Mediterranean diet. No studies have looked specifically at beets and erectile function, but many have found that beets have benefits linked to widening blood vessels—lowering blood pressure and boosting sports performance.

+ EAT PLENTY
Fresh fruits and vegetables (particularly beets), whole grains, legumes, fish, olive oil, nuts, seeds

− LIMIT
Sodium, meat, processed/fried foods

BENIGN PROSTATIC HYPERPLASIA

Benign prostatic hyperplasia, or BPH, becomes more common with age: an estimated 50 percent of 50-year-olds, 60 percent of 60-year-olds, and so on, develop prostate problems. In some cases, BPH causes no symptoms, but in others the enlarged prostate can squeeze the urethra and interfere with urinary flow and erections. Much research shows that diet may help, including nutrients such as vitamin C, zinc, lycopene, and beta-sitosterol.

+ EAT PLENTY
Soy, avocados, leafy greens, fish and shellfish, tomatoes, garlic, nuts, seeds

− LIMIT
Processed foods, meat, caffeine, alcohol, spicy foods

PROSTATE CANCER

Prostate cancer is the second most common cancer in men worldwide. There is a genetic element, and a family history increases your risk, as does being overweight or obese. Most prostate cancers arise in the outer parts of the gland, and as such have few if any symptoms and are difficult to diagnose. Some studies show that the antioxidant lycopene may have a role in prevention.

+ EAT PLENTY
Soy, avocados, leafy greens, fish and shellfish, tomatoes, garlic, nuts, seeds

− LIMIT
Processed foods, meat, caffeine, alcohol, spicy foods

Bibliography

While every effort has been made to ensure the materials in this book are accurate, the publisher apologizes for any errors or omissions and would be grateful to be notified about any corrections. Sources are given in order of appearance across the spreads. All links accessed December 2017.

10–11 Theories of aging

American Federation for Aging Research, "Theories of Aging."

12–15 What affects how we age?

G. Passarino, *et al*, "Human longevity: Genetics or Lifestyle? It takes two to tango," *Immunity & Ageing* (2016) 13:12.

S. Mizushima, *et al*, "The relationship of dietary factors to cardiovascular diseases among Japanese in Okinawa and Japanese immigrants, originally from Okinawa, in Brazil," *Hypertens Res* (1992) 15(1):45–55.

M. H. Forouzanfar, *et al*, "Global, regional, and national comparative risk assessment of 79 behavioural, environmental and occupational, and metabolic risks or clusters of risks in 188 countries, 1990–2013," *Lancet* (2015) 386(10010):2287–2323.

WHO, "Western Pacific Region Obesity. Fact sheet number 311" (2014).

A. Peeters, *et al*, "Obesity in adulthood and its consequences for life expectancy: a life-table analysis," *Ann Intern Med* (2003) 138(1):24–32.

WHO, "Report of a joint WHO/FAO expert consultation. Diet, nutrition and the prevention of chronic diseases" (2003).

I. Lee, "Effect of physical inactivity on major non-communicable diseases worldwide," *Lancet* (2012) 380(9838):219–229.

American Academy of Neurology, "Can exercising your brain prevent memory loss?," presented at the AAN's 61st meeting in Seattle, 25 April–2 May 2009.

A. Machado, *et al*, "Chronic stress as a risk factor for Alzheimer's disease," *Rev Neurosci* (2014) 25(6):785–804.

J. Choi, *et al*, "Reduced telomerase activity in human T lymphocytes exposed to cortisol," *Brain Behav Immun* (2008) May 22(4):600–605.

A. Steptoe and J. Wardle, "Positive affect measured using ecological momentary assessment and survival in older men and women," *Proc Nat Acad Sci* (2011) 108(45): 18244–18248.

J. Holt-Lunstad, *et al*, "Social relationships and mortality risk," *PLoS Medicine* (2010) 7(7):e1000316.

S. Cohen, *et al*, "Sleep habits and susceptibility to the common cold," *Arch Intern Med* (2009) 169(1):62–67.

F. Flament, *et al*, "Effect of the sun on visible clinical signs of aging in Caucasian skin," *Clin Cosmet Investig Dermatol* (2013) 6:221–232.

Cancer Research UK, " Skin cancer statistics".

NHS Choices, "How smoking affects your body."

WHO, "Tobacco fact sheet" (2017).

16–19 Diet lessons from around the world

WHO, "Life expectancy at birth 2000–2015."

UN, "World Population Prospects. Key findings and advance tables," 2017 review.

N. Roswall, *et al*, "Adherence to the healthy Nordic food index and total and cause-specific mortality among Swedish women," *Eur J Epidemiol* (2015) 30(6):509–517.

A. Olsen, *et al*, "Healthy aspects of the Nordic diet are related to lower total mortality," *J Nutr* (2011) 141:639–644.

M. C. Morris, *et al*, "MIND diet associated with reduced incidence of Alzheimer's disease," *Alzheimers Dement* (2015) 11(9):1007–1014.

22–23 Downsize your meals as the day goes on

S. Shi, *et al*, "Circadian disruption leads to insulin resistance and obesity," *Curr Biol* (2013) 23(5):372–381.

M. P. Carrasco-Benso, *et al*, "Human adipose tissue expresses intrinsic circadian rhythm in insulin sensitivity," *FASEB J* (2016) 30(9):3117–3123.

E. Van Cauter, *et al*, "Roles of circadian rhythmicity and sleep in human glucose regulation. *Endoc Rev* (1997) 18(5):716–738.

S. Almoosawi, *et al*, "Chrono-nutrition: a review of current evidence from observational studies on global trends in time-of-day of energy intake and its association with obesity," *Proc Nutr Soc* (2016) 75:487–500.

H. Kahleova, *et al*, "Meal frequency and timing are associated with changes in body mass index in Adventist Health Study 2," *J Nutr* (2017) 147(9):1722–1728.

M. St-Onge, *et al*, "AHA Scientific Statement. Meal timing and frequency: Implications for cardiovascular disease prevention," *Circulation* (2017) 135(9):e96–e21

Y. Kubota, *et al*, "Association of breakfast intake with incident stroke and coronary heart disease: The Japan public health center-based study," *Stroke* (2016) 47(2): 477–481.

L. E. Cahill, *et al*, "A prospective study of breakfast eating and incident coronary heart disease in a cohort of male US health professionals," *Circulation* (2013) 128(4): 337–343.

R. A. Mekary, *et al*, "Eating patterns and type 2 diabetes risk in men: breakfast omission, eating frequency and snacking," *Am J Clin Nutr* (2012) 95(5): 1182–1189.

D. Jakubowicz, *et al*, "High calorie intake at breakfast vs dinner differentially influences weight loss of overweight and obese women," *Obesity* (2013) 21(12):2504–2512.

24–25 Know how much is enough

Global BMI mortality collaboration, "Body-mass index and all-cause mortality," *Lancet* (2016) 388(10046):776–786.

Health and Social Care Information Centre, "Health Survey for England 2016. Table 4: body mass index (BMI) by survey year, age and sex."

OECD, "Obesity Update 2017."

B. Wansink, *Mindless Eating: Why we eat more than we think?,* New York, NY: Bantam Dell, 2006.

26–27 Eat more plants

C. Lassale, *et al*, "Abstract 16: A pro-vegetarian food pattern and cardiovascular mortality in the Epic study," *Circulation* (2015) 132:A16.

D. Aune, D, *et al*, "Fruit and vegetable intake and the risk of cardiovascular disease, total cancer and all-cause mortality," *Int J Epidemiol* (2017) 46(3):1029–1056.

P. Druesne-Pecollo, *et al*, "Beta-carotene supplementation and cancer risk: a systematic review and metaanalysis of randomized controlled trials," *Int J Cancer* (2010) 127(1):172–184.

E. A. Klein, *et al*, "Vitamin E and the risk of prostate cancer," *JAMA* (2011) 306(14):1549–1556.

D. E. Threapleton, *et al*, "Dietary fiber intake and risk of first stroke," *Stroke* (2013) 44(5):1360–1368.

WCRF, "Poor diet and cancer risk."

30–31 Swap red meat for fish

WHO, "Q&A on the carcinogenicity of the consumption of red meat and processed meat" (2015).

A. Pan, *et al*, "Red meat consumption and mortality," *Arch Intern Med* (2012) 172(7):555–563.

D. Mozaffarian, *et al*, "Plasma phospholipid long-chain omega-3 fatty acids and total and cause-specific mortality in older adults," *Ann Intern Med* (2013) 158(7):515–525.

L. G. Zhao, *et al*, "Fish consumption and all-cause mortality," *Eur J Clin Nutr* (2016) 70(2):155–161.

L. Schwingshackl, *et al*, "Food groups and risk of all-cause mortality," *Am J Clin Nutr* (2017) 105(6):1462–1473.

F. Marangoni, *et al*, "Role of poultry meat in a balanced diet aimed at maintaining health and wellbeing: an Italian consensus document," *Food Nutr Res* (2015) 59(1): 27606.

32–33 Eat as nature intended

J. Hutchinson, *et al*, "Evaluation of the effectiveness of the Ministry of Food cooking programme on self-reported food consumption and confidence with cooking," *Public Health Nutr* (2016) 19(18):3417–3427.

34–35 Choose naturally packaged fats

WHO, "Fact sheet number 394: healthy diet," (2015).

R. Micha, *et al*, "Global, regional, and national consumption levels of dietary fats and oils in 1990 and 2010," *BMJ* (2014) 350:h1702

WHO, "Cardiovascular disease. New initiative launched to tackle cardiovascular disease, the world's number one killer," (2016).

Heisei 20-year National Health and Nutrition Survey 2015.

What We Eat in America, NHANES 2013–2014.

S. S. Hammad, and P. J. Jones, "Dietary fatty acid composition modulates obesity and interacts with obesity-related genes," *Lipids* (2017). Published online 9 Sept 2017.

M. H. Laitinen, *et al*, "Fat intake at midlife and risk of dementia and Alzheimer's disease: a population-based study.," *Dement Geriatr Cogn Disord* (2006) 22(1):99–107.

N. D. Barnard, *et al*, "Saturated and trans fats and dementia: a systematic review," *Neurobiol Aging* (2014) 35 Suppl 2:S65–73.

V. Dhaka, *et al*, "Trans fats—sources, health risks and alternative approach—a review," *J Food Sci Technol* (2011) 48(5):534–541.

D. D. Wang, *et al*, "Association of specific dietary fats with total and cause-specific mortality," *JAMA Int Med* (2016) 176(8):11345–1145

S. Lockyer, and S. Stanner, "Coconut oil—a nutty idea," *Nutrition Bulletin* (2016) 41(1):42–54.

36–37 Dose up on the sunshine vitamin

BMJ, "Best practice: vitamin D deficiency," *Epidemiology*. Published 12 Jan 2017.

A. R. Martineau, *et al*, "Vitamin D supplementation to prevent acute respiratory tract infections," *BMJ* (2017) 356:i6583.

WHO and FAO of the UN, "Vitamin and mineral requirements in human nutrition: second edition," (2004).

38–39 Choose foods across the color spectrum

M. H. Carlsen, *et al*, "The total antioxidant content of more than 3100 foods, beverages, spices, herbs and supplements used worldwide," *Nutr J* (2010) 9:3.

40–41 Drink plenty of fluids

European Food Safety Authority, "Scientific opinion on dietary reference values for water," *EFSA Journal* (2010) 8(3):1459.

E. Saito, *et al*, "Association of green tea consumption with mortality due to all causes and major causes of death in a Japanese population: the Japan Public Health Center-based Prospective Study (JPHC Study)," *Ann Epidemiol* (2015) 25(7):512–518.

C. Santos, *et al*, "Caffeine intake and dementia," *J Alzheimers Dis* (2010) 20 Suppl 1:S187–204.

L. Wu, *et al*, "Coffee intake and the incident risk of cognitive disorders," *Clin Nutr* (2017) 36(3):730–736.

54 Breakfasts

J. S. Vander Wal, *et al*, "Egg breakfast enhances weight loss," *Int J Obes* (2008) 32:1545–1551.

56–57 Yogurt

L. J. Appel, "A clinical trial of the effects of dietary patterns on blood pressure," *New Engl J Med* (1997) 336:1117–1124.

R. A. Ralston, *et al*, "A systematic review and meta-analysis of elevated blood pressure and consumption of dairy foods," *J Hum Hypertens* (2012) 26(1):3–13.

J. R. Buendia, *et al*, "Abstract P169: Long term yogurt intake is associated with a lower risk of high blood pressure in middle-aged nurses and health professionals," *Circulation* (2016) 133:AP169

P. F. Jacques and H. Wang, "Yogurt and weight management," *Am J Clin Nutr* (2014) 99(5):1229S–1234S.

J. Eales, *et al*, "Is consuming yoghurt associated with weight management outcomes? Results from a systematic review," *Int J Obes* (2016) 40(5):731–746.

N. Kobyliak, *et al*, "Probiotics in the prevention and treatment of obesity: a critical view," *Nutr Metab* (2016) 13:14.

International Osteoporosis Foundation, "Facts and statistics. Osteoporosis—incidence and burden."

E. Laird, *et al*, "Greater yogurt consumption is associated with increased bone mineral density and physical function in older adults," *Osteoporosis Int* (2017) 28(8):2409–2419.

K. R. Pandey, *et al*, "Probiotics, prebiotics and synbiotics—a review," *J Food Sci Technol* (2015) 52(12):7577–7587.

M. Kechagia, *et al*, "Health benefits of probiotics: a review," *ISRN Nutr* (2013):481651.

L. M. O'Connor, *et al*, "Dietary dairy product intake and incident type 2 diabetes: a prospective study using dietary data from a 7-day food diary," *Diabetologia* (2014) 57(5):909–917.

D. Aune, *et al*, "Dairy products and the risk of type 2 diabetes: a systematic review and dose-response meta-analysis of cohort studies," *Am J Clin Nutr* (2013) 98(4):1066–1083.

60–61 Berries

R. Torronen, *et al*, "Berries modify the postprandial plasma glucose response to sucrose in healthy subjects," *Br J Nutr* (2010) 103(8):1094–1097.

A. J. Stull, "Blueberries impact on insulin resistance and glucose intolerance," *Antioxidants* (2016) 5(4):E44.

J. Mursu, *et al*, "Intake of fruit, berries, and vegetables and risk of type 2 diabetes in Finnish men: the Kuopio Ischaemic Heart Disease Risk Factor Study," *Am J Clin Nutr* (2014) 99(2):328–333.

E. E. Devore, *et al*, "Dietary intakes of berries and flavonoids in relation to cognitive decline," *Ann Neurol* (2012) 72(1):135–143.

A. Cassidy, *et al*, "High anthocyanin intake is associated with a reduced risk of myocardial infarction in young and middle-aged women," *Circulation* (2013) 127:188–196.

A. S. Kristo, *et al*, "Protective role of dietary berries in cancer," *Antioxidants* (2016) 5(4):37.

American Institute for Cancer Research, "Berries seem to burst with cancer protection," AICR Newsletter Number 119, Spring 2013.

H. D. Sesso, *et al*, "Strawberry intake, lipids, C-reactive protein, and the risk of cardiovascular disease in women," *J Am Coll Nutr* (2007) 26(4):303–310.

64–65 Bananas

L. Gougeon, *et al*, "Intakes of folate, vitamin B6 and B12 and risk of depression in community-dwelling older adults: the Quebec Longitudinal Study on Nutrition and Aging," *Eur J Clin Nutr* (2016) 70(3):380–385.

WHO, "WHO Global Health Day 2012: Control your blood pressure," (2013).

B. Rashidkhani, *et al*, "Fruits, vegetables and risk of renal cell carcinoma: a prospective study of Swedish women," *Int J Cancer* (2005) 113(3):451–455.

M. Maclure and W. Willett, "A case control study of diet and risk of renal adenocarcinoma," *Epidemiol* (1990) 1(6):430–440.

E. K. Mitsou, *et al*, "Effect of banana consumption on faecal microbiota: a randomised, controlled trial," *Anaerobe* (2011) 17(6):384–387.

70–71 Eggs

J. E. Kim, *et al*, "Effects of egg consumption on carotenoid absorption from co-consumed, raw vegetables," *Am J Clin Nutr* (2015) 102(1):75–83.

British Heart Foundation, "Eggs and cholesterol" (2015).

R. Fallaize, *et al*, "Variation in the effects of three different breakfast meals on the subjective satiety and subsequent intake of energy at lunch and evening meal," *Eur J Nutr* (2013) 52(4):1353–1359.

J. S. Vander Wal, *et al*, "Egg breakfast enhances weight loss," *Int J Obes* (2008) 32:1545–1551

74–75 Whole grains

D. Aune, *et al*, "Whole grain consumption and risk of cardiovascular disease, cancer, and all cause and cause specific mortality," *BMJ* (2016) 353:i2716.

D. Aune, *et al*, "Dietary fibre, whole grains, and risk of colorectal cancer," *BMJ* (2011) 343:d1167.

D. Aune, *et al*, "Whole grain and refined grain consumption and the risk of type 2 diabetes," *Eur J Epidemiol* (2013) 28(11):845-858.

Scientific Advisory Committee on Nutrition, "Carbohydrates and health" (2015).

J. P. Karl and E. Saltzman, "The role of whole grains in body weight regulation," *Adv Nutr* (2012) 3(5):697–707.

78 Lunches

R. E. Oldham-Cooper, *et al*, "Playing a computer game during lunch affects fullness, memory for lunch, and later snack intake," *Am J Clin Nutr* (2011) 93(2):308–313.

84–85 Legumes

A. Menotti, *et al*, "Food intake patterns and 25-year mortality from coronary heart disease," *Eur J Epidemiol* (1999) 15(6):507–515.

L. A. Bazzano, *et al*, "Legume consumption and risk of coronary heart disease in US men and women: NHANES I Epidemiologic Follow-up Study," *Arch Intern Med* (2001) 161(21):2573–2578.

D. Ramdath, *et al*, "The role of pulses in the dietary management of diabetes," *Can J Diabetes* (2016) 40(4):355–363.

R. Villegas, *et al*, "Legume and soy food intake and the incidence of type 2 diabetes in the Shanghai Women's Health Study," *Am J Clin Nutr* (2008) 87(1):162–167.

V. Ha, *et al*, "Effect of dietary pulse intake on established therapeutic lipid targets for cardiovascular risk reduction," *CMAJ* (2014) 186(8):E252–262.

S. S. Li, *et al*, "Dietary pulses, satiety and food intake," *Obesity* (2014) 22(8):1773–1780.

86 Mixed bean bowl with pita nachos

S. J. Kim, *et al*, "Effects of dietary pulse consumption on body weight," *Am J Clin Nutr* (2016) 103(5):1213–1223.

90–91 Bell peppers and chilies

American Chemical Society, "News releases. Hot pepper compound could help hearts," (2012).

R. H. Raghavendra and K. A. Naidu, "Spice active principles as the inhibitors of human platelet aggregation and thromboxane biosynthesis," *Prostaglandins, Leuko Essent Fatty Acids* (2009) 81(1):73–78.

S. Whiting, *et al*, "Capsaicinoids and capsinoids. A potential role for weight management?," *Appetite* (2012) 59(2):341–348.

S. Whiting, *et al*, "Could capsaicinoids help to support weight management?," *Appetite* (2014) 74:183–188.

M. Shareck, *et al*, "Inverse association between dietary intake of selected carotenoids and vitamin C and risk of lung cancer," *Front Oncol* (2017) 7:23.

B. S. Berthon and L. G. Wood, "Nutrition and respiratory health—feature review," *Nutrients* (2015) 7(3):1618–1643.

WHO, "Chronic respiratory diseases. Burden of COPD."

94–95 Root vegetables

A. J. Cooper, *et al*, "Fruit and vegetable intake and type 2 diabetes: EPIC-InterAct prospective study and meta-analysis," *Eur J Clin Nutr* (2012) 66 (10):1082–1092.

L. M. Oude Griep, *et al*, "Colours of fruit and vegetables and 10-year incidence of CHD," *Br J Nutr* (2011) 106(10):1562–1569.

X. X. Ge, *et al*, "Carotenoid intake and esophageal cancer risk: a meta-analysis," *Asian Pac J Cancer Prev* (2013) 14(3):1911–1918.

A. Ahluwalia, *et al*, "Dietary nitrate and the epidemiology of cardiovascular disease: report from a national heart, lung and blood institute workshop," *J Am Heart Assoc* (2016) 5(7):e003402

M. Siervo, *et al*, "Inorganic nitrate and beetroot juice supplementation reduces blood pressure in adults," *J Nutr* (2013) 143(6):818–826.

100–101 Soy

M. Chen, *et al*, "Association between soy isoflavone intake and breast cancer risk for pre- and post-menopausal women," *PLoS One* (2014) 9 (2): e89288.

K. Taku, *et al*, "Extracted or synthesized soybean isoflavones reduce menopausal hot flash frequency and severity," *Menopause* (2012) 19(7):776–790.

X. Zhang, *et al*, "Prospective cohort study of soy food consumption and risk of bone fracture among post-menopausal women," *Arch Intern Med* (2005) 165(16):1890–1895.

W. Koh, *et al*, "Gender-specific associations between soy and risk of hip fracture in the Singapore Chinese Health Study," *Am J Epidemiol* (2009) 170 (7): 901–909.

M. Messina, "Soy and health update: Evaluation of the clinical and epidemiologic literature," *Nutrients* (2016) 8(12):754.

Y. Kokubo, *et al*, "Association of dietary intake of soy, beans, and isoflavones with risk of cerebral and myocardial infarctions in Japanese populations: the Japan Public Health Center-based (JPHC) study cohort 1," *Circulation* (2007) 116(22):2553–2562.

X. Zhang, *et al*, "Soy food consumption is associated with lower risk of coronary heart disease in Chinese women," *J Nutr* (2003) 133(9):2874–2878.

V. Messina, "Soyfoods and heart disease," *Today's Dietitian* (2016) 18(4):18.

104–105 Avocados

M. B. Purba, *et al*, "Skin wrinkling: can food make a difference?," *J Am Coll Nutr* (2001) 20 (1):71–80.

N. Z. Unlu, *et al*, "Carotenoid absorption from salad and salsa by humans is enhanced by the addition of avocado or avocado oil," *J Nutr* (2005) 135(3):431–436.

Rejuvenation Science, "Lutein and lycopene can help prevent prostate cancer."

M. L. Dreher and A. J. Davenport, "Hass avocado composition and potential health effects," *Crit Rev Food Sci Nutr* (2013) 53(7):738–750.

V. L. Fulgoni, *et al*, "Avocado consumption is associated with better diet quality and nutrient intake, and lower metabolic syndrome risk in US adults," *Nutr J* (2013) 12:1.

107 Dinners

D. Jakubowicz, *et al*, "High caloric intake at breakfast vs. dinner differentially influences weight loss of overweight and obese women," *Obesity* (2013) 21(12):2504–2512.

108–109 Leafy green vegetables

J. A. Giaconi, *et al*, "The association of consumption of fruits/vegetables with decreased risk of glaucoma among older African American women in the study of osteoporotic fractures," *Am J Ophthalmol* (2012) 154(4):635–644.

J. Wu, *et al*, "Intakes of lutein, zeaxanthin, and other carotenoids and age-related macular degeneration during 2 decades of prospective follow-up," *JAMA Ophthalmol* (2015) 133(12):1415–1424.

M. C. Morris, *et al*, "Relations to cognitive change with age of micronutrients found in green leafy vegetables," *FASEB J* (2015) 29(1):Supplement 260.3

X. Zhang, *et al*, "Cruciferous vegetable consumption is associated with a reduced risk of total and cardiovascular disease mortality," *Am J Clin Nutr* (2011) 94(1):240–246.

Q. J. Wu, *et al*, "Cruciferous vegetables intake and the risk of colorectal cancer: a meta-analysis of observational studies," *Ann Oncol* (2013) 24(4):1079–1087.

111 Sumac fishcakes with greens

J. Zhang, *et al*, "Synergy between sulforaphane and selenium in the induction of thioredoxin reductase 1 requires both transcriptional and translational modulation," *Carcinogenesis* (2003) 24(3):497–503.

112–113 Fish and shellfish

P. Barberger-Gateau, *et al*, "Dietary patterns and risk of dementia," *Neurology* (2007) 69 (20):1921–1930.

British Heart Foundation, "Reducing your blood cholesterol."

Arthritis Research UK, "Fish oils."

115 Roasted haddock with a herby crumb

N. Azad, *et al*, "Neuroprotective effects of carnosic acid in an experimental model of Alzheimer's disease in rats," *Cell J* (2011) 13(1):39–44.

M. Moss and L. Oliver, "Plasma 1,8-cineole correlates with cognitive performance following exposure to rosemary essential oil aroma," *Ther Adv Psychopharmacol* (2012) 2(3):103–113.

118–119 Mushrooms

Mushroom Bureau, "Mushrooms The New Superfood."

M. Zhang, *et al*, "Dietary intakes of mushrooms and green tea combine to reduce the risk of breast cancer in Chinese women," *Int J Cancer* (2009) 124(6):1404–1408.

M. J. Feeney, *et al*, "Mushrooms and health summit proceedings," *J Nutr* (2014) 144(7):1128S–1136S.

L. J. Cheskin, *et al*, "Lack of energy compensation over 4 days when white button mushrooms are substitued for beef," *Appetite* (2008) 51 (1): 50–57.

S. R. Koyyalamudi, *et al*, "Vitamin D2 formation and bioavailability from Agaricus bisporus button mushrooms treated with ultraviolet irradiation," *J Agric Food Chem* (2009) 57(8):3351–3355.

R. Beelman and M. Kalaras, "Post-harvest vitamin D enrichment of fresh mushrooms," HAL Project #MU07018, Penn State University (2009).

122–123 Onions, garlic, and leeks

M. DeMartinis, M*, et al*, "Allergy and Aging: An old/new emerging health issue," *Aging & Disease* (2017) 8(2):162–175.

Z. Bahadoran, *et al*, "Allium vegetable intakes and the incidence of cardiovascular disease, hypertension, chronic kidney disease, and type 2 diabetes in adults," *J Hypertens* (2017) 35(9):1909–1916.

C. Galeone, *et al*, "Allium vegetable intake and risk of acute myocardial infarction in Italy. *Eur J Nutr* (2009) 48(2):120–123.

H. L. Nicastro, H L*, et al*, "Garlic and onions: Their cancer prevention properties," *Cancer Prev Res* (2015) 8(3):181–189.

Y. Zhou, *et al*, "Consumption of large amounts of Allium vegetables reduces risk for gastric cancer in a meta-analysis," *Gastroenterology* (2011) 141(1):80–89.

I. M. Taj Eldin, *et al*, "Preliminary study of the clinical hypoglycemic effects of *Allium cepa* (red onion) in type 1 and type 2 diabetic patients. *Environ Health Insights* (2010) 4:71–77.

126–127 Tomatoes

N. Z. Unlu, *et al,* "Carotenoid absorption from salad and salsa by humans is enhanced by the addition of avocado or avocado oil," *J Nutr* (2005) 135(3):431–436.

K. Canene-Adams, *et al,* "Combinations of tomato and broccoli enhance antitumor activity in dunning r3327-h prostate adenocarcinomas," *Cancer Res* (2007) 67(2):836–843.

P. Chen, *et al*, "Lycopene and risk of prostate cancer: a systematic review and meta-analysis," *Medicine* (2015) 94(33):e1260.

D. Cuevas-Ramos, *et al*, "Effect of tomato consumption on high-density lipoprotein cholesterol level," *Diabetes, Metab Synd Obes* (2013) 6:263–273.

X. Li and J. Xu, "Dietary and circulating lycopene and stroke risk: a meta-analysis of prospective studies," *Scientific Reports* (2014) 4:5031.

130–131 Olive oil

T. Psaltopoulou, *et al*, "Olive oil intake is inversely related to cancer prevalence," *Lipids Health Dis* (2011) 10:127.

C. Berr, *et al*, "Olive oil and cognition: results from the Three-City Study," *Dement Geriatr Cogn Disord* (2009) 28(4):357–364.

S. Lopez, *et al*, "Virgin olive oil and hypertension," *Curr Vasc Pharmacol* (2016) 14(4):323–329.

C. Samieri, *et al*, "Olive oil consumption, plasma oleic acid and stroke incidence: the Three-City Study," *Neurology* (2011) 77(5):418–425.

J. Weisenberger, "Heart-healthy fats: It's the type—not the amount—that matters," *Today's Dietitian* (2013) 15(9):14.

134–135 Citrus fruits

E. Yonova-Doing, *et al*, "Genetic and dietary factors influencing the progression of nuclear cataract," *Opthamology* (2016) 123(6):1237–1244.

M. C. Cosgrove, *et al*, "Dietary nutrient intakes and skin aging appearance among middle-aged American women," *Am J Clin Nutr* (2007) 86(4):1225–1231.

K. J. Joshipura, *et al*, "Fruit and vegetable intake in relation to risk of ischemic stroke," *JAMA* (1999) 282(13):1233–1239.

J. M. Roza, *et al*, "Effect of citrus flavonoids and tocotrienols on serum cholesterol levels in hypercholesterolemic subjects," *Altern Therap Health Med (*2007) 13(6):44–48.

N. P. Aptekmann and T. B. Cesar, "Long-term orange juice consumption is associated with low LDL-cholesterol and apolipoprotein B in normal and moderately hypercholesterolemic subjects," *Lipids Health Dis* (2013) 12:119.

S. Gorinstein, "Red grapefruit positively influences serum triglyceride levels in patients suffering from coronary atherosclerosis: studies in vitro and in humans," *J Agric Food Chem* (2006) 54(5):1887–1892.

S. Zhang, *et al*, "Citrus consumption and incident dementia in elderly Japanese: the Ohsaki cohort 2006 study," *Br J Nutr* (2017) 117(8):1174–1180.

K. Baghurst, "The health benefits of citrus fruits," CSIRO Health Sciences and Nutrition (2003).

140–141 Nuts

A. A. Tucker, "Consumption of nuts and seeds and telomere length in 5,582 men and women of the National Health and Nutrition Examination Survey (NHANES)," *J Nutr Health Aging* (2017) 21(3):233–240.

C. Yeh, *et al,* "Peanut consumption and reduced risk of colorectal cancer in women: A prospective study in Taiwan," *World J Gastroenterol* (2006) 12(2):222–227.

Y. Bao, *et al*, "Association of nut consumption with total and cause-specific mortality," *New Engl J Med* (2013) 369:2001–2011.

D. Aune, *et al*, "Nut consumption and risk of cardiovascular disease, total cancer, all-cause and cause-specific mortality," *BMC Med* (2016) 14:207.

M. Bes-Rastrollo, *et al*, "Prospective study of nut consumption, long-term weight change, and obesity risk in women," *Am J Clin Nutr* (2009) 89(6):1913–1919.

C. J. Tsai, *et al*, "Frequent nut consumption and decreased risk of cholecystectomy in women," *Am J Clin Nutr* (2004) 80(1):76–81.

C. J. Tsai, C J*, et al*, "A prospective cohort study of nut consumption and the risk of gallstone disease in men," *Am J Epidemiol* (2004) 160(1):961–968.

146–147 Spices

E. M. Bartels, "Efficacy and safety of ginger in osteoarthritis patients," *Osteoarthritis Cartilage* (2015) 23(1):13–21.

M. A. Shirvani, *et al,* "The effect of mefenamic acid and ginger on pain relief in primary dysmenorrhea: a randomized clinical trial," *Arch Gynecol Obstetr* (2015) 291(6):1277–1281.

A. K. Agarwal, "Spice up your life: adipose tissue and inflammation," *J Lipids* (2014) 182575.

M. Serafini and I. Peluso, "Functional foods for health: the interrelated antioxidant and anti-inflammatory role of fruits, vegetables, herbs, spices and cocoa in humans" *Curr Pharm Des* (2016) 22(44):6701–6715.

J. Zheng, "Spices for prevention and treatment of cancers" *Nutrients* (2016) 8(8): 495.

Cancer Research UK, "Turmeric."

C. A. Anderson, *et al*, "Effects of a behavioral intervention that emphasizes spices and herbs on adherence to recommended sodium intake: results of the SPICE randomized clinical trial," *Am J Clin Nutr* (2015) 102(3):671–679.

M. McCulloch, "Cinnamon's link to diabetes control," *Today's Dietitian* (2015) 17(11):12.

P. A. Davis and W. Yokoyama, "Cinnamon intake lowers fasting blood glucose: meta-analysis" *J Med Food* (2011) 14(9):884–889.

148 Turkey steak with kale and squash

C. S. Johnston, *et al*, "Vinegar: medicinal uses and antiglycemic effect," *Med Gen Med* (2006) 8(2):61.

150–151 Squashes

W. Koh, *et al*, "Plasma carotenoids and risk of acute myocardial infarction in The Singapore Chinese Health Study," *Nutr Metab Cardiovasc Dis* (2011) 21(9):685–690.

L. Gallicchio, *et al*, "Carotenoids and the risk of developing lung cancer," *Am J Clin Nutr* (2008) 88(2):372–383.

E. Leoncini, *et al*, "Carotenoid intake from natural sources and head and neck cancer," *Cancer Epidemiol Biomarkers Prev* (2015) 24(7):1003–1011.

American Academy of Opthamology, "What is vitamin A deficiency?" (2012).

158–159 Foods for the brain

M. M. Karnani, *et al*, "Activation of central orexin/hypocretin neurons by dietary amino acids," *Neuron* (2011) 72(4):616–629.

K. Kent, *et al*, "Food-based anthocyanin intake and cognitive outcomes in human intervention trials: a systematic review," *J Hum Nutr Diet* (2017) 30(3):260–274.

E. E. Devore, *et al*, "Dietary intakes of berries and flavonoids in relation to cognitive decline," *Ann Neurol* (2012) 72(1):135–143.

C. Cao, *et al*, "High blood caffeine levels in MCI linked to lack of progression to dementia," *J Alzheimers Dis* (2012) 30:559–572.

K. Ritchie, *et al*, "The neuroprotective effects of caffeine: a prospective population study (the Three City Study)," *Neurology* (2007) 69(6):536–545.

I. Driscoll, *et al*, "Relationships between caffeine intake and risk for probable dementia or global cognitive impairment: the Women's Health Initiative Memory Study," *J Gerentol A Biol Sci Med Sci* (2016) 71(12):1596–1602.

D. Smith, *et al*, "Homocysteine-lowering by B-vitamins slows the rate of accelerated brain atrophy in mild cognitive impairment," *PLoS One* (2010) 5(9):e12244.

M. Mathew and S. Subramanian, "In vitro evaluation of anti-Alzheimer effects of dry ginger (Zingiber officinale Roscoe) extract," *Indian J Exp Biol* (2014) 52:606–612.

V. Mani, *et al*, "Reversal of memory deficits by Coriandrum sativum leaves in mice," *J Sci Food Agric* (2011) 91(1):186–192.

S. Koppula and D. K. Choi, "Cuminum cyminum extract attenuates scopolamine-induced memory loss and stress-induced urinary biochemical changes in rats," *Pharm Biol* (2011) 49(7):702–708.

K. Mahdy, *et al*, "Effect of some medicinal plant extracts on the oxidative stress status in Alzheimer's disease induced in rats," *Eur Rev Med Pharmacol Sci* (2012) 16(Suppl 3):31–42.

T. P. Ng, *et al*, "Curry consumption and cognitive function in the elderly," *Am J Epidemiol* (2006) 164(9):898–906.

M. C. Morris, *et al*, "Dietary fats and the risk of incident Alzheimer's disease," *Arch Neurol* (2003) 60:194–200

160–161 Brain and mental health conditions

A. Oulhaj, *et al*, "Omega-3 fatty acid status enhances the prevention of cognitive decline by B vitamins in mild cognitive impairment," *J Alzheimers Dis* (2016) 50(2):547–557.

F. N. Jacka, *et al*, "A randomised controlled trial of dietary improvement for adults with major depression (the 'SMILES' trial)," *BMC Med* (2017) 15:23.

164–165 Foods for vision

American Optometric Association, "Essential fatty acids Omega-3: DHA and EPA."

American Optometric Association, "Vitamin C."

American Optometric Association, "Nutrition and cataracts."

I. I. Bussel and A. A. Aref, "Dietary factors and the risk of glaucoma: a review" *Ther Adv Chron Dis* (2014) 5(4):188–194.

American Optometric Association, "Age-related macular degeneration."

American Optometric Association, "Nutrition and AMD."

166–167 Hearing and balance

C. G. Le Prell, *et al*, "Free radical scavengers, vitamins A, C, and E, plus magnesium reduces noise trauma," *Free Radic Biol Med* (2007) 42(9):1454–1463.

168–169 Foods for hearing and balance

B. Gopinath, *et al*, "Dietary antioxidant intake is associated with the prevalence but not incidence of age-related hearing loss," *J Nutr Health Aging* (2011) 15(10):896–900.

J. Attias, *et al*, "Oral magnesium intake reduces permanent hearing loss induced by noise exposure," *Am J Otolaryngol* (1994) 15(1):26–32.

J. Attias, *et al*, "Reduction in noise-induced temporary threshold shift in humans following oral magnesium intake," *Clin Otolaryngol Allied Sci* (2004) 29(6):635–641.

S. G. Curhan, *et al*, "Carotenoids, vitamin A, vitamin C, vitamin E and folate and risk of self-reported hearing loss in women," *Am J Clin Nutr* (2015) 102(5):1167–1175.

J. Shargordsky, *et al*, "A prospective study of vitamin intake and the risk of hearing loss in men," *Otolaryngol Head Neck Surg* (2010) 142(2):231–236.

J. T. Glicksman, *et al*, "A prospective study of caffeine intake and risk of incident tinnitus," *Am J Med* (2014) 127(8):739–743.

A. McCormack, *et al*, "Association of dietary factors with presence and severity of tinnitus in a middle-aged population," *PLoS One* (2014) 9(12):e114711.

B. Gopinath, *et al*, "Consumption of omega-3 fatty acids and fish and risk of age-related hearing loss," *Am J Clin Nutr* (2010) 92(2):416–421.

S. G. Curhan, *et al*, "Fish and fatty acid consumption and the risk of hearing loss in women," *Am J Clin Nutr* (2014) 100(5):1371–1377.

B. Gopinath, *et al*, "Dietary glycemic load is a predictor of age-related hearing loss in older adults," *J Nutr* (2010) 140(12):2207–2212.

172–173 Foods for oral health

S. Najeeb, *et al*, "The role of nutrition in periodontal health: an update," *Nutrients* (2016) 8(9):E530.

G. F. Ferrazzano, *et al*, "Protective effect of yogurt extract on dental enamel demineralization in vitro," *Aus Dent J* (2008) 53:314–319.

A. Haukioja, "Probiotics and oral health," *Eur J Dent* (2010) 4(3):348–355.

K. Hojo, *et al*, "Abstract 920: Effects of yoghurt on the human oral microbiota and halitosis." Presented at the 83rd General session of the International Association for Dental Research, Baltimore, USA (2008). http://www.dent.niigata-u.ac.jp/prevent/ISBOR04/Baltimore.htm#0920

176–177 Foods for immunity

K. A. Kaspersen, *et al*, "Obesity and risk of infection: results from the Danish Blood Donor Study," *Epidemiology* (2015) 26(4):580–589.

178–179 Bones, muscles, and joints

NHS Choices, "Menopause and your bone health."

180–181 Foods for bones, muscles, and joints

National Osteoporosis Society, "A balanced diet for bones."

X. Zheng, *et al*, "Soy isoflavones and osteoporotic bone loss: a review with an emphasis on modulation of bone remodeling," *J Med Food* (2016) 19(1):1–14.

L. McCabe, *et al*, "Prebiotic and probiotic regulation of bone health: role of the intestine and its microbiome," *Curr Osteoporos Reports* (2015) 13(6):363–371.

P. D'Amelio and F. Sassi, "Gut microbiota, immune system and bone," *Calcified Tissue International.* Published online 30 Sep 2017.

F. L. Collins, *et al*, "The potential of probiotics as a therapy for osteoporosis," *Microbiol Spectr* (2017) 5(4).

A. Gioxari, *et al*, "Intake of omega-3 polyunsaturated fatty acids in patients with rheumatoid arthritis," *Nutrition* (2018). Published online 8 Jul 2017.

L. Skoldstam, *et al*, "An experimental study of a Mediterranean diet intervention for patients with rheumatoid arthritis," *Ann Rheum Dis* (2003) 62(3):208–214.

182–183 Skin and sensation

M. C. Cosgrove, *et al*, "Dietary nutrient intake and skin-aging appearance among middle-aged American women," *Am J Clin Nutr* (2007) 86(4):1225–1231.

184–185 Foods for skin and sensation

M. Br Purba, *et al*, "Skin wrinkling: can food make a difference?," *J Am Coll Nutr* (2001) 20(1):71–80.

A. E. Millen, *et al*, "Diet and melanoma in a case control study," *Cancer Epidemiol Biomarkers Prev* (2004) 13(6):1042–1051.

M. Rodavich, "CPE Monthly: Skin cancer and nutrition," *Today's Dietitian* (2015) 17(2):50.

M. Rizwan, *et al*, " Tomato paste rich in lycopene protects against cutaneous photodamage in humans in vivo," *Br J Dermatol* (2011) 164(1):154–162.

F. W. Danby, "Nutrition and aging skin: sugar and glycation," *Clin Dermatol* (2010) 28(4):409–411.

188–189 Foods for the lungs

K. B. Min and J. Y. Min, "Serum carotenoid levels and risk of lung cancer death in US adults," *Cancer Sci* (2014) 105(6):736–743.

L. G. Wood, *et al*, " Lycopene-rich treatments modify noneosinophilic airway inflammation in asthma: proof of concept," *Free Radic Res* (2008) 42(1):94-102.

B. S. Berthon and L. G. Wood, "Nutrition and Respiratory Health," *Nutrients* (2015) 7(3):1618–1643.

R. E. Foong and G. R. Zosky, "Vitamin D deficiency and the lung: disease initiator or disease modifier?," *Nutrients* (2013) 5(8):2880–2900.

Y. Zhu, *et al*, "Association of dietary vitamin E intake with risk of lung cancer: a dose-response meta-analysis," *Asia Pac J Clin Nutr* (2017) 26(2):271–277.

Cancer Research UK, "The safety of vitamins and diet supplements."

F. Hirayama, *et al*,"Folate intake associated with lung function, breathlessness and the prevalence of chronic obstructive pulmonary disease," *Asia Pac J Clin Nutr* (2010) 19(1):103–109.

192–193 Foods for the heart and blood

V. Ha, *et al*, "Effect of dietary pulse intake on established therapeutic lipid targets for cardiovascular risk reduction," *CMAJ* (2014) 186(8):E252–262.

H. Wu, *et al*, "Association between dietary whole grain intake and risk of mortality," *JAMA Intern Med* (2015) 175(3):373–384.

D. Aune, *et al*, "Fruit and vegetable intake and the risk of cardiovascular disease, total cancer and all-cause mortality," *Int J Epidemiol* (2017) 46(3):1029–1056.

S. Bulotta, *et al*, "Beneficial effects of the olive oil phenolic components oleuropein and hydroxytyrosol: focus on protection against cardiovascular and metabolic diseases," *J Trans Med* (2014) 12:219.

S. S. Leung Yinko, *et al*, "Fish consumption and acute coronary syndrome," *Am J Med* (2014) 127(9):848–857.

C. Chrysohoou, *et al*, "Long-term fish consumption is associated with protection against arrhythmia in healthy persons in a Mediterranean region–the ATTICA study," *Am J Clin Nutr* (2007) 85(5):1385–1391.

194–195 Heart and blood conditions

WHO, "Cardiovascular diseases (CVDs) fact sheet" (2017).

NIH U.S. National Library of Medicine. MedlinePlus. Aging changes in the heart and blood vessels.

198–199 Foods for gut health

E. K. Mitsou, *et al*, "Effect of banana consumption on faecal microbiota," *Anaerobe* (2011) 17(6):384–387.

D. Aune, *et al*, "Dietary fibre, whole grains, and risk of colorectal cancer," *BMJ* (2011) 343:d6617.

C. J. Tsai, *et al*, "Frequent nut consumption and decreased risk of cholecystectomy in women," *Am J Clin Nutr* (2004) 80(1):76–81.

C. J. Tsai, *et al*, "A prospective cohort study of nut consumption and the risk of gallstone disease in men," *Am J Epidemiol* (2004) 160(1):961–968.

A. M. Bode and Z. Dong, "The Amazing and Mighty Ginger." *Herbal Medicine: Biomolecular and Clinical Aspects. 2nd Edition.* CRC Press/Taylor and Francis, 2011.

R. Haniadka, *et al*, "A review of the gastroprotective effects of ginger (Zingiber officinale Roscoe)," *Food Func* (2013) 4(6):845–855.

British Dietetic Association, "Fact sheet: Probiotics" (2015).

J. Eales, *et al*, "Is consuming yoghurt associated with weight management outcomes?," *Int J Obes* (2016) 40(5):731–746.

P. J. Tarraga Lopez, *et al*, "Primary and secondary prevention of colorectal cancer," *Clin Med Insights Gastroenterol* (2014) 7:33–46.

200–201 Gut health conditions

W. C. Knowler, *et al*, "Reduction in the incidence of type 2 diabetes with lifestyle intervention or metformin," *New Engl J Med* (2002) 346(6):393–403.

Cancer Research UK, "Bowel cancer incidence statistics."

202–203 Urinary health

UCSF Medical Center, "Urinary tract infections."

R. G. Jepson, *et al*, "Cranberries for preventing urinary tract infections," *Cochrane Database Syst Rev* (2012) 10:CD001321.

C. Young Bearden, "Holistic nutrition: cranberries and UTI prevention," *Today's Dietitian* (2017) 19(2):18.

204–205 Foods for urinary health

WCRF International, "Continuous update project. diet, nutrition, physical activity and bladder cancer" (2015).

NHS Choices, "Urinary incontinence."

J. A. Nettleton, *et al*, "Associations between microalbuminuria and animal foods, plant foods, and dietary patterns in the multiethnic study of atherosclerosis," *Am J Clin Nutr* (2008) 87(6):1825–1836.

G. M. Herber-Gast, *et al*, "Consumption of whole grains, fruit and vegetables is not associated with indices of renal function in the population-based longitudinal Doetinchem study," *Br J Nutr* (2017) 118:375–382.

A. Chanson-Rolle, *et al*, "Systematic review and meta-analysis of human studies to support a quantitative recommendation for whole grain intake in relation to type 2 diabetes," *PLoS One* (2015) 10(6):e0131377.

National Kidney Foundation, "Diet and kidney stones."

D. Prezioso, *et al*, "Dietary treatment of urinary risk factors for renal stone formation. A review of CLU working group," *Arch Ital Urol Androl* (2015) 87(2):105–120.

G. C. Curhan, *et al*, "Intake of vitamins B6 and C and the risk of kidney stones in women," *J Am Soc Nephrol* (1999) 10 (4):840–845.

P. M. Grin, *et al*, "Lactobacillus for preventing recurrent urinary tract infections in women: meta-analysis," *Can J Urol* (2013) 20(1):6607–6614.

T. Kontiokari, *et al*, "Dietary factors protecting women from urinary tract infection," *Am J Clin Nutr* (2003) 77(3):600–604.

National Institute of Diabetes and Digestive and Kidney Diseases, "High blood pressure and kidney disease."

B. Haring, *et al*, "Dietary protein sources and risk for incident chronic kidney disease," *J Ren Nutr* (2017) 27(4):233–242.

206–207 Women's health

J. L. Gordon, *et al*, "Estradiol variability, stressful life events, and the emergence of depressive symptomatology during the menopausal transition," *Menopause* (2016) 23(3):257–266.

C. Zhang, *et al*, "Abdominal obesity and the risk of all-cause, cardiovascular, and cancer mortality: sixteen years of follow-up in US women," *Circulation* (2008) 117(13):1658–1667.

208–209 Foods for women's health

NHS Choices, "Menopause and your bone health."

H. K. Seitz, *et al*, "Epidemiology and pathophysiology of alcohol and breast cancer: Update 2012," *Alcohol Alcohol* (2012) 47(3):204–212.

Cancer Research UK, "Alcohol facts and evidence."

Cancer Research UK, "Breast cancer incidence (invasive) stats."

210–211 Men's health

A. S. Prasad, *et al*, "Zinc status and serum testosterone levels of healthy adults," *Nutrition* (1996) 12(5):344–348.

S. Pilz, *et al*, "Effect of vitamin D supplementation on testosterone levels in men," *Horm Metab Res* (2011) 43(3):223–235.

Cleveland Clinic, "Low testosterone (male hypogonadism)."

212–213 Foods for men's health

P. H. Lin, *et al*, "Nutrition, dietary interventions and prostate cancer: the latest evidence," *BMC Med* (2015) 13:3

National Cancer Institute, "PDQ cancer information summaries. Prostate cancer, nutrition and dietary Supplements (PDQ)" (2017).

X. Xu, *et al*, "Tomato consumption and prostate cancer risk," *Scientific Reports* (2016) 6:37091.

G. Maskarinec, *et al*, "Serum prostate-specific antigen but not testosterone levels decrease in a randomized soy intervention among men," *Eur J Clin Nutr* (2006) 60:1423–1429.

C. Lovegrove, *et al*, "Systematic review of prostate cancer risk and association with consumption of fish and fish-oils," *Int J Clin Pract* (2015) 69(1):87–105.

P. Christudoss, *et al*, "Zinc status of patients with benign prostatic hyperplasia and prostate carcinoma," *Indian J Urol* (2011) 27(1):14–18.

W. T. Clements, *et al*, "Nitrate ingestion: A review of the health and physical performance effects," *Nutrients* (2014) 6(11):5224–5264.

M. I. Maiorino, *et al*, "Lifestyle modifications and erectile dysfunction: what can be expected?," *Asian J Androl* (2015) 17(1):5–10.

S. Di Francesco and R. L. Tenaglia, "Mediterranean diet and erectile dysfunction: a current perspective," *Cen Eur J Urol* (2017) 70(2):185–187.

Cancer Research UK, "Prostate cancer incidence statistics."

P. Chen, *et al* (2015), "Lycopene and risk of prostate cancer: a systematic review and meta-analysis," *Medicine* 94(3):e1260.

Index

Recipes are *italicized* throughout.

Q

R

S

T

U

V

W

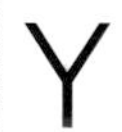

Z

The author

Juliette Kellow is a registered dietitian and has a passion for food, diet, nutrition, and health. She's worked in the NHS and for the food industry, and is the former editor of *Top Santé*. Juliette now works as a nutrition consultant and currently writes for many magazines and newspapers. She's regularly on UK radio as a nutrition expert and has advised many celebrities on their diet.

The consultant

Dr. Sarah Brewer is a Cambridge-educated doctor, medical nutritionist, and nutritional therapist, and the author of over 60 books. She has a specialist interest in the link between illness and diet. www.DrSarahBrewer.com

Acknowledgments

FROM THE AUTHOR A massive thank you to my two favorite boys—my husband Neil and son Sam—for "holding the fort" and providing such amazing support, not just while I've been writing this book, but with all my work. A special thanks to my lovely mom, who, at 85 years old, is an excellent example of how a lifetime of healthy choices really can result in longevity. Also, a mention for my dad, who lived happily and healthily to be 93—had he still been with us, he would have been a centenarian when this book was published and would have been so proud of me. Thank you to all my incredible friends who have offered endless support and spent hours listening to me talking about anti-aging—they will undoubtedly be grateful that the "B" word, as it's become affectionately known, is no longer a part of their (hopefully long-lived) lives. Finally, thanks to everyone at DK, especially editor Nikki Sims.

FROM THE PUBLISHER We would like to acknowledge the help of the following in the production of this book: Claire Cross, Alastair Laing, and Toby Mann for editorial assistance, Philippa Nash for design assistance, Charlotte Simpkins for recipe testing, Katie Hardwicke for proofreading, and Vanessa Bird for indexing.

DISCLAIMER

The authors provide information on a wide range of nutrition and health topics, and every effort has been made to ensure that the information in this book is accurate. The book is not a substitute for expert medical advice, however, and you are advised always to consult a medically qualified doctor or other health professional for specific information on your own personal health matters, including specialist dietary advice. All information given in this book is intended for those in good health. If you have a pre-existing medical condition or are taking any type of medication, you should consult your doctor before embarking on a radical change of diet, since some foods have interactions with medication and certain conditions prohibit the consumption of certain foods. If in doubt, check with your doctor first.